Adult Nurse Practitioner
Certification Review

Adult Nurse Practitioner Certification Review

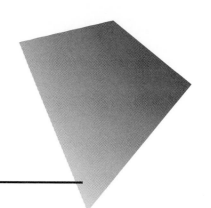

Second Edition

JoAnn Zerwekh, EdD, RN, FNP, APRN, BC
Faculty
University of Phoenix Online
Phoenix, Arizona

Executive Director
Nursing Education Consultants
Midlothian, Texas

Jo Carol Claborn, MS, RN, CNS
Executive Director
Nursing Education Consultants
Midlothian, Texas

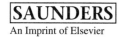
SAUNDERS
An Imprint of Elsevier

SAUNDERS

An Imprint of Elsevier

11830 Westline Industrial Drive
St. Louis, Missouri 63146

ADULT NURSE PRACTITIONER CERTIFICATION REVIEW ISBN 0-7216-8252-9

NOTICE

Nursing is an ever-changing field. Standard safety precautions must be followed, but as new research and clinical experience broaden our knowledge, changes in treatment and drug therapy may become necessary or appropriate. Readers are advised to check the most current product information provided by the manufacturer of each drug to be administered to verify the recommended dose, the method and duration of administration, and contraindications. It is the responsibility of the licensed health care provider, relying on experience and knowledge of the patient, to determine dosages and the best treatment for each individual patient. Neither the publisher nor the author assumes any liability for any injury and/or damage to persons or property arising from this publication.

Previous edition copyrighted 1999.

International Standard Book Number   0-7216-8252-9

Executive Publisher: Barbara Nelson Cullen
Senior Developmental Editor: Victoria Bruno
Publishing Services Manager: Deborah L. Vogel
Project Manager: Deon Lee
Design Manager: Amy Buxton

Printed in the United States of America

Last digit is the print number: 9 8 7 6 5 4 3 2 1

Dedication

We dedicate this book to our parents

CHARLES GRAHAM AND HAZEL COOPER, who have provided us a lifetime of unconditional love and support

Reviewers

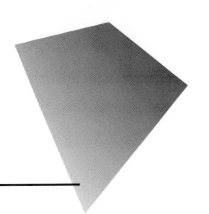

RHONDA LARIMORE RN, FNP-CERTIFIED, MSN
Western Carolina University
Asheville, North Carolina

BRENDA S. RAPP MSN, CS, FNP-C
Health Texas Provider Network (Baylor System)
Waxahachie, Texas

CATHERINE ELIZABETH COHILL TURNER, RN, MSN, FNP-C, CDR, USN
Halyburton Naval Hospital
Cherry Point, North Carolina

Contributors

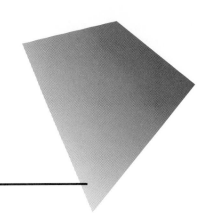

MARY ATTARDO
Easton, Massachusetts

KATHRYN A. BLAIR, PhD, RN, FNP
Professor
Graduate Coordinator FNP-Emphasis
University of Northern Colorado
Greeley, Colorado

MARY BOYLE, MSN, RN, FNP, BCADM, CDE, CS
Mayo Clinic
Scottsdale, Arizona

SUSAN CHANEY, EdD, APRN, FNP-C, BC
Professor/FNP Coordinator
College of Nursing
Texas Women's University
Dallas, Texas
Family Nurse Practitioner
Homeless Outreach Medical Services
Parkland Health & Hospital System
Dallas, Texas

SHARON G. CHILDS, MS, APRN-BC, CS, ONC
Adult Nurse Practitioner
Orthopedic Trauma/Critical Care–Clinical Nurse
Specialist
Baltimore, Maryland

CYNDY CHURGIN, RN-C, FNP, CNM
Casa Blanca Medical Group
Mesa, Arizona

SHARON DECKER, MSN, RN, CS, CCRN
Professor & Director of Clinical Simulations
School of Nursing
Texas Tech University Health Science Center
Lubbock, Texas

GAIL KOELKER, MSN, RN-C, FNP
Certified Family Nurse Practitioner
Good Shepherd Health System
Longview, Texas
Faculty, University of Phoenix
BSN Online Program
Phoenix, Arizona

ELA-JOY LEHRMAN, PhD, MS, MAED, RN, CNM
Professor & Chair, Nursing & Health Sciences
Southern Arizona Campus
University of Phoenix
Phoenix, Arizona

MARGARET A. LYNCH, MSN, BA
Family Nurse Practitioner
The Cambridge Hospital
Cambridge, Massachusetts

MARY D. MACKENBURG, MS, RN, CPNP
Assistant Professor, Department of Nursing
College of St. Catherine
St. Paul, Minnesota
Nurse Practitioner
Emergency Department
Children's Hospital and Clinics
St. Paul, Minnesota

JOYCE A. MEADOR, MSN, RN, ARNP-BC, GNP
University of Phoenix Online
BSN Program
Phoenix, Arizona

DIANE TODD PACE, PhD, APRN, BC
Nurse Practitioner/Researcher
University of Tennessee Health Science Department
Assistant Clinical Professor, College of Nursing
**Assistant Professor, Department of Preventative
  Medicine**
Memphis, Tennessee
Union University
Assistant Professor
Jackson, Tennessee
Online Faculty
University of Phoenix
Phoenix, Arizona

PATRICIA SHANNON, MS, MA, RN, CS, PNP
Faculty
University of Phoenix
Phoenix, Arizona
Adjunct Faculty
Grand Canyon University
Phoenix, Arizona

SCOTT W. SHIFFER, MSN, FNP
Head Family Practice Department
Naval Hospital
Rota, Spain

TAMARA R. TRIPP, MSN, ANP/GNP-C
Medical Plaza Family Physicians
Charlotte, North Carolina

Preface

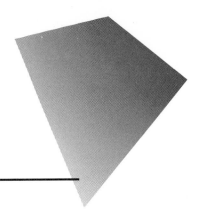

With the dawn of the role of the nurse practitioner, there is an increasing need for additional reference information and study materials for the certification examinations. Nurse practitioners are playing a vital role in the changing health care delivery system in the United States. The number of candidates for the certification examinations is rapidly increasing as more nursing programs implement the nurse practitioner curriculum in their graduate programs. *Adult Nurse Practitioner Certification Review,* second edition, has been developed to assist the advanced practice nurse to prepare for the ANP certification examination. Extensive efforts have been made to include current information that is representative of the content based on the blueprints for the certification exams. This book of questions is not intended to be an exhaustive review of the content, but an adjunct to the review process.

Test-taking strategies are included in Chapter 1. As a candidate prepares for the examination, it is vitally important for him or her to be familiar with and to practice good test-taking strategies. Good test-taking strategies can prevent the candidate from making mistakes and selecting the wrong answer. As the review process begins, a review of the test-taking strategies chapter and the practice of good test-taking strategies are critical. With many years of experience in the field of test-taking, we have consistently identified the importance practice test-taking plays in the review process. Practice questions give the candidate an opportunity to review questions written from different perspectives. To enhance the review process, answers along with complete rationales are provided at the end of each chapter. Not only does the candidate increase knowledge of the subject area, but also with more practice, test-taking skills become fine-tuned. Good test-taking skills make the candidate more comfortable and help to decrease the stress associated with certification exams.

This book also includes chapters reviewing important concepts related to Growth & Development and Health Promotion & Maintenance. These chapters provide questions that test information related to adult growth and development, general health supervision, and health maintenance. The clinical chapters are developed using a systems approach (cardiovascular, respiratory, endocrine, etc). In each of these chapters, the test questions are divided into three areas: Physical Examination & Diagnostic Tests, Disorders, and Pharmacology. This format assists the candidate to easily locate specific questions. The last three chapters in the text are on Research & Theory, Issues & Trends, and Legal & Ethical Issues, all aspects of nurse practitioner practice. The test questions in these chapters focus on professional competencies inherent in the role and function of the ANP.

Our thanks to the many nurse practitioners across the country who provided questions and insight into the role of the nurse practitioner. We wish to thank Victoria Bruno, our editor at Elsevier, for her support and suggestions in our preparation of the manuscript. Thank you also goes to the nurse practitioners who took time from their busy schedules to review the questions for content and clarity.

Acknowledgments

We are continually grateful for the contributions and efforts of our test item contributors, who provided their expertise and knowledge for this nurse practitioner certification review series.

We thank the staff at Elsevier: Barbara Nelson Cullen, Executive Publisher, and Victoria Bruno, Senior Developmental Editor, for their calmness and patience, and Deon Lee, Project Manager, who managed the book's production. What a job to keep track of thousands of questions!

Last, but certainly not least, we want to thank: Our children, Tyler and Ashley Zerwekh, Jaelyn Conway, Michael Brown, and Kim Aultman, for teasing their mothers about writing so many books!! Our parents, Charles Graham and Hazel Cooper, for their continued support and encouragement. Tom Gaglione and Robert Claborn for their encouragement, support, and love. We love you all.

Contents

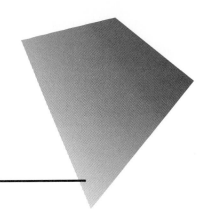

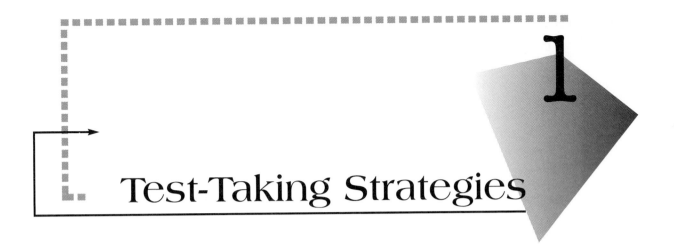

Test-Taking Strategies

Strategies

Knowing how to take an examination is a skill that is developed through practice and experience. Being able to take an examination effectively is almost as important as having the basic knowledge required to answer the questions. Everyone has taken an examination only to find, on review, that questions were answered incorrectly because of inadequate test-taking skills. Nurse practitioner programs provide the graduate student with a comprehensive base of knowledge; how you use this knowledge will determine your success on a certification examination. The certification examination is an objective test that covers knowledge, understanding, and application of professional nursing theory and practice. When you register for the examination, you will receive a "candidate handbook" or information materials from the certification board administering the examination. The handbook will have helpful information to assist you in preparing for the examination, including important registration information, a test content outline, sample test questions, and in some cases a bibliography. This important information can assist you in your review process.

Read the information in this chapter carefully and make sure you understand the strategies discussed. This chapter is designed to help you identify problem areas in test-taking skills and learn how to use strategy and judgment in selecting correct answers. It is important for you to practice test-taking skills if you are going to be able to use them on the certification examination.

Question Characteristics

A. Multiple-choice questions.
   1. Scene or scenario—establishes the setting of the question. Not all questions will have a scenario; if a scenario is included, consider the appropriateness of the answer to the information provided.
   2. Stem—states the question that is being asked.
   3. Options—there are four options from which to choose an answer.
      a. Distracters—designed to distract you from the correct answer.
      b. Correct answer—correctly answers the question asked in the stem.
      c. There are only four options in any item; there are no combinations of options to consider.
      d. There is only one correct response; no partial credit is given for another answer.
B. Questions are derived from clinical situations common in the practice setting.

Strategies for Multiple-Choice Questions

1. Cover the options with your hand or a piece of scratch paper. This strategy makes you focus on the content of the question and prevents your eyes from "darting" to look at the distracters. If you peruse the distracters before you completely understand the question, key words in the distracters will influence your interpretation of the question. If you practice this during your preparation for the examination, when you are taking the test on the computer, you will be less likely to go to the answers before you understand the question.

2. Do not read extra meaning into the question. The question is asking for specific information; if it appears to require simple "common sense," then assume it is simple. Do not look for a hidden meaning in what appears to be an easy question.

EXAMPLE

The nurse practitioner understands that the most common form of facial paralysis in the adult client is:

1. Facial nerve fasciitis.
2. Trigeminal neuralgia.
3. Bell's palsy.
4. Herpes zoster.

The correct answer is Option #3. Be careful not to "read into" the question and add pain to the facial paralysis symptom. The most common form of facial paralysis is Bell's palsy, which is a disorder affecting the facial nerve and characterized by muscle flaccidity of the affected side of the face. Trigeminal neuralgia is a disorder of cranial nerve V, characterized by an abrupt onset of pain in the lower and upper jaw, cheek, and lips. Herpes zoster affects the dermatomes and does not cause paralysis, but pain is possible with postherpetic neuralgia.

EXAMPLE

When administering skin tests to an immunocompromised client, the nurse practitioner must consider:

1. The importance of not applying more than one skin test at a time.
2. The possibility that the reaction may be more aggressive than expected.
3. The use of a known allergen for the client and its use as a control.
4. That the immunocompromised client should not be skin tested.

The correct answer is Option #3. Do not read into the question and make it more difficult by trying to make the client sicker (e.g., full-blown acquired immunodeficiency syndrome [AIDS]). It is important to remember to apply controls when skin testing the immunocompromised client. Ask clients what diseases they believe they have immunity to, such as measles. If the client is unable to mount an immune response at all, the known allergen will not cause a reaction. If the controls are not applied, the nurse practitioner may assume a skin test result is negative, when in fact, the client's immune system is unable to respond.

3. Read the stem carefully. Make sure you understand exactly what information the question is asking. It is important to understand the question before reviewing the options for the correct answer.

EXAMPLE

A client with a history of Parkinson's disease has a positive TB skin test and Isoniazid (INH) is ordered as a prophylactic medication. Before beginning administration of INH, it is important for the nurse practitioner to determine:

1. Whether the client's Parkinson's disease is being treated with levodopa (Larodopa).
2. How long the client has had Parkinson's disease.
3. How much respiratory compromise the client is currently experiencing.
4. The adequacy of urinary output and renal function.

The question asks you to determine whether giving the INH to a client with Parkinson's disease is a problem. The correct answer is Option #1. This question requires the nurse practitioner to critically think about other medications the client may be taking and whether they would interfere with the action or effectiveness of INH. In this case, INH requires concurrent administration of vitamin B_6 to prevent problems of optic neuritis. Vitamin B_6 will decrease the effectiveness of levodopa. If the client is to receive the INH, his antiparkinson medication needs to be reevaluated.

4. Before reviewing the options, think about characteristics of the condition and what critical concepts should be considered. Begin by assessing each option with regard to the characteristics of the condition.

EXAMPLE

The usual clinical presentation of an adult client with cystitis is:

1. No chills, fever, headache, malaise, or discomfort noted.
2. Acute onset of chills, fever, flank pain, headache, malaise, and costovertebral angle tenderness.
3. Complaints of dysuria, urgency, frequency, nocturia, and suprapubic heaviness.
4. Signs and symptoms of fever, irritability, decreased appetite, vomiting, diarrhea, constipation, dehydration, and jaundice.

Formulate in your mind possible answers to the question. Think to yourself "Which of these symptoms are normally seen with cystitis? What is different about pyelonephritis? Is the usual presentation without symptoms? Is there involvement of the gastrointestinal tract (as alluded to in Option #4). If you are unsure, go back and reassess the question. In this instance, Option #3 is correct. An adult with cystitis usually presents with dysuria, urgency, frequency, nocturia, and suprapubic heaviness. Acute onset of chills, fever, flank pain, headache, malaise, and costovertebral angle tenderness are common symptoms of pyelonephritis.

5. Identify the type of response the question requires. A positive stem requires identification of three false items and one correct answer.

E X A M P L E

Clients who believe they have been exposed to human immunodeficiency virus (HIV) should have an HIV antibody test how soon after the exposure?

1. The next day and 2 months later.
2. 6 months after exposure and again at 12 months.
3. 6 to 12 weeks after exposure and again at 6 months.
4. 4 weeks and 12 weeks.

The correct answer is Option #3. This question requires you to identify three incorrect responses and one correct response. The HIV antibody develops between 6 and 12 weeks after exposure. Because of the variability of antibody development, it is recommended that the test be repeated in 6 months to confirm the findings.

6. Questions may require identification of something the practitioner should not or would not do (e.g., unsafe action, contraindication, inappropriate action).

E X A M P L E

The nurse practitioner is prescribing astemizole (Hismanal) for a geriatric client's allergy problems. When the client's current medications are considered, which medication would be a contraindication to the administration of astemizole?

1. Erythromycin ethylsuccinate (EES).
2. Verapamil (Calan).
3. Propranolol (Inderal).
4. Captopril (Capoten).

The correct answer is Option #1. Macrolides and astemizole should not be administered concurrently. The nurse practitioner is required to identify a medication that should not be ordered.

7. Questions may also be analytical. Some questions may ask the nurse practitioner to identify findings or statements that are consistent or inconsistent with the client's presenting problem and/or to differentiate between them.

E X A M P L E

Dementia can be distinguished from delirium by:

1. Dementia lasts days to weeks compared with delirium, which lasts months to years.
2. Dementia is often associated with medications or systemic illness.
3. Dementia exhibits a disturbance in attention that is not present in delirium.
4. Dementia does not include altered perception such as hallucinations.

Before you examine the options in this question, it is important to think about the differences between dementia and delirium. The correct answer is Option #4. Adults with dementia do not usually have altered perceptions that include hallucinations. Dementia does last months to years. Delirium is often associated with medications or systemic illness and a disturbance in the ability to pay attention.

8. Identify key words that affect your understanding of the question. Make sure you understand exactly what information the question is seeking. Be wary of questions in which the stem includes words such as *except, contraindicated, avoid, least, not applicable,* and *does not occur.* These words change the direction of the question. It may help to rephrase the question in your own words to better understand what information is being requested.

E X A M P L E

Clients with arteriosclerotic heart disease (ASHD) go through several stages before becoming severely compromised. Which does not occur in the early stages of ASHD?

1. Decreased urine output.
2. Dyspnea during exercise.
3. Anginal pain relieved by rest.
4. Increased serum triglyceride levels.

Rephrase the question: In early stages of ASHD, which of the following does not occur? It is important that you identify the key point "early stages of ASHD" and the key words "does not occur." If you miss these essential points, you do not understand the question, and chances are you will not choose the correct answer. The correct answer is Option #1: a decrease in urine output occurs when cardiac disease is advanced enough to cause a severe decrease in cardiac output and renal perfusion.

9. As you read the options, eliminate those you know are not correct. Now that you understand the question, begin eliminating the incorrect answers. This will help narrow the field of choice. When you select an answer or eliminate a distracter, you should have a specific reason for doing so. Don't try to predict a correct answer; it is distressing if the answer you want is not a selection.

E X A M P L E

A 45-year-old female complains of knee pain when kneeling and a "clicking" noise when walking up steps. On physical examination, there is a slight knee effusion and tenderness when the patella is palpated against the condyles. The diagnosis for this client is:

1. Anterior cruciate tear. (No, the client generally cannot bear weight on the extremity without it buckling or giving way.)
2. Dislocated patella. (No, there would be considerable effusion and locking of the knee in flexion.)
3. Chondromalacia patella. (Yes, there is clicking and anterior knee pain around or under the kneecap exacerbated by knee extensor stress.)
4. Tendinitis. (No, there would be no clicking sound with movement.)

After systematic evaluation of the options, Option #3 is the correct answer.

10. Identify similarities in the distracters. Frequently, three options will contain similar information, and one will be different. The different one may be the correct answer.

E X A M P L E

An elderly client is to be encouraged to increase her intake of protein. The addition of which of these foods to 100 ml of milk will provide the greatest amount of protein?

1. 50 ml light cream and 2 tbsp corn syrup.
2. 30 g powdered skim milk and one egg.
3. 1 small scoop (90 g) ice cream and 1 tbsp chocolate syrup.
4. 2 egg yolks and 1 tbsp sugar.

Options #1, #3, and #4 all contain a simple sugar. The correct answer, Option #2, has more protein. Notice that three of the options are similar; the one that is different may be the correct answer. This strategy is not a substitute for basic knowledge but may help you figure out the answer.

11. Select the most comprehensive answer. All of the options may be correct, but **one** will include the other three options or need to be considered first.

E X A M P L E

Diagnostic studies used in the differential diagnosis of systemic lupus erythematosus (SLE) include:

1. CBC, SMA_{12}, and erythrocyte sedimentation rate (ESR).
2. Chest radiograph and coagulation profile.
3. Antinuclear antibody (ANA), ESR, and C-reactive protein.
4. CBC, urinalysis, chest radiograph.

The correct answer is Option #3. Although all of the tests included in the answer may be included in a complete physical examination, laboratory tests specific for or inclusive of the diagnosis of SLE include the ANA, ESR, and C-reactive protein. During flares, the ESR and C-reactive protein level are increased. The ANA titer in a client with SLE is positive at a ratio of 1:80.

12. Select the answer that is most specific to what the question asks. All of the options may be correct, but one is more specific or essential.

E X A M P L E

When you are taking the history of a client with known allergies, what is the most important information to determine?

1. Reaction associated with each allergen.
2. Drug allergies.
3. Food allergies.
4. Environmental exposure.

It is absolutely essential that the reaction to each allergen is known. The other options are important but are not most important during the taking of the history. Look for key words that indicate the question is asking for a priority of care—first, initial, best, most. The correct answer is Option #1. The other alternatives may be correct but should be prioritized. Often clients will indicate they have a reaction to a particular food or medication, such as nausea, stomach pain, or diarrhea and consider it an allergy. The signs and symptoms of the reaction, speed of onset, how long it lasts, and what successful treatment has been used in the past are important pieces of information. Both drug and food allergies should be explored.

13. Watch questions in which the options contain several items to consider. After you are sure you understand what information the question is requesting, evaluate each part of the distracter. Is it appropriate to what the question is asking? If an option contains one incorrect item, the entire option is incorrect. All of the items listed in the selection must be correct if it is to be the correct answer to the question.

EXAMPLE

When evaluating an electrocardiogram, which characteristics most clearly indicate atrial tachycardia?

1. Heart rate of 96 bpm, P waves present on each QRS complex, T wave every other beat.
2. P waves present on every other beat, heart rate of 100 bpm, and irregular.
3. Heart rate of 110 bpm, P waves present before each QRS complex, and regular.
4. P waves for every third QRS complex, adequate PR interval, heart rate of 90 bpm.

The correct answer is Option #3. In a methodical evaluation of the items in the distracters, you can eliminate items in Options #1, #2, and #4. Sinus or atrial tachycardia is characterized by a rate at or above 100 bpm, P waves are present for each QRS, the PR interval is below 0.20, the T wave occurs after each QRS complex, and the beat is regular.

14. Be alert to relevant information contained in previous questions. Sometimes as you are answering questions, you will find information similar to that in a question you already answered. Previous questions may assist you in identifying relevant information in the current question.

EXAMPLE

The American College of Physicians (ACP) recommends that healthy adults receive a tetanus diphtheria (Td) booster vaccination:

1. Every 5 years.
2. At age 75.
3. At age 65.
4. Every 10 years.

The ACP recommends that adults receive a Td booster every 10 years or a single booster at age 50 for clients who have completed full pediatric series, including teenage and young adult boosters. The correct answer to this question is Option #4. Another question involving immunizations, reads as follows:

EXAMPLE

In taking the history of an alert, older adult, the nurse practitioner determines that the client is an avid gardener and spends a great deal of time outside. He had a pneumococcal vaccination last year and states he cannot remember when he had a tetanus vaccination. A health maintenance recommendation for this client would be to obtain:

1. Pneumococcal vaccine.
2. Tetanus vaccine.
3. Hepatitis B vaccine.
4. No recommendation.

The correct answer is Option #2. A clue to the answer to this question may be found in the previous question. Older adults who enjoy gardening and outdoor activities should have a Td booster once every 10 years, because the ACP recommends this practice. Some professionals advocate that high-risk populations (e.g., gardeners, construction workers, or others who spend a lot of time outdoors) have a Td booster every 5 years. When you are taking the test on the computer, it is more difficult to remember previous questions, and you will not be able to go back and change answers.

15. Multiple-choice mathematical computations may be included in the examination. Mathematical computations may include calculations of IM, PO, and IV dosages; calculations of pediatric dosage; determination of creatinine clearance; and conversion of units of measurement.

EXAMPLE

The nurse practitioner is ordering digoxin (Lanoxin) 0.25 mg for a client who has difficulty swallowing pills. How would the order be written?

1. Digoxin 0.25 mg Sig: 1 cc elixir PO qd.
2. Digoxin 0.25 mg Sig: 1 tab PO qd.
3. Digoxin 0.25 mg Sig: 2.5 cc PO elixir qd.
4. Digoxin 0.025 mg/5 cc Sig: 5cc PO qd.

First, you must know that the digoxin dispensing dose for adults is 0.25 mg/cc. For a dose of 0.25 mg, the correct answer is Option #1.

16. Evaluate priority questions carefully.

Frequently, all of the answers are appropriate to the situation. You need to decide which of the actions you should do first.

EXAMPLE

While working in her garden, an older adult was bitten on the hand by a raccoon. Her last Td booster was 4 years ago. At the rural clinic, the nurse practitioner cleansed the wound. The next action is to:

1. Administer tetanus antitoxin.
2. Contact local animal control authorities.
3. Administer rabies immune globulin (RIG) and human diploid cell vaccine (HDCV).
4. Teach the client how to do hourly soaks of the hand with a normal saline and peroxide solution.

The correct answer is Option #3. Any type of bite from an animal that may harbor rabies (e.g., a skunk, bat, raccoon, fox, coyote, or rat) should be treated with both active and passive rabies immunization.

The priority action is to prevent rabies. Tetanus antitoxin would be indicated if the adult was not current on the immunization. Animal authorities would be called after the initial treatment to locate the animal and kill it, so that the brain could be examined for rabies.

Techniques to Increase Critical Thinking Skills

Memory aids and mindmapping™ are tools that assist in creating associations between ideas and images. Mnemonics are words, phrases, or other techniques that help you remember information. Imagery is a tool that helps you identify a problem and create a mental picture. Learning content by using these techniques will help you to recall information more effectively.

Mindmapping™ is a method of organizing important information that is in sharp contrast to the traditional outline format. A thought or concept is written in the center of the page, and images and color are added to information as ideas begin to flow from the focal point in the center (Figure 1–1).

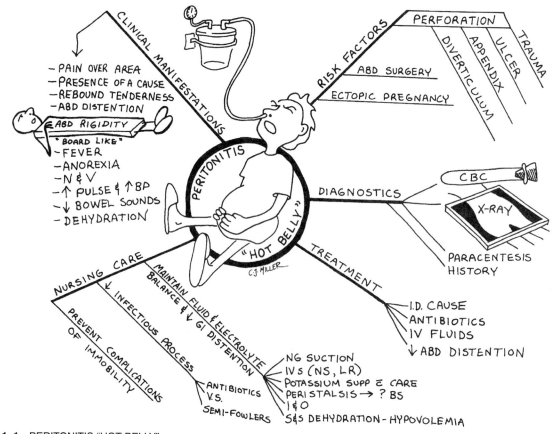

FIGURE 1–1 PERITONITIS "HOT BELLY"
With permission from Zerwekh J, Claborn J, Miller CJ: *Memory notebook of nursing*, Vol I, Dallas, Texas, 2000, Nursing Education Consultants Publishing, p 85.

Acronyms help you to recall information by means of word association or arrangements of letters to recall specific details. Examples of these are the 6 Ps of dyspnea (Figure 1–2), the 5 Ps of circulatory assessment (Figure 1–3), and the ABCs of malignant melanoma (Figure 1–4).

Acrostics are catchy phrases in which the first letter of each word stands for something to recall. For example, to remember the use of canes and walkers (Figure 1–5), think of "Wandering Wilma's Always Late" (**W**alker **W**ith **A**ffected **L**eg). Everyone remembers the cranial nerve mnemonic (Figure 1–6).

Memory aids or images are pictures or caricatures that help you to recall information more effectively (Figure 1–7).

Rhymes are phrases or words spoken in a rhythmic or musical manner that increase recall. A helpful musical rhyme for hypoglycemia versus hyperglycemia is "hot and dry, sugar high; cold and clammy, need some candy" (Figure 1–8). Another rhyme, "fingers, nose, penis, toes," identifies the areas where lidocaine with epinephrine is contraindicated as a local anesthetic. Or the short sentence, "two is too much," may help you remember toxic levels of the following three drugs, which have a narrow margin of safety: lithium, digoxin, and theophylline (Figure 1–9). *Note: These are just examples. There are entire books on these helpful aids (see the list of references).*

Test-Taking Skills for Paper-and-Pencil Tests

Although you will take the certification exams on the computer, the test-taking skills described in this chapter can also be applied to paper-and-pencil exams that you may encounter as a student in your program.

1. Go through the exam and mark all the answers that you know are correct. This ensures you have adequate time to answer the questions you know. Go back and evaluate those questions for which you did not readily recognize the answer.

2. Do not indiscriminately change answers. If you go back and change an answer, you should have a specific reason for doing so. Sometimes you remember information and realize you answered the question incorrectly. Frequently, test takers "talk themselves out of" the correct answer and change it to an incorrect one.

3. After you have completed the exam, go back and check your booklet and make sure all of the questions are answered. Answer all of the questions, even if you must guess.

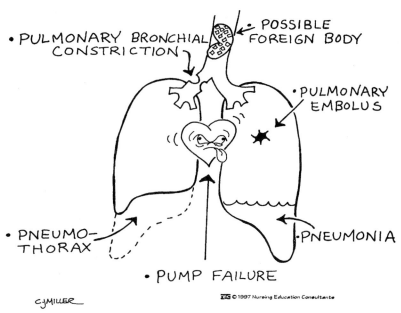

CJ MILLER   © 1997 Nursing Education Consultants

FIGURE 1–2   THE 6 PS OF DYSPNEA
With permission from Zerwekh J, Claborn J, Miller CJ: *Memory notebook of nursing*, Vol II, Dallas, Texas, 1997, Nursing Education Consultants Publishing, p 22.

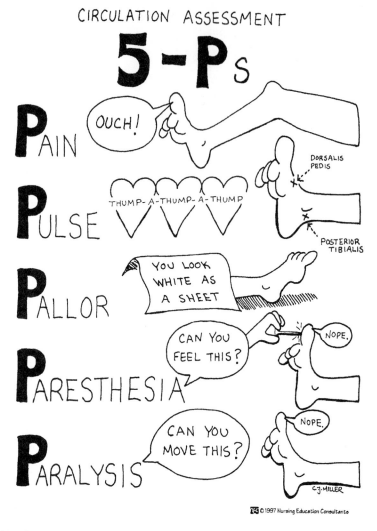

FIGURE 1-3 CIRCULATION ASSESSMENT: THE 5 PS
With permission from Zerwekh J, Claborn J, Miller CJ: *Memory notebook of nursing*, Vol II, Dallas, Texas, 1997, Nursing Education Consultants Publishing, p 27.

Successful Test Taking

1. Listen carefully to the instructions given at the beginning of the examination. Make sure you understand all of the information given and exactly how to mark your answers and/or how to use the keyboard.

2. Watch your timing. Do not spend too much time on one question. It is very important that you practice your timing on the practice exams. You will not be able to review your questions and answers on completion of the computer test. Do it right the first time, and there will be no need to review the entire test again. Watch your timing on computer tests; make use of a computer clock, if it is available.

3. Be aware of your "first hunch." It is frequently the correct answer. Sometimes information is processed by the brain without you being aware of it. If something about an answer "feels right" or you have a "gut-level feeling," pay attention to it.

4. Eliminate distracters that assume the client "would not understand" or "is ignorant" of the situation and those that "protect the client from worry." For example, "The client should not be told she has cancer because it would upset her too much."

5. Be wary of distracters that contain the words *always* and *never*.

6. There is no pattern of correct answers. Both computer and paper-and-pencil examinations are compiled by a computer, and the position of the correct answers is selected at random.

7. Check the length of the options to consider. The option in which the correct answer is adequately stated is *sometimes* longer than the other options.

HINTS TO MALIGNANT MELANOMA

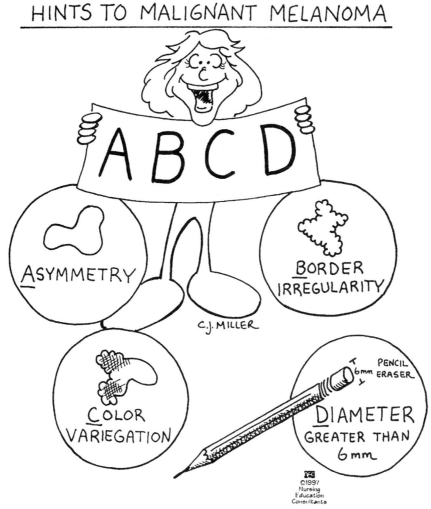

FIGURE 1–4   HINTS TO MALIGNANT MELANOMA (ABCD)
With permission from Zerwekh J, Claborn J, Miller CJ: *Memory notebook of nursing*, Vol I, Dallas, Texas, 1997, Nursing Education
Consultants Publishing, p 137.

Decrease Anxiety

Your activities on the day of the examination
strongly influence your level of anxiety. By carefully
planning ahead, you will be able to eliminate some
anxiety-provoking situations. If you are a diabetic or
have special needs, contact the certification agency
ahead of time to make arrangements to have food or
other accommodations that you might require.

1. Visit the examination site before the day of
   the exam. Evaluate travel time, parking, and
   time to get to the designated area. Get an
   early start to allow extra time.

2. If you have to travel some distance to the
   examination site, try to spend the night in the
   immediate vicinity.

3. Do something pleasant the evening before
   the examination. This is not the time to "cram."

4. Anxiety is contagious. If those around you are
   extremely anxious, avoid contact with them
   before the examination.

5. Make your meal before the test a light,
   healthy one.

6. Avoid eating highly spiced or different foods.
   This is not the time for a gastrointestinal
   upset.

7. Wear comfortable clothes. This is not a good
   time to wear tight clothing or new shoes.

8. Wear clothing of moderate weight. It is difficult to control the temperature to keep everyone comfortable. Take a sweater or wear
   layered clothes that can be removed if you get
   too warm.

9. Wear soft-soled shoes; this decreases the noise
   in the testing area.

10. Make sure you have the papers that are
    required to gain admission to the exam site.

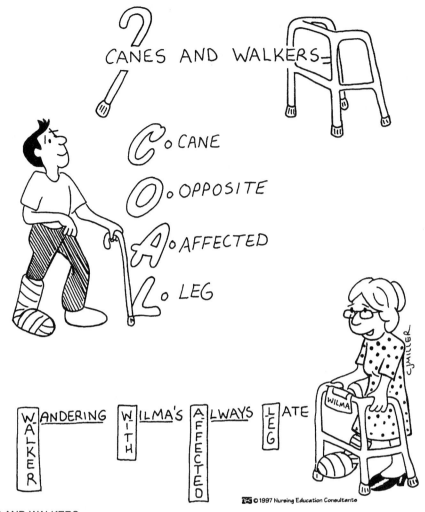

FIGURE 1–5 CANES AND WALKERS
With permission from Zerwekh J, Claborn J, Miller CJ: *Memory notebook of nursing*, Vol II, Dallas, Texas, 1997, Nursing Education Consultants Publishing, p 8.

Do not forget your reading glasses, if you wear them.

11. Do not take study material to the exam site. You cannot take it into the exam area, and it is too late to study.

12. Do not panic when you encounter content with which you are unfamiliar in a question. Use good test-taking strategies, select an answer, and continue. Remember, your time is limited and you may not know all of the right answers.

13. Reaffirm to yourself that you know the material. It is not time for any self-defeating behavior or negative self-talk. **YOU WILL PASS!!** Build your confidence by visualizing yourself in 6 months working in the area you desire. Create that mental picture of where you want to be and who you want to be—certified nurse practitioner. Use your past successes to bring positive energy and "vibes" to your certification. **WE KNOW YOU CAN DO IT!**

Study Habits

Enhancing Study Skills

- Decide on a realistic study schedule: write it down and stick with it.
- Divide the review material into segments—pediatrics, well woman, geriatric, and so forth.
- Prioritize the segments; review first the areas in which you feel you are deficient or weak.
- Identify areas that will require additional review.
- Establish a realistic schedule; study in short segments or "bursts." Avoid marathon sessions.
- Plan on achieving your study goal several days before the examination.
- Do not study when you are tired or when there are frequent distractions or interruptions.
- Review general concepts of practice from a variety of resources.

CRANIAL NERVE MNEMONIC

S = Sensory	M = Motor	B = Both

O	Olfactory	O	On	S	Some
O	Optic	O	Old	S	Say
O	Oculomotor	O	Olympus'	M	Marry
T	Trochlear	T	Tiny	M	Money
T	Trigeminal	T	Tops	B	But
A	Abducens	A	A	M	My
F	Facial	F	Finn	B	Brother
A	Acoustic	A	And	S	Says
G	Glossopharyngeal	G	German	B	Bad
V	Vagus nerve	V	Viewed	B	Business
S	Spinal	S	Some	M	Marry
H	Hypoglossal	H	Hops	M	Money

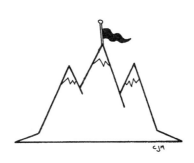 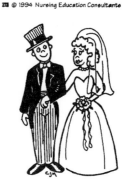

FIGURE 1–6   CRANIAL NERVE MNEMONIC
With permission from Zerwekh J, Claborn J, Miller CJ: *Memory notebook of nursing*, Vol II, Dallas, Texas, 1994, Nursing Education Consultants Publishing, p 91.

HYPERTHYROIDISM

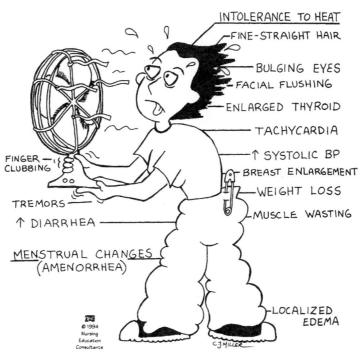

FIGURE 1–7   HYPERTHYROIDISM
With permission from Zerwekh J, Claborn J, Miller CJ: *Memory notebook of nursing*, Vol I, Dallas, Texas, 1994, Nursing Education Consultants Publishing, p 46.

BLOOD SUGAR MNEMONIC

Hot & Dry = Sugar High

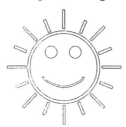

Cold & Clammy = Need Some Candy

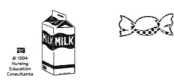

FIGURE 1–8 BLOOD SUGAR MNEMONIC
With permission from Zerwekh J, Claborn J, Miller CJ: *Memory notebook of nursing*, Vol I, Dallas, Texas, 1994, Nursing Education Consultants Publishing, p 50.

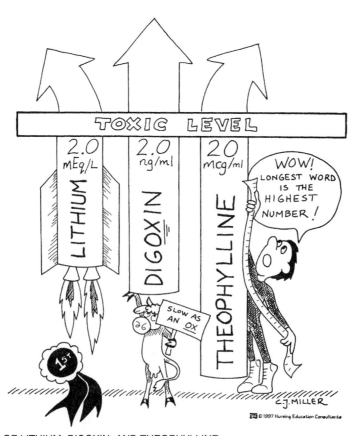

FIGURE 1–9 TOXIC LEVELS OF LITHIUM, DIGOXIN, AND THEOPHYLLINE
With permission from Zerwekh J, Claborn J, Miller CJ: *Memory notebook of nursing*, Vol II, Dallas, Texas, 1997, Nursing Education Consultants Publishing, p 43.

Group Study

- Keep the group limited to four or five people.
- Group members should be mature and serious about studying.
- The group should agree on the planned study schedule.
- If the group makes you anxious or you do not feel it meets your study needs, do not continue to participate.

Testing Practice

- Include testing practice in your schedule.
- Select about 50 questions for a practice testing session of 1 hour. This will allow you to evaluate the pace of the exam (i.e., approximately one question per minute).
- Try to answer the questions as if you were taking the real examination. Do not look up the right answer immediately after answering the question. Complete all of the questions you have selected, then go back and check your answers against the key.
- Use the testing strategies described in this chapter.

- Evaluate the practice exams for problem areas: test-taking skills and knowledge base.
- Evaluate the questions you answer incorrectly. Review the rationale for the right answer and understand why you missed it.
- Utilize the questions at a later point to review the information again.

References

Beitz J: Unleashing the power of memory: The mighty mnemonic, *Nurse Educator* 22(2):25-28, 1997.

Bloomingfield R: *Mnemonics, rhetorics, and poetics for medics*, Salem, NC, 1982, Harbinger Medical Press.

Rayfield S, Manning L: *Nursing made insanely easy*, Shreveport, La, 2002, ICAN, Inc. Publishing.

Zerwekh J, Claborn J: Test-taking strategies. In *NCLEX-RN™: A comprehensive study guide*, ed 5, Dallas, Texas, 2002, Nursing Education Consultants Publishing.

Zerwekh J, Claborn J, Miller CJ: *Memory notebook of nursing*, Vol I, ed 2, Dallas, Texas, 2000, Nursing Education Consultants Publishing.

Zerwekh J, Claborn J, Miller CJ: *Memory notebook of nursing*, Vol II, ed 2, Dallas, Texas, 2003, Nursing Education Consultants Publishing.

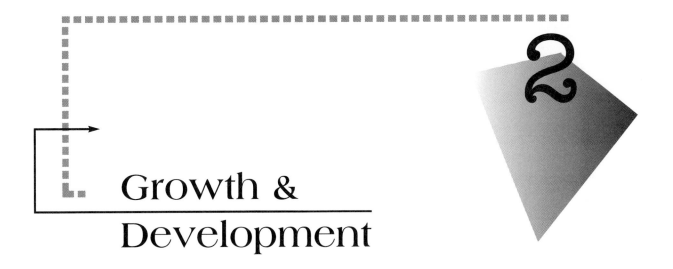

Growth & Development

2

Adult

1. The nurse practitioner understands that the growth of long bones and the myelinization and differentiation of the central nervous system continues until about the age of:

   1. 18.

   2. 20.

   3. 22.

   4. 25.

2. Visual acuity is affected in middle-aged individuals when going from a well-lighted place into a dark room because of:

   1. Diminishing pupil size caused by aging.

   2. Problems associated with myopia.

   3. Change in the ability to determine depth perception.

   4. Problems associated with presbycusis.

3. According to Erickson, early adulthood is the time for:

   1. Developing a stable self-concept.

   2. Forming close, intimate relationships.

   3. Finding security with a sexual identity.

   4. Breaking emotional and physical ties with parents.

4. According to the Holmes and Rahe Social Readjustment Rating Scale, the highest degree of adjustment is required after:

   1. Loss of a job.

   2. Death of a spouse.

   3. Marriage.

   4. Divorce.

Older Adult

5. As an individual ages, which physiologic change would affect responses to pharmacologic agents?

   1. Increased gastric emptying.

   2. Increased glomerular filtration rate.

   3. Decreased percentage of body fat.

   4. Decreased albumin concentration.

6. The number one cause of accidental death in clients older than 65 years is:

   1. Motor vehicle accidents.

   2. Poisoning.

   3. Falls.

   4. Drowning.

7. The nurse practitioner selects which assessment tool to evaluate balance and gait problems in the elderly?

   1. Lawton & Brody Balance and Coordination Scale.

   2. Tinetti Balance and Gait Evaluation.

   3. Instrumental Activities of Daily Living Scale.

   4. Index of Independence of Activities of Daily Living.

8. The nurse practitioner is assessing the nutritional status of an elderly client. The nurse practitioner identifies the common physiologic changes in the gastrointestinal (GI) system to be:

   1. Increased peristalsis.

   2. Decreased absorption of iron.

   3. Maintenance of normal fat metabolism.

   4. Increased drug metabolism.

9. What are the normal physiologic changes in the thyroid gland that occur with aging?

   1. Hypertrophy with a decrease in triiodothyronine (T_3) and thyroxine (T_4).

   2. Normal size with an increase in thyroid-stimulating hormone (TSH) and a decrease in T_4.

   3. Atrophy of the gland with a decrease in TSH, T_3, and T_4.

   4. Increase in nodularity with normal TSH and T_4.

10. The aging process causes what normal physiologic changes in the heart?

    1. Heart size stays the same, and the valves thicken and become rigid as a result of fibrosis and sclerosis.

    2. Cardiomegaly occurs along with prolapse of the mitral valve and regurgitation.

    3. Dilatation of the right ventricle occurs with sclerosis of pulmonic and tricuspid valves.

    4. Hypertrophy of the right ventricle occurs with decreasing capacity and compromised efficiency of the coronary arteries.

11. Which pulmonary physiologic change is commonly associated with the aging process?

    1. Increased cough response.

    2. Decrease in vital capacity.

    3. Decreased anteroposterior (AP) diameter of thorax.

    4. Increase in residual P_{CO_2}.

12. Which of these clinical findings would indicate a deviation from the normal age-related changes in the neurologic system and may have some diagnostic significance for the older client?

    1. Decreased sense of touch.

    2. Increased tolerance to pain.

    3. Decreased short-term memory.

    4. Decreased ability to maintain balance.

13. During a teaching session, the nurse practitioner instructs the client regarding normal skin lesions in the older population. These would include:

    1. Seborrheic dermatitis.

    2. Senile keratosis.

    3. Senile lentigines.

    4. Squamous cell carcinoma.

14. Which assessment is a normal physiologic change of the respiratory system that occurs with aging?

    1. Decreased residual lung volume (RV).

    2. Hyperresonance.

    3. Increased forced vital capacity (FVC).

    4. Increased tactile fremitus.

15. The nurse practitioner indicates an understanding of the normal aging process with which documentation of the GI system in the physical examination?

    1. Increase in the size of the liver (16 cm).

    2. Absent bowel sounds.

    3. Femoral bruit.

    4. Increased adipose tissue.

16. During the physical examination of an older client, the nurse practitioner indicates an understanding of deviations in the neurologic system from the normal aging process with which clinical finding?

    1. Decrease in short-term memory.

    2. Decrease in deep-tendon and superficial reflexes.

    3. Decreased sense of touch.

    4. Positive Romberg's sign.

17. Which functional assessment tool should the nurse practitioner use to evaluate the safety for a client who has had a cerebrovascular accident (CVA) and is planning to return to his or her home environment?

    1. Older Adults Resources and Services (OARS) ADL Scale.

    2. Bennet Social Isolation Scales.

    3. Mini Mental State Examination.

    4. Norton Scale.

18. The nurse practitioner understands which factor is most influential in the driving ability of an older adult?

    1. Ability to coordinate the transmissions.

    2. Acuity of vision.

    3. Comprehension of the details of the road rules.

    4. Reaction times.

19. As an individual ages, which physiologic change would affect sleep?

    1. Decreased rapid eye movement (REM) sleep.

    2. Increased delta or stage IV sleep.

    3. Decreased nocturnal awakenings.

    4. Decreased sleep latency.

20. When treating an infection in the older adult, the nurse practitioner must consider which of the following?

    1. Thymus-derived immunity is increased.

    2. Immune function declines with age.

    3. Immune function increased with age.

    4. Antibody production increases.

21. The diminished immunity of the older adult can be attributed to a decline in:

    1. B-cell function.

    2. T-cell production.

    3. B-cell production.

    4. T-cell function.

22. Which physiologic factor of aging contributes to incontinence in the elderly?

    1. Decreased vascularity of the bladder mucosa.

    2. Increased urethral closing pressure.

    3. Increased ability to concentrate urine.

    4. Decreased bladder capacity.

23. The nurse practitioner understands that as the client ages,

    1. The cells of the immune system are able to proliferate as they would in the younger client.

    2. The total number of remaining T cells is decreased.

    3. The elderly client is able to respond to infections with previously produced "remembered" antibodies.

    4. The immune system is able to respond to antigenic stimulation as in the younger client.

Answers & Rationales

Adult

1. **(4)** The growth of the long bones and the myelinization and differentiation of the central nervous system continue until about the age of 25 years. An adult may add ⅛ to ¼ inch to height, with men growing more in stature than women, but women's skulls tend to grow more than men's skulls do. In reality, some bones and the skull continue to grow throughout life. Muscles strengthen and reach peak efficiency between 25 and 30 years of age.

2. **(1)** With aging, there is a shrinking of the pupil size along with a weakening of the muscles that cause the pupil to dilate and constrict. Option #2 refers to nearsightedness. Depth perception may decrease slightly. Option #4 refers to high-frequency hearing loss.

3. **(2)** Intimacy versus isolation is the developmental task of early adulthood (ages 18-40). Options #1, #3, and #4 apply to adolescence.

4. **(2)** The Holmes and Rahe Social Readjustment Rating Scale indicates that death of a spouse is the most stressful life event, followed by divorce, marital separation, and loss of a job.

Older Adult

5. **(4)** Medications often bind to protein (not fat); albumin decreases with age. A low albumin level decreases the number of protein-binding sites, causing an increase in the amount of free drug in the plasma. Drug overdose may occur in the elderly. Gastric emptying and glomerular filtration rate *decrease* with aging.

6. **(3)** Falls are the major cause of morbidity and mortality in the elderly. A fall is often the precipitating event for a cascade of problems leading to death. Complications from falls include fractures, pneumonia, pressure ulcers, pain, and immobility.

7. **(2)** The Tinetti Balance and Gait Evaluation is an activity-based test that asks the client to perform tasks, such as sitting and rising from a chair, turning, and bending. It requires no more than 15 to 20 minutes to perform. Another appropriate test for assessment of risk for falls is the timed "Up and Go" test, which assesses balance and gait speed. Lawton and Brody are the authors of the Instrumental Activities of Daily Learning, which assesses the ability to perform complex tasks such as shopping, doing laundry, preparing food, and so forth. The Index of Independence of Activities of Daily Living helps to identify activities of daily living (ADL) with which the client needs assistance.

8. **(2)** Decreased hydrochloric acid, which occurs with aging, leads to decreased absorption of iron and vitamin B_{12}. Fat absorption would decrease, as would peristalsis and drug metabolism.

9. **(4)** There is usually adequate secretion of thyroid-stimulating hormone (TSH) and a normal serum concentration of thyroxine (T_4). Aging may produce fibrosis and increased nodularity, but overall, thyroid function remains within normal limits.

10. **(1)** The heart does not increase in size with normal aging. An enlarged heart is a result of cardiac dysfunction. Dilatation of the left

ventricle occurs with myocardial infarctions and altered cardiac functioning associated with cardiac disease, not normal aging. The aging process does cause fibrosis and sclerosis of the cardiac valves; all valves are equally affected.

11. **(2)** A decrease in the vital capacity, along with a 50% increase in residual volume, occurs during the aging process. Other age-related changes include a less effective cough, impaired ciliary action, and weaker respiratory muscles. Increased anteroposterior (AP) diameter is associated with aging and is found in clients with chronic obstructive pulmonary disease (COPD). Po_2 usually decreases, but Pco_2 usually remains unchanged.

12. **(4)** Decreased ability to maintain balance may indicate a cerebellar complication. The first three findings are normal age-related changes.

13. **(3)** Senile lentigines are gray-brown, irregular, macular lesions on sun-exposed areas of the face, arms, and hands and are normal skin lesions. The other lesions are commonly occurring abnormal skin lesions in the older adult.

14. **(2)** A normal age-related change is an increase in the AP diameter that results in hyperresonance. Age-related changes result in an increase in the residual volume (RV) and decrease in the forced vital capacity (FVC). An increased tactile fremitus is a deviation that is of diagnostic significance.

15. **(4)** Common age-related changes within the gastrointestinal (GI) system include increased adipose tissue, decrease in liver size, reduced motility and peristalsis, decrease in acid secretions and motor activity of stomach, and decrease in the glomerular filtration rate. Absence of bowel sounds after 5 full minutes and bruits are deviations of clinical significance.

16. **(4)** Romberg's sign indicates the inability to maintain balance, which indicates a need for further evaluation. Options #1, #2, and #3 are normal age-related changes. A decrease in short-term memory that affects functional ability would then be considered a deviation.

17. **(1)** The OARS ADL Scale is the more appropriate screening tool for identifying at-risk populations. The Bennet Social Isolation Scale would be appropriate for evaluation of social interactions and resources. The Mini Mental State Examination is used to evaluate memory, orientation, and attention. The Norton Scale is used to evaluate pressure ulcer risk.

18. **(2)** The most age-dependent driving factor is sensory change, and the elderly driving client being assessed for driving capacity should use any corrective devices for optimal performance. Poor hearing alone is generally not a limiting factor for motor vehicle operation. Visual acuity has received the greatest emphasis in assessment of older drivers. Documenting the best corrected binocular visual acuity, color perception, and dark vision are basic elements in assessing driving visual acuity. The other factors have not been clearly demonstrated as highly applicable from laboratory performance to on-the-road skills for the elderly driver.

19. **(1)** Rapid eye movement (REM) sleep begins approximately 120 minutes from sleep onset and recurs in three to four regularly spaced, 10- to 15-minute cycles. REM sleep is associated with skeletal muscle atonia, rapid eye movements, and dreaming. This is decreased with aging. Delta or stage IV is deep sleep and is also decreased with aging. There is increased nocturnal awakening along with increased sleep latency. Sleep is generally less efficient in the older client. More time is spent in bed but time spent sleeping is decreased.

20. **(2)** Immune function declines with age, making the older adult more susceptible to infection. The older adult has less thymus-derived immunity as a result of the shrinking of the thymus gland, thus making it more difficult for the older adult to produce antibodies.

21. **(4)** The older adult has a diminished cell-mediated immunity because of a decline in T-cell function. The T cells have a decreased ability to produce cytokines, which are needed to facilitate B-cell growth and maturation, and a decreased ability to proliferate in response to an antigen.

22. **(4)** A decreased bladder capacity along with the decreased ability to concentrate urine and the decreased urethral closing pressure after menopause lead to incontinence. Other factors include depression, decreased mobility, decreased vision, and lack of attention to bladder cues of fullness.

23. **(3)** The elderly client is able to respond to infections with previously produced "remembered" antibodies; however, the antibodies are less able to respond to new antigens. In the elderly client, the cells of the immune system are unable to proliferate as in the younger client. The total number of T cells remains the same, but the cell function is decreased and cells are less likely to proliferate and may have decreased cytotoxicity. Because of the changes of aging, the immune system of the elderly client is less able to respond to antigenic stimulation than that of the younger client.

Health Promotion & Maintenance

1. What are the current American Cancer Society dietary recommendations for cancer prevention?

    1. Maintain a desirable body weight and eat a variety of foods, including fruits and vegetables and foods that are high in fiber.

    2. Increase the amount of protein in the diet.

    3. Use alcohol in small to moderate amounts.

    4. Increase servings of fresh fruits, fish, and dairy products.

2. In the presence of dyslipidemia and diabetes, the National Cholesterol Education Program guidelines set the goal for lipid levels as:

    1. Low-density lipoprotein (LDL) <130 mg/dl and triglyceride levels <200 mg/dl.

    2. LDL <160 mg/dl and triglyceride levels <240 mg/dl.

    3. LDL <100 mg/dl and triglyceride levels <180 mg/dl.

    4. LDL <150 mg/dl and triglyceride levels <220 mg/dl.

3. The American Diabetes Association recommends screening adults starting at age 45 with a fasting plasma glucose (FPG) test every:

    1. 1 year.

    2. 3 years.

    3. 5 years.

    4. 10 years.

4. What is a tertiary prevention activity for an elderly woman who has had a cerebrovascular accident (CVA)?

    1. An annual influenza vaccination.

    2. A physical therapy program.

    3. An annual mammogram.

    4. An annual ophthalmologic examination to evaluate for glaucoma.

5. A client is continuing his recovery at home after extensive surgery. The practitioner would instruct the client to increase his intake of what foods to promote healing?

   1. Tomatoes, rice, whole-grain cereal.

   2. Milk, poultry, yellow vegetables.

   3. Red meat, oranges, green beans.

   4. Liver, corn, eggs.

6. When an elderly client has an alteration in the sensory/perceptual function of hearing, which plan would be most appropriate for the nurse practitioner to implement during a health promotion session?

   1. Increase the pitch of the voice.

   2. Stand behind the client when speaking.

   3. Speak in a tone that does not include shouting.

   4. Use typical complex sentences to prevent insulting the client.

7. Which of the following management plans demonstrates an understanding of primary prevention of falls among the elderly?

   1. Evaluate need for assistive devices for ambulation after the client has been injured in a fall.

   2. Provide resources to correct hazards contributing to risk for falls in the home environment.

   3. Reinforce the need to use prescribed eyeglasses to prevent further injury from falls.

   4. Provide information about medications, side effects, and interactions.

8. Which of these health promotion screenings should be completed annually for the elderly client older than 65 years?

   1. Chest x-ray examination.

   2. Pneumococcal vaccination.

   3. Sigmoidoscopy.

   4. Stool guaiac test.

9. While teaching a class to a group of senior citizens, which would be most important for the nurse practitioner to do during the presentation?

   1. Provide increased overhead lighting to enhance visualization.

   2. Provide handouts on blue paper with black print.

   3. Show a video narrated by a woman.

   4. Recognize that past life experiences are beneficial in learning new information.

10. What is the most common occupationally related health problem?

    1. Repetitive motion injury.

    2. Hearing loss.

    3. Lung disease.

    4. Cancer.

11. Which of the following best describes the benefit of sports screening physicals in the college student?

    1. Screening for undiagnosed cardiomyopathy.

    2. Assessment of drug and alcohol use.

    3. Estimation of aerobic capacity.

    4. Identification of unresolved injuries.

12. A 48-year-old man comes to the clinic after having his cholesterol checked at a health fair. He states that they told him it was greater than 300 and that he needed to see his primary care provider for further testing. Appropriate interventions for the nurse practitioner include:

    1. Prescribing a cholesterol-lowering agent.

    2. Ordering an electrocardiogram (ECG) and an exercise stress test.

    3. Starting the client on an exercise program.

    4. Performing a thorough history and physical and drawing blood for a lipid profile.

13. In preparing a client who is to have a colorectal screening, the nurse practitioner should instruct the client to:

    1. Eat at least two servings of meat daily before collecting samples.

    2. Avoid antibiotics, aspirin, iron, and antiinflammatory medications.

    3. Avoid taking extra vitamin and mineral supplements before the test.

    4. Eat extra servings of high-fiber foods and water to ensure good samples.

14. Which age group should be targeted to be taught testicular self-examination?

    1. 10 to 14 years.

    2. 15 to 25 years.

    3. 30 to 40 years.

    4. 45 to 65 years.

15. According to the American Dietetics Association, how many servings of the bread/cereal/pasta/rice group should be eaten each day?

    1. 6 to 11 servings.

    2. 2 to 4 servings.

    3. 3 to 5 servings.

    4. 2 to 3 servings.

16. At what age should routine screening mammography begin for women who have no increased risk of breast cancer?

    1. 30 years old.

    2. 35 years old.

    3. Begin at age 40.

    4. Before the age of 50.

17. Which of the following components should be included when taking a history from a client who is new to the clinic?

    1. Medical and surgical histories, family medical and surgical histories, psychosocial history, diet and exercise habits, chemical use, sexual practices, review of systems.

    2. Interval history, medical history, family medical history, dietary habits, substance use, and sexual practices.

    3. Medical and surgical histories, family medical history, psychosocial history, physical activity, tobacco and other substance use, and sexual practices.

    4. The history listed on the form provided to clients for completion before the physical examination is sufficient, and no interview needs to be done.

18. A 50-year-old woman comes to the clinic for a first-visit checkup. She states that she is in good health and takes no medications. She does not know her family history, because she was adopted. She is 62 inches tall and weighs 175 lb. She admits to a sedentary lifestyle. She does not smoke and admits to drinking 4 to 5 alcoholic beverages per week. Which of the following interventions would be most appropriate for the nurse practitioner to recommend in this client's plan of care?

    1. An exercise program that includes jogging and weight training.

    2. Addition of vitamin supplements to her diet and elimination of alcoholic beverages.

    3. Possible job changes that will increase the amount of exercise she gets daily.

    4. Keeping a daily record of her food intake and bringing it to her next visit.

19. Which group is at greatest risk for alterations in immune function related to nutritional status?

    1. Young adults.

    2. Adults.

    3. Adolescents.

    4. Older adults.

20. The nurse practitioner is discussing making lifestyle changes that will decrease the geriatric client's risks for cardiovascular disease. Which of the following is most important to include in this discussion?

    1. Decrease smoking, increase vitamin supplements, and increase protein intake.

    2. Control hypertension, stop smoking, maintain normal weight, and exercise regularly.

    3. Maintain normal levels of serum blood sugar and decrease cholesterol intake.

    4. Get a yearly physical examination, increase fiber in diet, and exercise regularly.

21. Which lifestyle modifications are most effective in controlling hypertension in the older client?

    1. Maintain normal weight, decrease sodium diet, and exercise regularly.

    2. Increase dietary protein, decrease weight, and use stress reduction techniques.

    3. Consume a high–complex-carbohydrate, low-sodium diet; decrease stress.

    4. Reduce weight, increase vitamin supplements, and exercise regularly.

22. Which of the following is an example of a community health promotion activity?

    1. A high school–based family planning clinic.

    2. A worksite urgent care clinic.

    3. An asthma follow-up clinic in an elementary school.

    4. Employer-sponsored multiphasic health screening.

23. Which of the following guidelines should the nurse practitioner follow when developing educational materials?

    1. Present the most important material first in all capital letters for emphasis.

    2. Provide the information in English and in three other languages.

    3. Keep sentences short and to the point and use graphic images for clarification.

    4. Maintain an eighth-grade reading level.

Immunizations

24. The influenza vaccination is recommended annually for high-risk groups. The nurse practitioner knows that the group with the greatest need for this vaccination would be:

    1. Adults with chronic disease.

    2. Residents of long-term care facilities.

    3. Clients undergoing dialysis.

    4. Health care employees.

25. The nurse practitioner understands that the only contraindication to hepatitis B vaccination is:

    1. Pregnancy and lactation.

    2. History of poliomyelitis.

    3. Prior anaphylaxis or severe hypersensitivity.

    4. Mild viral illness.

26. Immunizations and chemoprophylaxis offered routinely to clients who are 65 years of age or older are:

    1. Diphtheria, tetanus toxoid, and pertussis absorbed (DPT); influenza; and Pneumovax.

    2. Tetanus toxoid and diphtheria (Td), influenza, and pneumococcal vaccine.

    3. Td and influenza; to those with chronic diseases, offer the pneumococcal vaccine.

    4. Influenza and pneumococcal pneumonia and Td for those who have not had a booster in the last 10 years.

27. The nurse practitioner understands that the following is considered an attenuated live-virus vaccination:

    1. Rubella and measles.

    2. Mumps and hepatitis B.

    3. Poliomyelitis and hepatitis B.

    4. Rubella and rabies.

28. Which of the following client situations requires the use of inactivated (not live) vaccines?

    1. History of nonspecific allergies.

    2. Immunocompromised adult.

    3. Concurrent antimicrobial therapy.

    4. Mild acute illness.

29. In taking the history of a healthy 50-year-old adult, the nurse practitioner determines that the client is an avid gardener and spends a great deal of time enjoying the outdoors. A health maintenance recommendation for this client is to obtain a:

    1. Pneumococcal vaccine.

    2. Tetanus vaccine.

    3. Hepatitis B vaccine.

    4. Varicella vaccine.

30. The Advisory Committee on Immunization Practices (ACIP) recommends that healthy adults receive a Td booster vaccination:

    1. Every 5 years.

    2. Every 8 years.

    3. At age 60.

    4. Every 10 years.

31. Which statement most correctly describes tetanus toxoid?

    1. Tetanus toxoid induces persistent antitoxin antibody titers.

    2. DPT and diphtheria and tetanus toxoids absorbed (DT) are safe to give to adults.

    3. The recommended dose for the adult is 0.75 ml IM.

    4. Tetanus toxoid fluid provides the same antitoxin antibody titers as tetanus toxoid.

32. Immunizations recommended for healthy young adults include:

    1. Measles, rubella, varicella, and hepatitis B.

    2. Pneumovax, influenza, and rubella.

    3. Tetanus, influenza, varicella, Pneumovax, and hepatitis B.

    4. Influenza, hepatitis B, rubella, measles, and tetanus.

Answers & Rationales

1. **(1)** The American Cancer Society recommends the maintenance of a desirable body weight; research has shown an association between increased deaths from various cancers and varying degrees of being overweight. Another recommendation is to eat a wide variety of foods, consistent with the Food Guide Pyramid put out by the U.S. Department of Agriculture and the U.S. Department of Health and Human Services. A variety of fruits and vegetables should be included in the daily diet (five to nine servings per day), because research has shown that there is an association between lower cancer rates and high fruit and vegetable consumption. High-fiber foods are also recommended; a lower risk of colon cancer is seen in those individuals who consume a high-fiber diet. There are no recommendations to increase the amount of protein in the diet at this time; because of the high consumption of red meat in the American diet, many people are already getting large quantities in their current diets. The American Cancer Society recommends limiting the daily consumption of alcohol to two drinks for males, one drink for females, and no drinks for pregnant females. They also state that ideally, no alcohol should be consumed; regular alcohol consumption has been shown to increase the risk of various cancers.

2. **(1)** The recommendation is low-density lipoprotein (LDL) <130 mg/dl and triglyceride levels <200 mg/dl. All other choices have inaccuracies in goals.

3. **(2)** The American Diabetes Association recommends screening adults, starting at the age of 45, every 3 years.

4. **(2)** The physical therapy program will assist her in restoring her optimum level of functioning after a cerebrovascular accident (CVA). Option

#1 is a primary prevention activity that is not specific to a CVA. Options #3 and #4 are examples of secondary prevention activities that are not specific to a CVA.

5. **(3)** The client needs an increased intake of protein and vitamin C to promote healing. Red meat, citrus fruits, and green vegetables will provide the highest amounts of these elements from the selections offered.

6. **(3)** Shouting increases the pitch of the voice. In presbycusis, which is a hearing loss in the elderly, high-pitched consonant sounds are the first to be affected, and the change may occur gradually. The nurse practitioner should face the client when speaking. If there is a need to stand behind the client, then touch can be used to get the client's attention. Simple sentences should be used to facilitate understanding.

7. **(4)** This information will prevent complications that may result in a fall. Options #1 and #2 are appropriate for tertiary prevention. Option #3 is appropriate for secondary prevention, that is, preventing the client from experiencing another fall.

8. **(4)** This evaluation will assist in identifying any problems with bleeding. Option #1 is not necessary. Option #2 is not a screening and would not be administered annually. A sigmoidoscopy is recommended every 3 to 5 years for clients older than 50 years.

9. **(4)** Using past life experiences applies the concept of adult educational principles. Overhead lighting may produce an increase in the glare, which can decrease visualization. There is an alteration in color perception (e.g., blue appears green-blue) as an individual ages. As individuals age, the ability to hear women's

and children's voices decreases, since these are high-pitched voices. This video would not enhance the program if the clients frequently have presbycusis as a result of the normal aging process.

10. **(3)** All of these disorders can be associated with workplace exposure, but currently, lung disease is still the most common occupationally related disease. Musculoskeletal injuries are on the rise.

11. **(4)** The only proven benefit of a sports screening examination is to identify athletes at risk for orthopedic injuries associated with previously unresolved injuries. A thorough history with the screening exam will increase the likelihood of detecting underlying health problems but has not been shown to be very effective.

12. **(4)** The client's history and findings on physical examination will reveal the presence of any coronary heart disease (CHD) risk factors (e.g., age, family history of CHD, diabetes, current cigarette smoking, blood pressure, height/weight, cardiovascular exam). A lipid profile is also recommended to assess the level of risk; it consists of measurement of total cholesterol, high-density lipoprotein (HDL), LDL, and triglyceride levels. It would be prudent to have a precise cholesterol level determined, because the previous result was from a screening health fair and there is no written record of the result. These parameters should be assessed first before a cholesterol-lowering agent, electrocardiogram (ECG), or stress test is ordered. An exercise program is also important but should only be initiated after the client's history and physical and lipid profile results are known; if the lipid profile results are exam findings are abnormal, stress testing may be appropriate before a new exercise program is undertaken.

13. **(2)** Screening for colorectal cancer includes annual fecal occult blood screening for individuals older than 50 years. Avoiding medications that can cause gastrointestinal irritation and bleeding can help prevent false-positive results. Rare meat and vegetables that are high in peroxidase (such as the ones listed) will cause false-positive results, whereas vitamin C can cause false-negative results.

14. **(2)** The 15- to 25-year age group is most commonly affected by testicular cancer.

15. **(1)** The recommended servings for each of the food groups are as follows:

Food Group	Servings
Bread/cereal/rice/pasta	6-11 servings
Fruit	2-4 servings
Vegetable	3-5 servings
Meat/poultry/fish, dry beans, eggs, nuts	2-3 servings
Fats/oils/sweets	Use sparingly

16. **(3)** In the summer of 1997, the National Institutes of Health (NIH) and the American Cancer Society changed the recommendation to begin yearly mammography at age 40.

17. **(1)** All of these areas are important to cover in the initial interview of a new client. The history will help determine the necessary components of the physical examination, laboratory or radiologic studies that are ordered, and counseling that is done during the appointment.

18. **(4)** An account of the client's usual intake is necessary, so that problem areas can be identified. Before any exercise program is started, a physical examination should be done to assess the client's physical condition and to aid in the proper selection of a specific exercise plan. A dietary assessment needs to be completed before vitamin and protein supplements are recommended; the client may already be receiving adequate amounts in her diet. A more active job would be ideal; however, most people do not have options regarding their choice of job, so increasing her activity outside of work would be most appropriate.

19. **(4)** The older adult is at greatest risk for altered immune function related to nutrition. The older adult often does not receive adequate nutrition for a variety of reasons: altered taste, eating alone, inability to prepare meals, malabsorption. Adequate nutrition in the older adult has been shown to improve immune status and antibody response to influenza vaccine.

20. **(2)** Hypertension, smoking, and hyperlipidemia are the major risk factors for the development of cardiovascular disease. Controlling hyperglycemia, high dietary fiber intake, and vitamin supplements assist in maintaining a healthy lifestyle; however, they are not as important in preventing cardiovascular disease.

21. **(1)** These three modifications are the most effective in maintaining normal blood pressure.

22. **(4)** Multiphasic health screening is a form of periodic health surveillance in which participants undergo a battery of laboratory or diagnostic tests to determine risk factors and detect disease. The other three settings described are not examples of community health promotion activities; they are secondary care settings. The locations of the two clinics are community settings.

23. **(3)** Printed materials must be written at a reading level that most people can understand. Do not use all capital letters, because words so written are difficult to read. In addition, it is helpful to write in the active versus the passive voice, to use one-and two-syllable words, to avoid complex grammatical structures, and to express only one idea in each sentence. Well-chosen and easily understood graphics can significantly enhance the literature.

Immunizations

24. **(2)** Influenza outbreaks may affect 60% of those in long-term care, and fatality rates are high. All the other groups listed are appropriate target populations for the influenza vaccine but are not as high a priority.

25. **(3)** Prior anaphylaxis and severe hypersensitivity would be considered a contraindication; a mild viral illness would not. The client who is pregnant or lactating may be immunized.

26. **(4)** Pneumococcal and annual influenza immunizations are recommended for those who are 65 years of age and older. Adult tetanus toxoid and diphtheria (Td) is offered to those who have not had a booster in the last 10 years.

27. **(1)** Attenuated live-virus vaccines are available for the following communicable diseases: measles, mumps, rubella, poliomyelitis, yellow fever, and smallpox. Rabies vaccine contains a killed virus, and hepatitis B vaccine contains a purified viral antigen obtained from the blood of an infected human being and then inactivated when manufactured into a vaccination.

28. **(2)** Live vaccine can produce serious disseminated disease in a client with an immunocompromising illness such as leukemia, lymphoma, human immunodeficiency virus (HIV) infection, or acquired immunodeficiency syndrome (AIDS) and in clients undergoing cancer chemotherapy. Mild acute illness, concurrent antimicrobial therapy, and a history of nonspecific allergies are not contraindications for use of a live vaccine.

29. **(2)** Adults who enjoy gardening and outdoor activities should have a tetanus vaccine at least every 10 years because of the high-risk activities. A pneumococcal vaccine is recommended for adults age 65 or older and for those who have a chronic illness or who are immunosuppressed. Most older adults have had chickenpox as a child and do not require the vaccine.

30. **(4)** The ACIP recommends that adults receive a Td booster every 10 years or a single booster at age 50 for clients who have completed full pediatric series, including teenage and young adult boosters.

31. **(1)** Tetanus toxoid induces more persistent antitoxin antibody titers than tetanus toxoid fluid. Diphtheria, tetanus toxoid, and pertussis absorbed (DPT) and diphtheria and tetanus toxoids absorbed (DT) are for use in children younger than of 7 years; however, they should *not* be used in adults. The recommended dose of DT for an adult is 0.5 ml IM.

32. **(4)** Five percent to 20% of young adults are susceptible to measles and/or rubella. Influenza and hepatitis B vaccines are recommended for students who are exposed to a large number of people. Tetanus immunization is recommended every 10 years, especially in high-risk situations (young adults who participate in outdoor sports). Pneumovax is indicated for a young adult who has a chronic disease, such as diabetes, chronic pulmonary disease, or chronic cardiovascular disease and is also indicated for young adults who are immunocompromised.

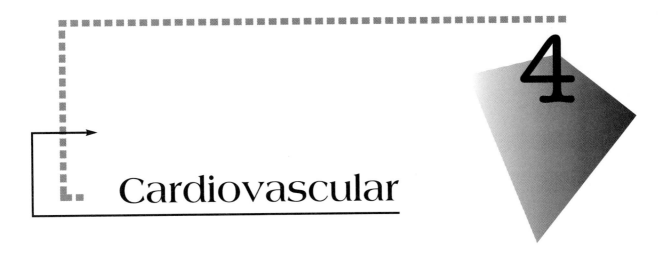

Cardiovascular

Physical Examination & Diagnostic Tests

1. The practitioner is performing a physical examination on a healthy male adult. On auscultation with a stethoscope, which statement describes the areas where the characteristic heart sounds S_1 and S_2 can be heard most clearly?

   1. S_1 is best heard at the apex and S_2 at the base of the heart.

   2. Both are heard equally well at the right midclavicular line.

   3. On the left side, S_1 is at the area of pulmonic valve and S_2, at the aortic valve.

   4. Both sounds are best heard at Erb's point.

2. During a general assessment of an adult client, the practitioner determines the presence of the apical impulse at the point of maximal impulse (PMI) on the client's chest wall. Where on the chest wall is the PMI normally found?

   1. Second intercostal space at the midclavicular line on the left side.

   2. Right lower sternal border, fifth intercostal space.

   3. Left side at the fifth intercostal space on the midclavicular line.

   4. Left fifth intercostal space, lateral to the midclavicular line.

3. The nurse practitioner is auscultating the carotids. What is the correct procedure?

   1. Use the diaphragm of the stethoscope.

   2. Use the bell of the stethoscope.

   3. Place the stethoscope 1 inch off the area above the sternocleidomastoid muscle.

   4. Position the client at a 30-degree angle; press firmly with the bell of the stethoscope.

4. When inspecting the precordium, the nurse practitioner is checking for:

   1. Scars and anatomic landmarks.

   2. Pulsations and retractions.

   3. Heaves and cardiac dullness.

   4. Pericardial friction rub and lifts.

5. While examining a client in a left lateral decubitus position, the nurse practitioner auscultates a third heart sound (S$_3$). The nurse practitioner knows that:

   1. This sound is considered normal in children and young adults.

   2. This sound is rarely associated with myocardial failure in the older adult.

   3. The client should be immediately referred to a cardiologist for evaluation.

   4. This sound is considered a normal splitting of the S$_2$ during inspiration.

6. The nurse practitioner knows that the correct auscultatory site for the aortic area is the:

   1. Midclavicular line, fifth interspace, left side.

   2. Left fourth interspace close to the sternum.

   3. Right second interspace close to the sternum.

   4. Midclavicular line, second interspace, left side.

7. The nurse practitioner should include which statement in his/her teaching when ordering a lipid profile for a client? Eat a typical diet over the next week, and

   1. Consume a normal breakfast on the morning of the exam.

   2. Fast for 12 hours before the exam.

   3. There are no restrictions on alcohol for this test.

   4. Take any current medications with a few sips of water before the test.

8. When auscultating the heart sounds of a 72-year-old client with a history of hypertension, the nurse practitioner notes an S$_4$. This finding could indicate:

   1. A normal variant in people 65 years or older.

   2. The beginning of ventricular failure.

   3. A decreased resistance to ventricular filling.

   4. A rapidly failing heart.

9. A 55-year-old client has a blood pressure (BP) of 168/100 mm Hg. This is classified as:

   1. Moderate hypertension.

   2. Mild hypertension.

   3. High-normal BP.

   4. Severe hypertension.

10. The nurse practitioner is examining a client with a history of rheumatic fever who is being monitored for the development of carditis. During the cardiac auscultation, where on the chest wall is the stethoscope placed to determine the most common murmurs associated with this condition?

   1. At the left sternal border, fourth left intercostal space.

   2. Fifth intercostal space, left side, at the midclavicular line.

   3. Second or third intercostal space at the left of the sternal border.

   4. Second intercostal space on the right of the sternal border.

11. A client presents with unusual coolness in the left hand as compared with the right hand. What is the next step in the examination?

   1. Palpate the radial pulse on both hands for a full minute.

   2. Perform the Allen test on both hands.

   3. Feel the forearms with the backs of the fingers.

   4. Hold the hand in a dependent position then reexamine.

12. S$_1$ and S$_2$ are identified when the nurse practitioner auscultates for cardiac sounds. The physiology responsible for the production of these heart sounds is:

   1. Closure of the atrioventricular (AV) valves produces S$_1$; closure of the semilunar valves forms S$_2$.

   2. Closure of the aortic valve produces S$_2$; opening of the mitral valve produces S$_1$.

   3. Opening of the AV valves produces S$_1$; closure of the semilunar valves produces S$_2$.

   4. Opening of the tricuspid valve produces S$_1$; closure of the pulmonic valve forms S$_2$.

13. The nurse practitioner is assessing a client with heart disease who is experiencing an atrial dysrhythmia. The pulse rate is irregular at 110 bpm and there is concern regarding a pulse deficit. How is a pulse deficit determined in this client?

    1. A 12-lead electrocardiogram (ECG) is necessary to determine the presence and length of the P-R intervals.

    2. The apical pulse is counted and then the radial pulse is counted; the pulse deficit is determined by the difference between the two rates.

    3. The apical pulse is counted, and an increase or decrease is correlated with the phases of the respiratory cycle.

    4. The apical pulse and radial pulse are determined simultaneously; a pulse deficit is established if the apical rate is higher than the radial rate.

14. The nurse practitioner notes a grade V systolic murmur while examining a client's precordium. Which characteristics describe this type of murmur?

    1. Barely audible; faintly heard with the bell of the stethoscope.

    2. Heard only with the diaphragm of the stethoscope.

    3. Heard with the stethoscope partly off the chest.

    4. Heard without the aid of the stethoscope.

15. Normal physiology changes in the geriatric population that affect conductivity and contractility of the myocardium include:

    1. Increased automaticity and excitability.

    2. Increased contractility and conductivity.

    3. Decreased excitability and conductivity.

    4. Decreased automaticity and contractility.

16. When determining temperature of an extremity as part of a peripheral vascular assessment on a client, which part of the hand is the most sensitive?

    1. Palm.

    2. Fingertips.

    3. Back of the wrist.

    4. Back of the fingers.

17. A 45-year-old man's lipid profile results are sent to the nurse practitioner. They are as follows: total cholesterol = 287 mmol/L; high-density lipoprotein (HDL) = 30 mg/dl; low-density lipoprotein (LDL) = 165 mg/dl; triglycerides = 238 mg/dl. The nurse practitioner interprets these results as:

    1. Abnormal; the elevated triglyceride level is of the most concern.

    2. Borderline; this is considered to be a borderline risk lipid profile.

    3. Abnormal; the total cholesterol and LDL levels are elevated, and the HDL is too low.

    4. Normal; these results are of no concern; follow up with client in 1 year.

18. A client returns to the chest pain clinic 3 weeks after a myocardial infarction (MI), complaining of pericardial pain and elevated temperature. Physical examination reveals a pericardial friction rub. What diagnostic studies are indicated?

    1. 24-hour Holter monitoring.

    2. Echocardiogram.

    3. Complete blood count (CBC) with differential.

    4. Cardiac enzymes with myoglobin.

19. On assessment of a geriatric client, the nurse practitioner notes bilateral pulsations and distention of the jugular veins when the client's head is elevated 45 degrees. What further assessment needs to be done at this time?

    1. Estimate the level of venous pressure by measuring from the sternal angle to the highest level of venous pulsations.

    2. Place the client in the supine position and determine effect of position change on distention and pulsations of jugular vein.

    3. Measure carotid pulses because of the increased left ventricular pressure.

    4. Have the client hold his/her breath to facilitate evaluation for the presence of carotid bruits.

20. The nurse practitioner is examining a woman with a known history of mitral valve disease. What type of murmur heard on auscultation supports a history of mitral stenosis?

   1. Diastolic murmur, heard loudest at the apex with the client on her left side.

   2. Midsystolic ejection murmur, heard loudest over the left lower sternal border.

   3. Holosystolic murmur, heard loudest over the apex and left auxiliary area.

   4. Diastolic murmur, heard loudest with client in sitting position leaning forward.

21. The nurse practitioner is doing an assessment of a client who had an MI affecting the left ventricle 2 weeks ago. The nurse practitioner would pay particular attention to what area of the physical assessment?

   1. The lower extremities and the jugular vein.

   2. The area on the chest where the PMI is heard.

   3. The presence of dyspnea and auscultation of crackles in the lungs.

   4. The level of dependent edema and fluid intake over the past 24 hours.

22. Which symptoms would indicate to the nurse practitioner that the client is experiencing intermittent claudication?

   1. Petechiae and itching of the lower part of the leg.

   2. Extensive discoloration and edema of the upper leg.

   3. Profuse rash and discoloration from the trunk down to the feet.

   4. Complaints of pain on walking, relieved by sitting down.

23. Stress testing, or the exercise tolerance test, is the most widely used diagnostic test for ischemic heart disease. It is most accurate, up to 98%, in what type of client?

   1. Males younger than 40 years with atypical angina pectoris.

   2. Asymptomatic premenopausal women without risk factors.

   3. Men older than 50 years with typical angina pectoris.

   4. Men with typical angina pectoris who are receiving digitalis.

24. When palpating for the apical impulse of a 46-year-old woman, the nurse practitioner feels a hyperkinetic impulse. The nurse would auscultate for which additional finding?

   1. A pericardial friction rub.

   2. A pansystolic murmur.

   3. Pulsus paradoxus.

   4. Decreased intensity of heart sounds.

25. While assessing a patient with a history of recent MI, the nurse practitioner notes pulsus alternans. The nurse practitioner would assess for other changes caused by:

   1. Unstable angina.

   2. Cardiogenic shock.

   3. Recurrent myocardial infarction.

   4. Left-sided congestive heart failure (CHF).

Disorders

26. A 70-year-old woman comes to the clinic with the complaint of severe aching of her legs after standing for 10 minutes. What other finding(s) in the lower extremities would support the nurse practitioner's tentative diagnosis of chronic venous insufficiency?

   1. 3+ pitting edema and cyanosis on dependency.

   2. Skin shiny and dusky red on dependency.

   3. Minimal hair; pallor on elevation.

   4. 1+ pulses and ulceration involving the toes.

27. The diagnosis of hypertension should be established on the basis of:

   1. At least three hypertensive readings in a week.

   2. At least five readings 1 month apart.

   3. One reading of 140 mm Hg systolic and 90 mm Hg diastolic or greater.

   4. One reading taken in three different positions.

28. A client has a 2-year history of hypertensive heart disease. The nurse practitioner expects the major pathophysiologic change to be:

    1. Right ventricular hypertrophy.

    2. Left atrial dilation.

    3. Left ventricular hypertrophy.

    4. Right atrial dilation.

29. Among the following descriptions, what data most clearly describe atrial tachycardia?

    1. Heart rate of 96 bpm, P waves present on each QRS complex, T wave every other beat.

    2. P waves present on every other beat, heart rate of 100 bpm and irregular.

    3. Heart rate of 110 bpm, P waves present before each QRS complex, and regular.

    4. P waves for every third QRS complex, adequate P-R interval, heart rate of 90 bpm.

30. What clinical manifestation of an MI is frequently **not** present in the geriatric client with heart disease?

    1. Prolonged severe chest pain.

    2. Diaphoresis, pallor, syncope.

    3. Dyspnea, increasing anxiety.

    4. Gastrointestinal distress, orthopnea.

31. The nurse practitioner is performing an assessment of a client who is having difficulty controlling his left-sided CHF. The nurse practitioner understands that the primary symptoms associated with this type of heart failure are:

    1. Systemic venous congestion.

    2. Dyspnea and pulmonary congestion.

    3. Increased peripheral edema and anorexia.

    4. Atrial fibrillation with a heart rate around 110 bpm.

32. The nurse practitioner is concerned that a client who has had an MI is experiencing constrictive pericarditis. What is a characteristic finding and how is it evaluated?

    1. Cardiac tamponade occurs; it is identified by the presence of muffled heart sounds and the presence of a paradoxic pulse.

2. Pericarditis with a pericardial triphasic friction rub is common; it is best heard at the apical area of the heart.

3. There is a mitral valve prolapse that is characterized by a late systolic murmur heard at the apex and the left sternal borders.

4. There are altered waves on the jugular venous pulse; this is determined with a light that is directed tangentially to illuminate the shadows of the pulsations.

33. A geriatric client has a diagnosis of left-sided CHF. The nurse practitioner would identify what common condition frequently associated with CHF?

    1. Peripheral vascular disease.

    2. Untreated hypertension.

    3. Ventricular dysrhythmias.

    4. Chronic obstructive pulmonary disease (COPD).

34. In evaluating the effectiveness of cardiopulmonary resuscitation (CPR) on the adult client, the nurse practitioner would note:

    1. Dilated pupils.

    2. Palpable carotid pulse.

    3. Capillary refill.

    4. Pink and warm skin.

35. The nurse practitioner is evaluating an ECG of a client who came to the clinic with complaints of weakness and fainting. His ECG reveals a heart rate of 68 bpm, absent P waves, regular QRS complex, and T waves present after each QRS complex. What is the best interpretation of this information?

    1. A normal ECG; need to further evaluate client's complaints of weakness.

    2. Third-degree block with junctional rhythm; transfer client to emergency department for cardiology consult.

    3. First-degree block; need to further evaluate client's cardiac medications.

    4. Administer sublingual nitroglycerin and refer client for a cardiology consult.

36. The nurse practitioner is conducting a follow-up examination on a client with coronary artery disease (CAD) and a history of pericarditis. What is one of the characteristic physical findings in pericarditis and how is it evaluated?

    1. A paradoxical pulse is common; it is identified by evaluating the changes in the amplitude of arterial pulse pressure associated with the respiratory cycle.

    2. There is a pulse deficit, which is determined by counting the radial pulse and the apical pulse at the same time and evaluating the difference.

    3. A pericardial friction rub is present; it is best heard with the diaphragm of the stethoscope and is loudest to the left of the sternum at the fourth or fifth intercostal space.

    4. There is an S_4 present; it is commonly heard at the apex with the bell of the stethoscope and the client in a left lateral position.

37. The typical symptoms of an MI usually experienced by the elderly include:

    1. Dyspnea and diaphoresis.

    2. Back pain and muscle cramping.

    3. Numbness and tingling of the left arm.

    4. Epigastric pain and nausea.

38. What are the risk factors that predispose women to cardiovascular disease?

    1. Absence of estrogen adversely affects lipoprotein metabolism.

    2. Fat deposited on the hips mobilizes, raising the serum cholesterol level.

    3. Coronary arteries are longer and wider in diameter.

    4. Resting ejection fraction is lower.

39. The nurse practitioner is planning the treatment for a geriatric client who has been given a new diagnosis of hypertension. What is the most appropriate action by the nurse practitioner in determining management of this client?

    1. Determine medications and dosage based on the client's weight, age, and drug availability.

    2. Begin step method by using diuretics and β-adrenergic blockers.

    3. Initiate lifestyle changes before beginning administration of medications.

    4. Determine other medical conditions for which the client is being treated.

40. Which statement accurately describes CAD in geriatric clients?

    1. Cardiovascular disease is increased in the female client who is receiving estrogen replacement.

    2. A major risk factor for cardiovascular disease in females and males is chronic hypertension.

    3. The majority of geriatric clients with CAD also have type II diabetes.

    4. Men older than 60 years continue to experience the highest level of CAD.

41. A client with a history of COPD comes to the clinic for his annual checkup with complaints of increasing difficulty breathing. Assessment findings include S_3 gallop, early systolic ejection click, and increased P-wave amplitude in leads II, III, and aVF of the ECG. The nurse practitioner would expect to observe which change on the chest x-ray film?

    1. Hypertrophy of the left ventricle.

    2. Hypertrophy of the right ventricle.

    3. Hypertrophy of the left atrium and ventricle.

    4. Hypertrophy of the right atrium and ventricle.

42. When cardiac output falls in CHF, the body attempts to compensate. What electrolyte imbalances occur as a result of this response?

    1. Hypernatremia and hyperkalemia.

    2. Hyponatremia and hypokalemia.

    3. Hypophosphatemia and hypercalcemia.

    4. Hyperphosphatemia and hypocalcemia.

43. When assessing the carotid pulse of a 72-year-old client at a community-based clinic, the nurse practitioner notes a bounding pulse with rapid rise and sudden collapse. The nurse practitioner would include which additional assessment to support this finding?

    1. Auscultation for a diastolic murmur.

    2. Auscultation for paradoxical pulse.

3. BP in both arms lying, sitting, and standing.

4. BP for an auscultatory gap.

44. The nurse practitioner understands that the pain experienced with angina pectoris or an MI is caused by irritation of the myocardial nerve fibers by the increase in:

1. Blood glucose.

2. Lactic acid.

3. Serum potassium.

4. Serum magnesium.

45. In obtaining the history and performing the physical examination of a client with suspected early CHF, which is the most prominent finding?

1. Moist crackles in the lung bases bilaterally.

2. Anorexia with weight loss of 3 lb in 1 week.

3. Increased urinary output and peripheral edema.

4. Facial edema and distended neck veins.

46. Chest pain that is sudden and severe, described as tearing, and accompanied by a decrease in peripheral pulses may indicate a diagnosis of:

1. Angina.

2. Acute MI.

3. Aortic dissection.

4. Pericarditis.

47. Dietary therapy for hyperlipidemia occurs in two steps, a step I and step II diet. A step I diet includes as daily intake:

1. Total fat ≤30% of total calories, <300 mg cholesterol, 8% to 10% saturated fat.

2. Total fat ≤30% of total calories, <200 mg cholesterol, <7% saturated fat.

3. Total fat ≤40% of total calories, <400 mg cholesterol, <15% saturated fat.

4. Total fat ≤30% of total calories, <2000 total calories, <3 g sodium.

48. The most frequent life-threatening dysrhythmia experienced by a client with an acute MI is:

1. Atrial fibrillation.

2. Ventricular tachycardia.

3. Third-degree heart block.

4. Ventricular fibrillation.

49. In an overweight, older adult female client with an elevated cholesterol level and abnormal lipoprotein profile, the first step in treatment includes:

1. Prescribing a bile acid sequestrant agent.

2. Initiation of a diet and exercise program.

3. Estrogen replacement therapy.

4. Referral to a cardiologist.

50. Clients with chronic atrial fibrillation are at risk for which condition?

1. Sudden cardiac death.

2. Cerebrovascular accident.

3. Ventricular tachycardia.

4. Acute myocardial infarction.

51. The nurse practitioner understands that the most common symptom of CHF in adults is:

1. Anorexia.

2. Dependent edema.

3. Dyspnea.

4. Weakness.

52. The nurse practitioner teaches the client with heart disease to avoid foods high in saturated fats, which include:

1. Nuts, legumes, and seeds.

2. Fish, shellfish, and mussels.

3. Palm oil, coconut oil, and butter.

4. Peanut oil, soybean oil, and olive oil.

53. An elderly male client is complaining of chest pain. A guideline to assist the nurse practitioner in differentiating the chest pain of angina from that of an infarction is:

1. Myocardial pain with an infarction is more severe.

2. Angina is more substernal and does not radiate to other areas.

3. Angina is frequently relieved by nitroglycerin.

4. Pain from an infarction is always associated with other symptoms.

54. The nurse practitioner is evaluating a client in the office who is complaining of chest pain and has a BP of 86/52 mm Hg. The ECG shows some signs of ischemia, and the client is to be transferred to the emergency department. What drug might the nurse practitioner give the client while awaiting transport to the emergency department?

    1. Furosemide (Lasix) 40 mg IV.

    2. Morphine sulfate 25 mg IV.

    3. Nitroglycerin SL.

    4. Acetylsalicylic acid (ASA; aspirin) 81 mg PO.

55. Which would **not** be considered as contributing to the development of thrombophlebitis?

    1. Excessive use of oral anticoagulants.

    2. Blow to the leg or arm.

    3. Recent IV therapy.

    4. Pregnancy.

56. An elderly client is being evaluated for a complaint of dizziness. What symptom/observation will make the nurse practitioner consider that this is a life-threatening event?

    1. The dizziness occurs in certain positions.

    2. Dizziness is accompanied by tinnitus.

    3. The symptoms worsen when standing.

    4. Dizziness is preceded by rapid breathing.

57. A 28-year-old man presents to the nurse practitioner with a history of chest pain that has been increasing over the past several days. The client states that the pain worsens on lying down. He denies any shortness of breath, cough, or radiation of the pain. He does give a history of a recent infection with coxsackievirus. On exam, the nurse notes that the client has a cardiac friction rub. One probable diagnosis considered by the nurse practitioner is:

    1. Acute MI.

    2. Pleural effusion.

    3. Pericarditis.

    4. Esophageal reflux.

58. The nurse practitioner would most likely suspect which differential diagnosis for an elderly client presenting with atrial fibrillation and functional decline?

    1. Hyperthyroidism.

    2. Hypothyroidism.

    3. Sick sinus syndrome.

    4. CHF.

59. Which finding in an older client would represent a deviation from normal aging changes?

    1. Decreased exercise tolerance.

    2. Grade II/VI systolic ejection murmur.

    3. Prolongation of the PR intervals on the ECG.

    4. Jugular venous pressure (JVP) of 4 cm.

60. During cardiac auscultation of an older adult, a grade II/VI murmur, heard best at the second right intercostal space, is noted. The murmur is auscultated louder with squatting. There is a small carotid pulse with a delayed upstroke. The client's history is benign, and his activity tolerance is within normal limits for his age. The nurse practitioner would interpret this murmur to be indicative of:

    1. Aortic regurgitation.

    2. Aortic stenosis.

    3. Mitral valve prolapse.

    4. Mitral regurgitation.

61. What is the most frequently diagnosed valvular heart problem in the elderly?

    1. Aortic stenosis.

    2. Mitral stenosis.

    3. Mitral regurgitation.

    4. Aortic regurgitation.

62. A middle-aged man with no known coronary artery risk factors presents with a cholesterol level of 255 mg/dl. The nurse practitioner would:

    1. Begin administering an HMG Co A reductase inhibitor.

    2. Start him on a step I diet, since all clients should be given a trial on a diet.

    3. Repeat cholesterol and determine HDL and calculated LDL levels.

4. Do nothing, since he has no coronary risks other than maleness.

Pharmacology

63. A 75-year-old client presents to the office complaining of "not feeling well." He has a history of chronic lung disease and CHF. His vital signs are pulse 78 bpm and irregular, respirations 26 breaths/min, and BP 158/100 mm Hg. An ECG indicates sinus rhythm and confirms the rate. The P-R interval is 0.28 seconds, P waves are present, and each is followed by a QRS complex. There are frequent premature atrial beats. The client is receiving digitalis, potassium, theophylline, hydrochlorothiazide, and a calcium channel blocker. What is the next best action to take?

    1. Determine serum theophylline, digitalis, and potassium levels.

    2. Increase dosage of calcium blocker and diuretic.

    3. Order pulmonary function studies.

    4. Refer client to a cardiologist.

64. A 49-year-old woman began receiving a thiazide diuretic for hypertension 1 month ago. She arrives in the clinic complaining of muscle cramps and dizziness. Physical exam findings are as follows:

    - BP 132/88 mm Hg (previous BP, 186/112 mm Hg)
    - Pulse 112 bpm
    - Respirations 24 breaths/min
    - Tenting positive
    - Skin turgor decreased
    - Neck veins flat
    - STAT serum electrolytes:
      Sodium 114 mEq/L
      Chloride 92 mEq/L
      Potassium 3.0 mEq/L
    - STAT blood glucose 201 mg/dl

    Initial treatment for this client should include fluid replacement:

    1. Orally with free water and a potassium supplement.

    2. Intravenously with normal saline solution and regular insulin administered subcutaneously.

    3. Intravenously with 1000 ml of normal saline solution with 40 mEq potassium chloride (KCl) at 50 ml/hr.

    4. Intravenously with 1000 ml of Ringer's lactate solution at 250 ml/hr.

65. A client is recovering from an acute episode of thrombophlebitis and is being treated with warfarin (Coumadin) 5 mg PO daily. In reviewing medication information, the nurse practitioner would include what information in her teaching?

    1. Do not take a multivitamin supplement.

    2. Limit dairy products.

    3. Aerobic exercises are the most effective.

    4. Maintain a daily record of intake and output.

66. The nurse practitioner is evaluating a client who is complaining of "not feeling good." He has a history of CAD and CHF. Vital signs are pulse 72 bpm, respirations 20 breaths/min, BP 130/88 mm Hg, temperature normal. There are no complaints of chest pain or difficulty breathing, and client has had some nausea but no vomiting over the past 2 days; lower extremities are negative for edema. The client states that he has been able to take his medications. His current medications are digoxin (Lanoxin) 0.25 bid, hydrochlorothiazide (HydroDIURIL) 100 mg bid, potassium (Micro-K) 10 mEq daily, and nitroglycerin transdermal patches. What is the priority of care for this client?

    1. Obtain a STATE ECG and white blood cell (WBC) count.

    2. Arterial blood gases and oxygen at 4 L/min.

    3. Determine serum digoxin and potassium levels.

    4. Serial cardiac enzymes now and q6h ×2.

67. The nurse practitioner has prescribed losartan (Cozaar) 50 mg PO qd. This medication promotes vasodilation by:

    1. Inhibiting conversion of angiotensin I to angiotensin II.

    2. Promoting the release of aldosterone.

    3. Promoting the synthesis of prostaglandin.

    4. Inhibiting calcium influx into smooth muscle cells.

68. A client with a history of hypertension begins receiving Aldactone 50 mg PO qd. The nurse practitioner instructs the client to call the clinic if which symptoms are experienced?

   1. Increased irritability, abdominal cramping, and lower extremity weakness.

   2. Decreased reflex response, nausea, and vomiting.

   3. Muscle twitching, numbness of the limbs, and depression.

   4. Weight gain, excessive thirst, and fever.

69. A client with a history of unstable angina is seen in the cardiac clinic for a checkup. The assessment reveals increased weight of 10 lb, distended jugular neck veins, and an S_3. What changes in the pharmacologic treatment should be initiated?

   1. Discontinue β-blockers and calcium channel blockers.

   2. Initiate thrombolytic therapy.

   3. Discontinue nitrate and aspirin therapy.

   4. Initiate diuretic and vasoconstrictor therapy.

70. A client arrives in the emergency department of a small rural hospital complaining that he "feels like my heart is racing." He is connected to a cardiac monitor, which reveals supraventricular tachycardia at a rate of 184 bpm, QRS complex <0.10 second, and BP 112/62 mm Hg. Which treatment modality is indicated?

   1. Synchronized cardioversion with 50 joules.

   2. Defibrillation with 100 joules.

   3. Adenosine 6 mg IV push.

   4. Lidocaine 1 mg/kg IV push.

71. An 80-year-old client with a history of glaucoma experiences unstable angina. He begins receiving diltiazem (Cardizem) 30 mg PO qid and aspirin 324 mg PO qd in addition to timolol ophthalmic solution (Timoptic) i gtt OD bid. This client would have an increased risk for:

   1. Bleeding episodes.

   2. Fainting episodes and falls.

   3. Rebound supraventricular tachycardia.

   4. Blurred vision.

72. A client with a serum cholesterol level of 256 mg/dl, HDL level of 38 mg/dl, and LDL level of 172 mg/dl is instructed on dietary modifications and niacin (nicotinic acid) 1 g PO tid. Specific instructions include:

   1. Limit daily fluid intake.

   2. Take measures to minimize orthostatic hypotension.

   3. Administer the drug an hour after eating.

   4. Avoid exposure to direct sunlight.

73. When monitoring for the therapeutic effects of verapamil (Calan SR), the nurse practitioner would assess for a(n):

   1. Increase in heart rate.

   2. Decrease in systemic vascular resistance.

   3. Increase in BP.

   4. Decrease in ventricular premature beats.

74. An adult male client with essential hypertension was treated by the nurse practitioner with sodium restriction and hydrochlorothiazide (Diuril) 25 mg PO daily. After 3 months of therapy, the BP was measured at 160/110 mm Hg. At this point, the nurse practitioner would:

   1. Begin enalapril (Vasotec) 5 mg qd.

   2. Begin 50 mg of metoprolol (Toprol XL) qd.

   3. Add 25 mg of hydrochlorothiazide (Diuril) daily.

   4. Discontinue Diuril and change to captopril (Capoten) 50 mg tid.

75. When prescribing antihypertensive drug therapy for elderly clients, the nurse practitioner recognizes that which class of antihypertensive agents should be avoided?

   1. Calcium entry antagonists.

   2. Diuretics.

   3. β-blockers.

   4. Angiotensin-converting enzyme (ACE) inhibitors.

76. Medications used in managing ischemic heart disease include:

   1. β-blockers, sedatives, aspirin.

   2. Nitrates, β-blockers, calcium channel blockers, aspirin.

3. Vasoconstrictors, aspirin, anxiolytics.

4. Nitrates, ACE inhibitors, aspirin, lipid-lowering drugs.

77. The nurse practitioner is following a middle-aged nonsmoking male who is being treated for hypertension. The client returns for a follow-up visit and complains of a recurrent dry cough since he began taking the medications. This is most likely a side effect of a(n):

1. β-Blocker.

2. Thiazide diuretic.

3. ACE inhibitor.

4. Calcium channel blocker.

78. The role of digoxin in the management of CHF is indicated:

1. With atrial fibrillation.

2. With mitral stenosis.

3. With normal ejection fraction.

4. With acute pericardial disease.

79. The nurse practitioner should monitor the elderly client for which of the most common adverse reactions to digoxin?

1. Blurred vision.

2. Confusion.

3. Diarrhea.

4. Eating disorder.

80. The nurse practitioner has been successfully treating an older client's hypertension with diet, exercise, and Hydrodiuril 25 mg PO qd for 5 months. During today's clinic visit, the client's BP was 154/90 mm Hg and temperature was 99.9° F (37.2° C). The physical examination revealed clear breath sounds, S_1 and S_2 with no murmurs, gallops, or rubs; and no jugular vein distention (JVD). The client denied syncope, headaches, or visual changes; there was a tender and edematous right ankle. Which laboratory values would be most appropriate for evaluation?

1. Blood urea nitrogen and sodium.

2. Serum cholesterol and serum calcium.

3. Serum potassium and blood count.

4. Serum uric acid and complete blood count.

81. An elderly white man with a long history of COPD has recently been given a diagnosis of hypertension. Which class of antihypertensive agents should the nurse practitioner avoid for this client?

1. ACE inhibitors.

2. β-Blockers.

3. Calcium channel blockers.

4. Diuretics.

82. Which class of pharmacologic agents would the nurse practitioner select for an elderly client with hypertension and a new diagnosis of CHF?

1. ACE inhibitors.

2. β-Blockers.

3. Calcium channel blockers.

4. Diuretics.

83. A male client with mild hypertension presents with red, painful swelling of the great toe. In addition to treating the gout, the nurse practitioner also knows he/she must:

1. Order laboratory studies for diabetes.

2. Explore for possible alcohol abuse.

3. Advise him to lose weight.

4. Change his thiazide antihypertensive.

84. An elderly man given a diagnosis of systolic hypertension 3 months previously presents for follow-up care. He is on a no-added-salt diet and has lost 8 lb in 3 months. Weekly BP checks at a senior center average 180s/70s. The health history includes benign prostatic hyperplasia, diet-controlled type II diabetes, and CAD with an MI 8 years ago. His chief complaints include periodic angina, occasional heartburn, slowed urinary stream with some dribbling, and decreasing energy level. The BP today is 188/78 mm Hg. Current medications are cimetidine (Tagamet) 200 mg prn, ASA 325 mg qd, nitroglycerin, and Maalox prn. The client is married and sexually active. Which medication would the nurse practitioner initiate after a complete physical, including ECG, and all indicated blood work had been done?

1. ACE inhibitor.

2. Diuretic.

3. α_1-Blocker.

4. β-Blocker.

85. A geriatric client has been receiving procainamide (Pronestyl) for 4 years to control his cardiac dysrhythmias. The nurse practitioner would evaluate for what side effect in the long-term use of this medication?

    1. Elevated liver enzyme levels.

    2. Appearance of antinuclear antibodies.

    3. Shortened AV interval.

    4. Tachycardia.

86. Secondary prophylaxis for acute rheumatic fever (ARF) in a 25-year-old schoolteacher includes:

    1. Penicillin V 125 to 250 mg PO bid indefinitely.

    2. Erythromycin 800 mg PO bid.

    3. One-time dose of 2.0 million units benzathine penicillin G combined with penicillin G procaine (Bicillin C-R) IM.

    4. No medication prophylaxis is needed after client reaches the early twenties.

87. A client has been prescribed lisinopril (Prinivil) 5 mg, PO, qd for his hypertension. An intractable cough that is unrelated to heart failure has developed. Which of the following medications can be substituted for this ACE inhibitor?

    1. Calcium channel blocker.

    2. Digoxin.

    3. Another ACE inhibitor (e.g., hydralazine-nitrate combination).

    4. An angiotensin receptor blocker (ARB).

88. A 60-year-old man with a history of unstable angina comes to the clinic complaining of increased pain that is not relieved by his nitroglycerine. During the assessment, the nurse practitioner notes elevation of the ST segment on the ECG. Oxygen therapy is administered and an IV line is inserted. What other therapy should be initiated while arranging transfer to an acute-care facility?

    1. Lidocaine drip at 2 mg/min.

    2. Metoprolol (Toprol XL) 100 mg PO.

    3. Morphine 2 mg IV push.

    4. Aspirin 160 mg PO.

89. A 54-year-old client with type II diabetes has been given a diagnosis of hypertension. Which antihypertensive drug is the recommended for treatment of hypertension in clients with diabetes?

    1. β-Blockers.

    2. Diuretics.

    3. Calcium channel blockers.

    4. ACE inhibitors.

90. A 68-year-old with a history of an MI who has experienced atrial fibrillation for 2 years comes to the clinic with a complaint of "increasing difficulty breathing, occasionally awakening at night with feeling of smothering." Which pharmacologic therapy would be appropriate for this client?

    1. Digitalis and an ACE inhibitor.

    2. Loop diuretic and β-blocker.

    3. Thiazide diuretic and calcium channel blocker.

    4. α₁-Blocker and nitrate.

91. A client with CAD has a cholesterol level of 278 mg/dl and a triglyceride level of 300 mg/dl. The nurse practitioner initiates therapy with lovastatin (Mevacor) 20 mg daily. The client is instructed to take the Mevacor daily

    1. In the morning with breakfast.

    2. 30 minutes before eating breakfast.

    3. In the evening.

    4. Around noon.

92. A 70-year-old white woman is a resident of a long-term care facility where the nurse practitioner makes rounds on a weekly basis. The nurse practitioner is reviewing recent laboratory results and notices the following: serum potassium: 5.9 mEq/L, serum sodium: 144 mEq/L, serum chloride: 111 mEq/L; blood urea nitrogen (BUN): 28 mg/dl; creatinine: 1.8 mg/dl. There have been no changes to her medications. Her current medications include: furosemide (Lasix) 20 mg, PO, qd; potassium chloride (K-Dur), 16 mEq, PO, qd; captopril (Capoten), 25 mg, PO, qd; and citalopram (Celexa), 10 mg, PO, qd. What is the likely cause of the elevated serum potassium level?

    1. Furosemide (Lasix).

    2. Potassium chloride (K-Dur).

    3. Captopril (Capoten).

    4. Citalopram (Celexa).

Answers & Rationales

Physical Examination & Diagnostic Tests

1. **(1)** S$_1$ is heard loudest at the apex; and S$_2$, at the base. Each sound should be carefully assessed for its intensity in each area.

2. **(3)** The point of maximal impulse (PMI) represents the thrust and contraction of the left ventricle (LV). The LV lies behind the right ventricle (RV) and extends to the left, forming the left border of the heart.

3. **(2)** The correct procedure is to listen for carotid bruits with the bell of the stethoscope, which brings out low-frequency sounds and filters out high-frequency sounds. It should be placed very lightly on the neck with just enough pressure to seal the edge.

4. **(2)** The purpose of inspection and palpation of the precordium is to determine the presence and extent of normal and abnormal pulsations. A slight retraction of the chest wall just medial to the midclavicular line in the fifth interspace is a normal finding, whereas marked or active retraction of the rib is abnormal and may indicate pericardial disease. Pericardial friction rubs are heard by auscultation.

5. **(1)** The splitting during inspiration refers to S$_1$ and S$_2$. The S$_3$ is normal in children, young adults, and pregnant women. In the older adult with heart disease, this often signifies myocardial failure.

6. **(3)** The right side of the chest close to the sternal border at the second intercostal space is the correct area in which to auscultate the aortic valve. The mitral valve is auscultated at the fifth left intercostal space at the midclavicular line. The tricuspid value is auscultated at the fourth left intercostal space at the sternal border. The pulmonic valve is auscultated at the second left intercostal space at the sternal border.

7. **(2)** A 12-hour fast is recommended because of the influence of intake on cholesterol levels (they may increase). A normal diet for the 7 days before the exam is recommended so that an accurate picture of the client's normal life is obtained. Alcohol should not be consumed for 48 hours before the test, because it may increase cholesterol, high-density lipoprotein (HDL), low-density lipoprotein (LDL), and triglyceride levels. If possible, all medications should be withheld until the test is over, especially corticosteroids, diuretics, β-blockers, oral contraceptives, and estrogens.

8. **(1)** An S$_4$ is a normal variant in people 65 years or older and may result from increased resistance to ventricular filling during atrial contraction.

9. **(1)** According to the classification of hypertension, a blood pressure (BP) of 168/100 mm Hg is within the moderate range.

10. **(2)** The fifth intercostal space at the midclavicular line on the left side is the best place to auscultate the closure sounds of the mitral valve. Option #1 describes the area of the tricuspid valve, Option #3 describes the area of the pulmonic valve, and Option #4 describes the aortic valve area.

11. **(3)** It is important to determine whether the coolness extends proximally from the hand. Then, palpation of pulses would be appropriate.

12. **(1)** Closure of the atrioventricular (AV) valves, which allows the filling of both ventricles simultaneously, produces the first heart sound (S_1); closure of the aortic and pulmonic valves produces the second heart sound (S_2).

13. **(4)** The apical and peripheral (radial) pulses must be evaluated simultaneously to determine whether all of the apical beats are being reflected in the radial pulse. If there is an apical rate of 100 bpm and a radial rate of 94 bpm, the client is said to have a pulse deficit of 6 points. This is usually done with two people counting during the same period.

14. **(3)** A grade V heart murmur is very loud and can be heard with the stethoscope partly off the chest wall. A grade VI murmur is the loudest, is audible with the stethoscope just removed from contact with the chest wall, and is accompanied by a thrill. A grade I murmur is barely audible or very faintly heard with the bell of the stethoscope.

15. **(4)** The normal aging process impairs automaticity, conductivity, and contractility. Ischemic changes and degeneration decrease sinus node automaticity and conduction velocity, resulting in bradycardic rhythms or atrial fibrillation. The poor myocardial contractility, usually related to hypertension or valvular disease, causes decreased ventricular emptying and increased filling pressures. These changes predispose the elderly to congestive heart failure (CHF).

16. **(4)** The most sensitive area on the examiner's hand is the back of the fingers.

17. **(3)** Desired levels for a lipid profile are total cholesterol <200 mg/dl, HDL >35 mg/dl, LDL <130 mg/dl, and triglycerides <250 mg/dl. A high total cholesterol level coupled with a low HDL level is a positive risk factor for coronary heart disease, the greatest concern for this client. In addition, this client has an elevated LDL level. These values, taken as a whole, would mandate intervention in this client.

18. **(3)** Dressler's syndrome (postmyocardial infarction syndrome) may develop 1 to 4 weeks after myocardial infarction (MI) and is characterized by pericarditis with effusion and fever. Dressler's syndrome is caused by antigen-antibody reactions. Laboratory findings include elevations in the white blood cell count and the erythrocyte sedimentation rate. Treatment includes corticosteroids.

19. **(1)** Jugular vein distention (JVD) is common in geriatric clients. When it is present with the client's head elevated at a 45-degree angle, further examination needs to be conducted regarding the venous pressure, which is reflective of pressure in the right heart chambers. The supine position will increase venous pressure and does not provide valid information in this situation. Auscultation for carotid bruits is an important part of assessment but does not have significant value in evaluating JVD.

20. **(1)** Mitral valve stenosis is a diastolic murmur of low intensity heard at the apex of the heart. Option #2 describes characteristics of a murmur with aortic stenosis. Option #3, a holosystolic murmur, is characteristic of mitral regurgitation, which allows for backflow of blood from ventricles into the atrium. Option #4 best describes aortic regurgitation.

21. **(3)** The client had a left ventricular MI. One of the most common complications is left-sided heart failure resulting in CHF. This would be first manifested as pulmonary congestion and difficulty breathing.

22. **(4)** Classically, intermittent claudication is described as pain in the lower extremity on activity that is relieved by stopping the activity.

23. **(3)** A positive result on stress testing indicates the likelihood of coronary artery disease (CAD) with 98% accuracy in men older than 50 years. Results are progressively less accurate in asymptomatic persons; and false-positive results are increased in asymptomatic men younger than 40 years, premenopausal women without risk factors, and clients receiving digitalis.

24. **(2)** A hyperkinetic impulse (increased amplitude) is caused by pressure overload of the left ventricle. Causes include hyperthyroidism, severe anemia, and mitral regurgitation. A pansystolic murmur is a classic finding of mitral regurgitation.

25. **(4)** Pulsus alternans (a weak pulse alternating with a strong one) is caused by left ventricular failure and is usually accompanied by an S_3 heart sound.

Disorders

26. **(1)** This assessment finding reflects changes caused by chronic venous insufficiency. The other findings are reflective of chronic arterial insufficiency.

27. **(1)** A diagnosis of hypertension should not be made on the basis of a single measurement of BP elevation. A minimum of three readings with an average systolic BP of 140 mm Hg and a diastolic BP of 90 mm Hg establishes the diagnosis. An average of two or more readings taken at each of two or more visits should follow an initial screening. The client should be seated with the arm at heart level. No caffeine or nicotine ingestion should be allowed 30 minutes before the reading. The room should be quiet for a minimum of 5 minutes, and an appropriate cuff should be used. Another high reading should be confirmed within 2 months.

28. **(3)** In the early stages of hypertensive heart disease, when there is an increased peripheral resistance to blood flow, the most significant change occurring in the heart is left ventricular hypertrophy. This is associated with an increase in the size of the myocardial cells without a corresponding increase in cell number (i.e., hyperplasia). After some time, all of the other options listed occur in the heart.

29. **(3)** Sinus or atrial tachycardia is characterized by a heart rate at or above 100 bpm, P waves present for each QRS complex, a P-R interval below 0.20, a T wave occurring after each QRS complex, and a regular rhythm.

30. **(1)** The classic chest pain of an infarction may not be present in the geriatric client as a result of altered pain perception and diminished pain sensation.

31. **(2)** Respiratory symptoms are predominant in clients with left-sided heart failure. Venous congestion and peripheral edema are associated with right-sided heart failure.

32. **(1)** Cardiac tamponade occurs as a complication of pericarditis. An excessive accumulation of fluids between the pericardium and the myocardium interferes with effective cardiac contraction and produces a paradoxical pulse. The triphasic friction rub is common to pericarditis but is not indicative of a complication of constrictive pericarditis. Jugular venous pressure (JVP) is used to determine levels of venous distention.

33. **(2)** Untreated hypertension causes significant increased work of the left ventricle, eventually causing CHF.

34. **(2)** Palpable carotid pulse with each compression is the best sign of effective cardiopulmonary resuscitation (CPR). The other answers are appropriate but not the best indicators of effective resuscitation efforts.

35. **(2)** This is a description of complete block with hemodynamic consequences. The client should be seen immediately by a cardiologist for possible pacemaker insertion. First-degree block has characteristic P waves and a long P-R interval. The client should not just be referred for followup; he should be seen by a cardiologist as soon as possible.

36. **(3)** A triphasic friction rub or a pericardial rub occurs in the majority of clients with pericarditis. Paradoxical pulse may occur if constrictive pericarditis and cardiac tamponade are present. Pulse deficits and the presence of S_4 are not characteristic of problems with pericarditis.

37. **(1)** Elderly individuals experience atypical symptoms of an MI including dyspnea, diaphoresis, vomiting, syncope, confusion, and weakness.

38. **(1)** Cardiovascular risk factors predisposing women to cardiovascular disease include smaller body size, declining estrogen level, heart and thoracic cavity smaller and lighter in size, coronary arteries smaller in diameter, shorter P-R interval, and higher resting ejection fraction. Increased body fat percentage and fat distributed in the abdomen may be mobilized more easily in response to stress and may increase serum cholesterol and blood glucose levels.

39. **(4)** The nurse practitioner must consider the geriatric client's other medical problems and treatment before prescribing medications for hypertension. Frequently, geriatric clients cannot take β-blockers because of chronic pulmonary conditions; the client may already be receiving diuretics for problems of fluid retention. Step therapy is appropriate if there is no other significant medical history. Lifestyle changes should be initiated, and medication should be adjusted as changes are made.

40. **(2)** Hypertension is considered a major factor in the development of CAD in the geriatric client. Female clients have an increased incidence of CAD after menopause; estrogen replacement appears to have cardioprotective effects on the heart, thus decreasing the incidence of CAD. Clients with diabetes have an increased incidence of CAD; however, the majority of clients with CAD do not have diabetes.

41. **(4)** Cor pulmonale is characterized by hypertrophy of the right ventricle caused by pulmonary hypertension (resistance). The increased P-wave amplitude (P pulmonale) occurs as the right atrium enlarges.

42. **(2)** Excess secretion of aldosterone predisposes to potassium excretion. Total body sodium content will be above normal, but the excessive secretion of antidiuretic hormone causes greater retention of water, diluting the serum level.

43. **(1)** Water-hammer pulse (bounding with a rapid rise and sudden collapse) is produced by an increase in pulse pressure and may be caused by an increased stroke volume, a decrease in peripheral resistance, or both. Because the nurse practitioner suspects either aortic regurgitation or a patent ductus arteriosus (primarily in children), auscultation for a diastolic murmur is indicated.

44. **(2)** Occlusion of the coronary arteries deprives the myocardial cells of glucose needed for aerobic metabolism. Anaerobic metabolism occurs, which causes the accumulation of lactic acid. Lactic acid irritates the myocardial nerve fibers, sending pain messages to the cardiac nerves and upper thoracic posterior roots located in the left shoulder and arm.

45. **(1)** The moist crackles (rales) heard in the bases of the lung(s) are the most prominent physical examination findings of early CHF. They are caused by transudation of fluid into the alveoli and airways. Later findings include distended neck veins, peripheral edema, hepatomegaly, and ascites (rather than weight loss).

46. **(3)** Aortic dissection almost invariably begins with sudden onset of severe chest pain that is tearing or ripping in quality and is accompanied by loss of or decrease in peripheral pulses and neurologic deficits. The pain of angina and acute MI is usually described as a pressure. Pericarditis produces pain that is more gradual in onset.

47. **(1)** A step I diet involves daily intake of ≤30% total calories made up of fat, <300 mg/day cholesterol intake, and 8% to 10% daily saturated fat intake. A decrease to <200 mg/day of cholesterol and 7% saturated fat is a step II diet, prescribed if step I is ineffective. The third selection is closer to the current average American's diet. Although watching calorie and sodium intake is important for weight and BP control, it is not part of a step I diet plan for hyperlipidemia.

48. **(4)** Although the other dysrhythmias may be experienced by a client after an MI, the most life-threatening is ventricular fibrillation. The vast majority of deaths caused by ventricular fibrillation happen within the first 24 hours, and of these deaths, more than half occur in the first hour. The majority of out-of-hospital deaths from MI are due to ventricular fibrillation.

49. **(2)** Diet and exercise are the mainstay of any treatment program and would be used initially in all cases. A bile acid sequestrant agent or estrogen replacement therapy may eventually be necessary if no improvement is seen with diet and exercise therapy. Referral to a cardiologist is not necessary, unless the client has symptoms or shows resistance to treatment.

50. **(2)** A cerebrovascular accident is often the outcome of chronic atrial fibrillation caused by blood pooling in the quivering atria. This is the reason that warfarin (Coumadin) is recommended to be maintained at an international normalized ratio (INR) of 2:3. Some trials suggest aspirin may provide adequate anticoagulation in doses of 160 to 325 mg/day.

51. **(3)** Dyspnea is the most common symptom of CHF. Initially, it is present only with moderate exertion, but as severity of CHF increases, the dyspnea may occur with mild exertion or at rest. Fatigue is another common complaint. Right-sided heart failure is associated with weakness, anorexia, nausea, and dependent edema. Chronic left ventricular failure usually leads to right ventricular failure.

52. **(3)** Palm and coconut oils, along with butter, are very high in saturated fats and should be avoided. The other selections are moderately high in fat content but consist of mostly unsaturated fats.

53. **(3)** Angina is difficult to differentiate from that of an infarction. One of the most characteristic symptoms is the relief of the angina with the administration of sublingual nitroglycerin.

54. **(4)** Aspirin helps prevent the formation of platelet-aggregating substances and may help prevent the occlusion of narrowed coronary arteries. Although Lasix and morphine both have their place in treating acute myocardial infarction, ASA is given first in the primary care physician's office. Nitroglycerin should not be given because the client's systolic BP is less than 90 mm Hg.

55. **(1)** Superficial inflammation of a vein can be caused by trauma, such as a blow to the arm or leg or recent IV therapy with irritating fluids, or it can occur secondary to pregnancy, especially during the postpartum period because of the increase in clotting factors (thromboplastin). Excessive use of oral anticoagulants can lead to bleeding, but not thrombophlebitis. Deep venous thrombosis (DVT) associated with thrombophlebitis is due to prolonged bed rest, major surgical procedures, injury to the blood vessel wall, and hypercoagulable states (use of oral contraceptives, especially by women who smoke, have cancer, and polycythemia vera).

56. **(3)** Dizziness that improves when lying down and worsens when standing is symptomatic of cardiac involvement and may indicate serious cardiac dysrhythmias. If dizziness occurs in certain positions, it is indicative of benign positional vertigo, which is common in the elderly. Dizziness accompanied by tinnitus is common in acute labyrinthitis and, if preceded by rapid breathing, may be caused by hyperventilation.

57. **(3)** The stated history of a recent coxsackievirus infection, pain that worsens in the supine position, and a friction rub is classic for viral pericarditis. The client's age makes an acute myocardial infarction unlikely, and the pain is not typical of pleural effusion or reflux.

58. **(1)** Signs and symptoms of hyperthyroidism in the older adult include progressive functional decline, atrial fibrillation, MI, tachycardia, weakness, fatigue, weight loss, anorexia, diarrhea, nervousness, tremor, pruritus, memory loss, and heat intolerance. Symptoms of hypothyroidism include arthralgia, weakness, decreased mental function, depression, constipation, weight loss, dry coarse skin with yellowish cast, dry sparse hair, and mask-like, puffy face with periorbital edema. Bradycardia would be assessed with both sick sinus syndrome and CHF. Sick sinus syndrome is often associated with the "bradycardia-tachycardia" syndrome.

59. **(4)** A JVP of 4 cm is a sign of CHF. Option #1 is a normal sign of aging. Option #2 is a result of sclerosing of the aorta, which occurs with aging. Option #3 is expected with the aging process.

60. **(2)** The findings are consistent with aortic stenosis. Aortic regurgitation is a diastolic murmur associated with rheumatic heart disease. No history of rheumatic heart disease is given. Mitral valve disease is one of the most common valvular disorders. A small percentage of clients with mitral valve prolapse do have autonomic dysfunction and complain of palpitations, atypical chest pain, orthostatic dizziness, near-syncope, cold extremities, throbbing headaches, and neurasthenia and manifest tachyarrhythmias. Mitral regurgitation may remain asymptomatic for many years, because the left ventricle dilates and adjusts well to the increase in volume load. Onset of dyspnea and fatigue may not occur for decades.

61. **(1)** Aortic stenosis is most common and caused by calcification. The symptoms would include syncope, angina, and dyspnea on exertion.

62. **(3)** The nurse practitioner needs to repeat the cholesterol determination and determine HDL and LDL levels before initiating any treatment. The HDL and LDL levels will help stratify risks and guide aggressiveness of intervention.

Pharmacology

63. **(1)** This client is presenting with symptoms of digitalis toxic effects—first-degree block and increasing cardiac irritability. If the potassium level is low, it may be precipitating the toxic effects. Also, it is important to determine that serum theophylline levels remain within the therapeutic range. There is no evidence presented to indicate that the pulmonary disease is progressing. The BP may be adequately controlled for this client; further information should be obtained before adjustment of the medications. According to the information presented, referral to a cardiologist is not appropriate at this time.

64. **(3)** Thiazide diuretics inhibit sodium reabsorption, promoting the excretion of sodium, chloride, and water. As the extracellular fluid volume decreases, plasma renin activity and aldosterone levels increase, resulting in potassium loss. Treatment is to restore the volume with normal saline solution and correct the potassium depletion. If the sodium concentration is increased too rapidly, irreversible neurologic damage can occur.

65. **(1)** Vitamin K is an antidote for Coumadin. Increased intake of green leafy vegetables could cause an increase in vitamin K levels and decrease the effectiveness of the medication. Also, multivitamin supplements may contain additional vitamin K.

66. **(3)** The client presents with the classic profile of digitalis toxic effects, which is frequently related to hypokalemia, especially since the potassium replacement is rather low for an adult and there is history of poor eating and nausea. The actions listed in the other options may be taken; however, it is important to determine the presence of hypokalemia and digitalis toxic effects, so that these conditions may be addressed immediately.

67. **(1)** ACE inhibitors such as losartan (Cozaar) decrease the conversion of angiotensin I to angiotensin II, a potent vasoconstrictor, and inhibit the release of aldosterone.

68. **(1)** Aldactone is a potassium-sparing diuretic. Clients should be instructed about signs of hyperkalemia. Leg cramps, general fatigue, nausea, and vomiting are significant in hypokalemia.

69. **(1)** β-Blockers are myocardial depressants that suppress heart rate and contraction (negative inotropic). Calcium channel blockers decrease AV conduction, which suppresses heart rate. Both drugs are contraindicated with the onset of left ventricular dysfunction. The presence of an S_3 indicates left ventricular function, especially when associated with signs and symptoms of right-sided failure. The increase in JVD and 10-pound weight gain are indicative of right-sided failure.

70. **(3)** The American Heart Association's Advanced Cardiac Life Support (ACLS) guidelines recommend adenosine as the drug of choice for emergent treatment of supraventricular tachycardia, when a client is hemodynamically stable.

71. **(2)** The combination of calcium channel blockers and β-adrenergic blocking agents, systemic or ophthalmic, may result in hypotension.

72. **(2)** Niacin can cause vasodilatation, leading to orthostatic hypotension. Antihyperlipidemic drugs may cause constipation. The effectiveness of antihyperlipidemic agents is enhanced when they are taken before or with meals.

73. **(2)** Calcium channel blockers depress the rate of discharge from the sinoatrial node and conduction velocity through the AV node, causing a decrease in heart rate; relax the coronary and systemic arteries, producing vasodilation (decrease in afterload and BP); and decrease myocardial contractility (negative inotropic effect).

74. If lifestyle modifications (low-salt diet, weight loss, smoking cessation, exercise, etc.) fail to reduce the client's blood pressure, it is recommended that the client continue lifestyle modifications and start drug therapy. The preferred drugs (unless contraindicated) for uncomplicated hypertension are diuretics or β-blockers. Depending on comorbid conditions, other drugs might be preferable (i.e., for type I diabetes with proteinuria, you would use ACE inhibitors rather than a β-blocker). It is important to start with a low dose of a long-acting, once-daily drug and slowly titrate the dose. In this situation, a diuretic was started first with the next logical progression to a β-blocker because no comorbid conditions were listed.

75. **(3)** Blood pressure should be lowered cautiously by using smaller doses of calcium entry antagonists, ACE inhibitors, or diuretics in the elderly. β-Blockers are not appropriate in normal doses for the elderly because of decreased β-adrenergic receptor sensitivity in these clients. Larger doses also result in depression, impotence, fatigue, and declining mental function. Elderly clients are especially likely to experience CHF and peripheral vascular insufficiency from β-adrenergic blocker toxic effects.

76. **(2)** Nitrates are venous and arterial dilators that decrease myocardial oxygen demand. β-Blockers have an antianginal effect and reduce myocardial oxygen demand. Calcium channel blockers relieve myocardial ischemic by reducing myocardial oxygen demand and dilate coronary arteries. Aspirin is effective for primary and secondary prevention of MI. Unless contraindicated, small doses of aspirin (162-325 mg daily) should be prescribed for clients with angina. Clients remaining symptomatic when treated with nitrates, β-blockers, or calcium channel–blocking drugs should be treated with a β-blocker plus another agent. Appropriate combinations are a nitrate or a β-blocker plus a calcium channel blocker other than verapamil. Combination therapy does not include sedatives, vasoconstrictors, ACE inhibitors, or lipid-lowering drugs.

77. **(3)** Adverse effects of ACE inhibitors include cough (1%-30%), headache, and dizziness. Adverse effects of calcium channel blockers include peripheral edema, dizziness, headache, nausea, and tachycardia. Adverse effects of thiazide diuretics include nausea, vomiting, diarrhea, dizziness, and headache. Adverse effects of β-blockers include fatigue, impotence, depression, and shortness of breath.

78. **(1)** Digoxin, once a first-line drug for all clients with CHF, is now prescribed for clients with atrial fibrillation, other tachycardias, and left ventricular dysfunction. When the ventricular rate is controlled in the client with atrial fibrillation or tachycardias, cardiac output increases. In cases of diastolic dysfunction with a sinus rhythm, digitalis is of no benefit. Digoxin is of relatively little value in most forms of cardiomyopathy, myocarditis, mitral stenosis, and chronic constrictive pericarditis.

79. **(2)** Noncardiac adverse reactions include a change in mental status. Although visual disturbances, diarrhea, and anorexia, nausea, or vomiting are also adverse reactions, they are not the most common in the elderly.

80. **(4)** The findings point to gout. A side effect of thiazide is hyperuricemia. Blood should be drawn for a CBC before therapy is started. The other options do not address the finding of a tender and edematous right ankle. The results of the cardiac assessments were benign. There are no indications of a concern for hyponatremia or hypernatremia or hypokalemia or hyperkalemia.

81. **(2)** β-Blockers increase peripheral vascular resistance, a phenomenon that already occurs with normal aging, so these drugs can precipitate or worsen symptoms of asthma, chronic obstructive pulmonary disease (COPD), peripheral vascular disease, sexual dysfunction, or CHF. The other classes have no effect or decrease the effect on peripheral resistance.

82. **(1)** ACE inhibitors have been shown to prolong life in clients with CHF by improving overall cardiac function. Options #2 and #3 are contraindicated in CHF. Although Option #4 may be correct, it is not a priority, as is Option #1.

83. **(4)** The most likely precipitating cause of his gout is the thiazide diuretic used to control his hypertension, since it blocks the excretion of uric acid. Although gout may be more common in obese clients and clients with alcoholism and diabetes, these conditions are not indicated here.

84. **(1)** The ACE inhibitor will preserve renal function and have less impact on sexual functioning. The nurse practitioner must monitor potassium levels and carefully monitor renal status for change. The ACE inhibitor has fewer negative side effects or interactions with the other medical conditions of this client.

85. **(2)** Eighty percent of the clients who take procainamide on a long-term basis have antinuclear antibodies. Twenty percent of these clients have a lupus-like syndrome.

86. **(1)** Secondary prevention or preventing the recurrent attacks of acute rheumatic fever (ARF) is controversial. Some authorities

identify reaching the early twenties and 5 years since the last ARF attack as the criteria for stopping the use of prophylactic penicillin, unless the client is at increased risk of exposure to streptococcal infections, as are schoolteachers or health professionals. Other authorities recommend lifelong prophylactic drug therapy. Although erythromycin is an alternative medication for penicillin-sensitive individuals, the dose in Option #2 is for a client having a dental or surgical procedure. The secondary prophylaxis dose for erythromycin is 250 mg PO bid.

87. **(4)** An annoying untoward effect of ACE inhibitors is an intractable cough. Angiotensin receptor blockers (ARBs) can be substituted, as long as the cough is not related to heart failure. A hydralazine-nitrate combination can be substituted if there is significant renal insufficiency or angioedema present. Use of antiarrhythmic agents, calcium channel blockers, and nonsteroidal antiinflammatory drugs (NSAIDs) should be avoided.

88. **(4)** The American Heart Association recommends administration of acetylsalicylic acid (ASA) as soon as possible whenever a client is believed to have had an MI. The decreased platelet aggregation effect of ASA helps limit the amount of myocardial damage.

89. **(4)** ACE inhibitors enhance renal function in patients with diabetes.

90. **(1)** The client who has atrial fibrillation is exhibiting symptoms of left ventricular (LV) failure. Treatment recommendations include enhancing contractility with a positive inotropic agent, and ACE inhibitors have been shown to slow LV dilation.

91. **(3)** Because most cholesterol is synthesized between midnight and 3 AM, HMG-CoA reductase inhibitors are best taken in the evening.

92. **(2)** The likely cause of the elevated serum potassium level is the K-Dur (potassium chloride). The nurse practitioner should hold the K-Dur (potassium chloride) and order daily measurement of serum potassium levels until levels return to normal. The client is taking Lasix (furosemide), which is a potassium-wasting diuretic, and it appears that the amount of potassium she was given to compensate for the anticipated losses was too much, and this often occurs as a result of the changes of aging. Once her serum potassium level returns to normal, it should be monitored again at 1 week. It is possible that with the low dose of furosemide (Lasix) and the captopril (Capoten), which is an ACE inhibitor and sometimes retains potassium, she may not need administration of the potassium chloride (K-Dur) restarted.

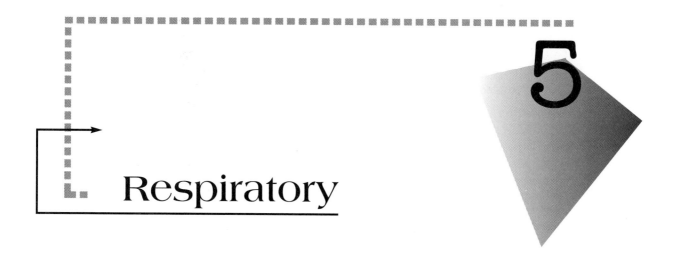

Respiratory

Physical Examination & Diagnostic Tests

1. The nurse practitioner knows that normal breath sounds that have a low pitch and soft intensity and are heard better on inspiration are called:

   1. Bronchial.

   2. Vesicular.

   3. Bronchovesicular.

   4. Rhonchi.

2. When auscultating for vocal resonance in a client with possible consolidation of lung tissue, the nurse practitioner hears "a-a-a" when the client says "e-e-e." This is called:

   1. Tactile fremitus.

   2. Bronchophony.

   3. Whispered pectoriloquy.

   4. Egophony.

3. The nurse practitioner understands the following about hyperresonance in percussion of the lungs:

   1. It is a normal finding in the adult client.

   2. It occurs commonly in pediatric clients.

   3. It is characterized by soft intensity, high pitch, short duration, and extreme dullness in quality.

   4. It is characterized by loud intensity, high pitch, medium duration, and dull quality.

4. What is the correct procedure for percussing the chest?

   1. Percuss the entire right side of the anterior chest and move to the left side.

   2. Begin at the upper left side of the posterior chest and compare with the respective anterior side, moving from front to back.

   3. Percuss the anterior chest systematically and symmetrically, moving from left to right side; then percuss the posterior chest.

   4. Percuss the posterior chest and then measure for diaphragmatic excursion on the anterior chest.

5. The nurse practitioner understands that pleural friction rubs are:

   1. Auscultated in the lower anterolateral chest.

   2. Heard best at the end of expiration.

   3. Characterized by a continuous, low-pitched, snoring sound heard early in inspiration.

   4. Noted when the client says "e-e-e" and the examiner hears "a-a-a" through the stethoscope.

6. Normal physiologic changes in the respiratory system of the geriatric client include:

   1. Increased rigidity of the rib cage and an increase in the anteroposterior (AP) diameter of the chest.

   2. Increased ciliary action resulting in a more forceful and recurrent cough.

   3. Increase in number of smaller alveoli with a decrease in residual capacity.

   4. Decrease in AP diameter of rib cage with decrease in lung expansion.

7. When assessing for tactile fremitus, where would the nurse practitioner place her hands on the client's chest?

   1. On the anterior chest at the level of the sixth intercostal space.

   2. At the level of bifurcation of the bronchi on the posterior chest wall.

   3. On the scapula and sternum.

   4. At the level of the diaphragm on the posterior chest wall.

8. On assessment of the client's respiratory status, crepitation is felt over the third rib at the midaxillary line on the left side. What is the interpretation of this finding?

   1. There is consolidation of fluid in the left lower lobe of the lung.

   2. Severe inflammation is present on the visceral pleural surfaces of the left lung.

   3. An increase in pressure has occurred in the pleural cavity of the right lung.

   4. Air is present in the subcutaneous tissue from an air leak in the respiratory system.

9. An important anatomic landmark on the anterior thoracic wall is the angle of Louis. Where on the thorax is this landmark present?

   1. The mid-nipple line on either side of the manubrium.

   2. Bilaterally at the manubriosternal junction.

   3. Midline at the base of the suprasternal notch.

   4. Just below the clavicle but above the manubrium.

10. During assessment of a geriatric client's respiratory status, the nurse practitioner determines the presence of coarse tactile fremitus posteriorly at the second intercostal space. The best interpretation of this finding is:

    1. Increased air trapping in the alveoli on the affected side.

    2. Presence of fluid or solid mass within the lungs.

    3. Increased pressure in the bronchial tree.

    4. Presence of hyperactive airway disease.

11. When the lateral diameter of the chest is the same size as the AP diameter, the nurse practitioner correctly documents this finding as a:

    1. Biot deviated chest.

    2. Pigeon chest.

    3. Funnel chest.

    4. Barrel chest.

12. The nurse practitioner is planning a community screening program for lung cancer in geriatric clients. The current evidence-based practice suggests:

    1. Bronchoscopy with biopsy for cytologic examination is recommended every 2 to 3 years for smokers.

    2. Primary prevention (through discouraging tobacco use) is more effective than screening.

    3. Evidence indicates that routine screening for lung cancer decreases mortality rates.

    4. Comparison of current and previous chest x-ray films is a sensitive test for lung cancer.

13. An adult male client comes to the clinic with the chief complaint of "coughing up blood" and night sweats. He has no history of respiratory or cardiac problems. His vital signs are pulse 96 bpm, respirations 28 breaths/min, blood pressure 140/92 mm Hg, and oral temperature of 99° F (37.2° C). The initial diagnostic evaluation of this client includes:

    1. Electrocardiogram (ECG), pulmonary function studies, sputum cytologic examination.
    2. Purified protein derivative (PPD) skin test, chest x-ray, sputum smear for acid-fast bacillus.
    3. Arterial blood gas (ABG) studies, complete blood count (CBC), chest x-ray film.
    4. Direct bronchoscopy with biopsy and complement fixation antibody titer.

14. In assessment of pulmonary function studies of a client, which finding is seen in chronic airflow limitation such as emphysema?

    1. Decreases in forced vital capacity (FVC) and forced expiratory volume in 1 second (FEV_1).
    2. Increases in functional residual capacity (FRC) and residual volume (RV).
    3. Decrease in RV and increase in total lung capacity (TLC).
    4. Increase in both FEV_1 and total lung capacity (TLC).

15. When interpreting PPD skin tests for clients at a long-term care facility, the nurse practitioner identifies positive results in individual with:

    1. Redness or erythema at the site.
    2. An induration reaction of ≥5 mm.
    3. An induration reaction of ≥10 mm.
    4. An induration reaction extending to 15 mm.

16. A client comes to the clinic complaining of difficulty breathing, lethargy, and coughing up blood in his sputum. He has no history of chronic illness or major health problems. The nurse practitioner orders diagnostic tests to determine the problem. What diagnostic test results would require immediate treatment of this client?

    1. Positive sputum smear for acid-fast bacillus.
    2. Sputum culture positive for *Pneumocystis carinii.*

    3. Presence of hemolysis on complement fixation test.
    4. Oxygen saturation 94%, leukocyte count >5000 white blood cells (WBCs)/mm^3.

Disorders

17. A client has received a blunt trauma injury to his chest. Which finding would be most indicative of further respiratory complications?

    1. Complaints of increased pain over the affected area.
    2. Oximetry readings consistently around 90%.
    3. Decreased breath sounds on the affected side.
    4. Fever of 102° F (39° C) and increased sputum production.

18. The nurse understands that the following characteristic is more likely to occur when the adult client has pneumonia (caused by *Streptococcus pneumoniae*) rather than bronchitis:

    1. Rusty sputum.
    2. Cough.
    3. Dyspnea.
    4. Wheezing.

19. A child is recovering from tuberculosis (TB). What information should be included in a teaching plan for his or her home care?

    1. It is critical for the child to take medications at the prescribed time; doses should not be skipped and the supply should not be allowed to run out.
    2. Respiratory isolation procedures need to be carried out at home; the child should avoid contact with immediate family members.
    3. It will be necessary for the parent to return to the clinic every week to have the child's sputum checked for viable bacteria.
    4. The child may experience a rash along with nausea and vomiting from the medications, and the parent should decrease the dosage if this occurs.

20. What would be a priority intervention for a client experiencing a respiratory arrest?

    1. Start chest compressions at 15 compressions and two breaths.

    2. Open the airway with a head tilt and chin lift.

    3. Give oxygen through a rebreathing mask at 10 L/min.

    4. Pinch the nose and give two breaths.

21. A client comes to the emergency department complaining of difficulty breathing. What is most important to establish initially in this client?

    1. What type of activity produces the dyspnea.

    2. The presence of consolidation by means of a chest x-ray film.

    3. ABG levels with respect to oxygen pressure.

    4. Presence of bilateral breath sounds over the lower lobes.

22. A client has severe dyspnea, and the history strongly suggests the possibility of a foreign body in the bronchi. What observation would contribute to the documentation of this problem?

    1. Unilateral retraction of the right chest wall.

    2. Presence of crepitation on the anterior chest wall.

    3. Retraction of the lower chest wall.

    4. A friction rub heard over the area of the bronchi.

23. The nurse practitioner is assessing a client who is complaining of shortness of breath and chest discomfort. His respirations are shallow and at a rate of 26 breaths/min. When the diaphragmatic excursion is evaluated, it is determined that the diaphragm is slightly higher on the right side than on the left side. The best interpretation of this finding is:

    1. This is normal because the liver is on the right side.

    2. There may be atelectasis in the right lower lobe.

    3. Consolidation is present in the right lower lobe.

    4. This indicates the presence of early stages of chronic obstructive lung disease.

24. A 22-year-old man comes to the office complaining of chest pain and shortness of breath. He states that the problems started suddenly after he ran sprints during basketball practice. He states that he has no history of pulmonary problems. He is about 72 inches tall and weighs approximately 145 lb. Pulse rate is 118 bpm, respiratory rate is 30 breaths/min, decreased breath sounds are heard, and there is hyperresonance over the left lung. According to the findings, what is the best diagnosis for this client?

    1. Spontaneous pneumothorax.

    2. Exercise-induced asthma.

    3. Pulmonary edema.

    4. Acute bronchiectasis.

25. A young woman comes to the clinic with complaints of tingling in her face and hands, sudden shortness of breath, and vague chest discomfort. She appears very anxious and denies any history of respiratory problems. On examination, her hands are cool to touch; her vital signs are respirations 34 breaths/min, pulse regular at a rate of 100 bpm, blood pressure 110/76 mm Hg, and normal temperature. Respiratory examination reveals bilateral breath sounds with tachypnea and no adventitious sounds. Percussion and visual examination of the chest reveal no abnormalities. What is the best immediate treatment?

    1. Rebreathing into a paper bag and encouraging controlled diaphragmatic breathing.

    2. Two puffs of a short-acting bronchodilator with a metered-dose inhaler (MDI) (inhaled β_2-adrenergic agonist, short-acting).

    3. Oxygen at 4 L and ABGs after 30 minutes.

    4. Establish an IV line; infuse 500 ml of normal saline solution for volume depletion.

26. A client with newly diagnosed chronic obstructive pulmonary disease (COPD) is being discharged from the hospital. The nurse practitioner is discussing home care with the client. What information is important for the practitioner to include in the home care teaching?

    1. Use the bronchodilator before exercising.

    2. Maintain bed rest for the first few days at home.

    3. Decrease amount of fluid intake to prevent fluid overload.

    4. Maintain flow rate of oxygen at around 5 to 7 L.

27. A client is brought to a rural emergency department by ambulance. Primary assessment reveals:

    - Respirations: 38 breaths/min with use of accessory muscles, prolonged expiration and wheezes
    - ECG: Sinus tachycardia rate 140 bpm.
    - Blood pressure: 192/98 mm Hg.
    - Lethargic: Responds to name only by opening eyes
    - Cyanosis of lips

    Therapeutic interventions initiated by emergency medical technicians include:

    - IV therapy with D_5W at 30 ml/hr
    - Oxygen therapy at 48% by Venturi mask

    STAT ABGs indicate:

    - pH = 7.24
    - $PaCO_2$ = 82 mm Hg
    - HCO_3 = 36
    - PaO_2 = 76 mm Hg

    Before obtaining a second set of ABGs, the nurse practitioner would:

    1. Assist respirations with bag-valve mask with 100% oxygen.
    2. Administer 1 ampule of sodium bicarbonate.
    3. Change oxygen delivery to nasal cannula at 2 L.
    4. Disconnect the supplemental oxygen.

28. Instructions to the elderly client with COPD concerning nutritional therapy would include foods that are:

    1. High calorie, high protein, low carbohydrate.
    2. High calorie, low protein, high carbohydrate.
    3. Low calorie, high protein, low carbohydrate.
    4. Low calorie, low protein, high carbohydrate.

29. Age-associated changes that increase the risk for pneumonia in the elderly client include an increase in:

    1. Compliance of the chest wall.
    2. Diameter of the trachea and bronchi.

    3. Lung parenchyma.
    4. Cough forcefulness.

30. An adult client arrives at the clinic complaining of difficulty breathing, a cough, and chest pain. History indicates the client was discharged from the hospital 2 days ago after a cesarean delivery and has a 15–pack-year smoking history. Diagnostic studies should include:

    1. Sputum for culture and sensitivity.
    2. Cardiac troponin proteins.
    3. Pulse oximetry.
    4. ABGs.

31. The nurse practitioner is aware that the flu or influenza:

    1. Can be caused by receiving a flu vaccine when one's resistance is low.
    2. Is characterized by a slow, insidious onset of chills, fever, and muscle aches.
    3. In older adults may persist for several weeks with symptoms of lack of energy and extreme fatigue.
    4. Is primarily contagious in the early autumn and spring, and children are at greatest risk.

32. An adult client with a history of asthma calls to tell the nurse practitioner that she is "blowing 55%" on the peak flowmeter. What advice would the nurse practitioner give this client?

    1. Call an ambulance immediately.
    2. Use a bronchodilator now and come in for evaluation in the office today.
    3. Come in for office evaluation this week.
    4. See a pulmonary physician.

33. An elderly client is evaluated by the nurse practitioner because of complaints of cough, fever, chest pain, and sputum production. In obtaining a history from this client, it is important to know whether the client has:

    1. Received the pneumococcal vaccine.
    2. Traveled out of the country.
    3. Pets in the household.
    4. Recently started new medications.

34. An elderly client presents with signs and symptoms that make the nurse practitioner suspect the diagnosis of pneumonia. Which of the following would the nurse practitioner most likely find during the examination?

    1. Chest pain with inspiration.

    2. Confusion with a low-grade temperature.

    3. Congested, productive cough.

    4. Fever with leukocytosis.

35. In developing a plan for an older client with pneumonia, the nurse practitioner understands that 30% to 40% of community-acquired pneumonia is caused by which organism?

    1. *Haemophilus influenzae.*

    2. *Klebsiella pneumoniae.*

    3. *Mycobacterium tuberculosis.*

    4. *Streptococcus pneumoniae.*

36. What would be most appropriate to include in the health promotion plan for an older client who is at risk for pneumonia?

    1. Annual pneumococcal vaccination.

    2. Annual pneumococcal and influenza immunization.

    3. Annual sputum culture and chest x-ray examination.

    4. PPD test done every 3 to 5 years.

37. The nurse practitioner evaluates an older client with a current history of alcoholism. The client presents with an elevated temperature, congested cough that produces rusty sputum, and occasional chills. The suspected diagnosis is bacterial pneumonia. The Gram-stained sputum smear would most likely reveal which organism?

    1. *Haemophilus influenzae.*

    2. *Klebsiella pneumoniae.*

    3. *Staphylococcus aureus.*

    4. *Streptococcus pneumoniae.*

38. An elderly client residing in a nursing home has recently been exposed to TB. The nurse practitioner interprets the initial PPD test result to be negative. Which plan would be most appropriate at this time?

    1. Evaluate client in another year.

    2. Repeat PPD test in 1 week.

    3. Ignore results and immediately begin administration of ethambutol.

    4. Evaluate client in 6 months, since there are no symptoms at this time.

39. The nurse practitioner knows that Horner's syndrome is commonly associated with:

    1. Chronic bronchitis.

    2. Pulmonary TB.

    3. Pancoast's syndrome of lung cancer.

    4. Pulmonary embolism.

40. An adult client who smokes presents with complaints of breathlessness. The nurse practitioner notes, on examination, dilated blood vessels on the chest and mild edema of the head and supraclavicular area. The nurse recognizes this condition as:

    1. Thyroid abnormality.

    2. Chronic bronchitis with mild congestive failure.

    3. Asthma with fluid retention.

    4. Superior vena cava obstruction.

41. An elderly client presents with postural hypotension; laboratory studies reveal hyponatremia. What is the most likely cause of these findings?

    1. Diabetic ketoacidosis.

    2. Severe trauma.

    3. Bronchogenic carcinoma.

    4. Antacid overuse.

42. The nurse practitioner knows the following about asthma in the elderly:

    1. Subcutaneous epinephrine is standard therapy.

    2. It is usually of the allergic type.

3. Attacks are usually preceded by viral infections.

4. Clinical presentation is usually dyspnea, costal retraction, and fever.

43. Clinical signs and symptoms of late-phase asthma include:

    1. Bronchoconstriction refractory to bronchodilator therapy.

    2. Sneezing, watery eyes, and cough.

    3. Wheezing and increased sputum production.

    4. Bronchodilation caused by release of histamine.

44. The nurse practitioner is assessing a client for asthma. What is a common clinical manifestation of asthma?

    1. Pruritus.

    2. Diffuse crackles.

    3. Nocturnal exacerbation.

    4. Chronic hypoxemia.

45. During a routine follow-up visit, a client with asthma states that she has been doing fine except that when she goes out for dinner, she notices she has increased bronchospasm and wheezing. Which would be an appropriate response?

    1. "Have you been taking your medication?"

    2. "Do you usually have wine with dinner?"

    3. "I recommend that you do not go out for dinner."

    4. "Does going out to dinner make you stressed?"

46. The practitioner is evaluating a 60-year-old man who presents with symptoms characteristic of obstructive sleep apnea. An overnight polysomnogram (PSG) is ordered. What is the characteristic result of this study that would confirm sleep apnea?

    1. Loud snoring all night long.

    2. Oxygen desaturation and 10-second periods of apnea.

    3. Frequent brief arousals during sleep.

    4. 5-second periods of apnea with brief arousals.

47. The practitioner is screening geriatric clients for problems related to sleep apnea. What risk factors are commonly associated with this condition?

    1. Male, older than 55 years, and obese.

    2. Obese, female, older than 35 years.

    3. Female, history of respiratory problems, loud snoring.

    4. Male, history of chronic respiratory disease, increased daytime sleeping.

48. A male client comes into the clinic complaining of increased fatigue, increased irritability, and depression. He reports having difficulty sleeping and waking up frequently during the night. On the basis of these symptoms, what else should be determined?

    1. Presence of ongoing daytime sleepiness.

    2. History of depression.

    3. Fluctuations in blood pressure.

    4. Recent changes in medications.

Pharmacology

49. The nurse practitioner is following up with a client who is experiencing acute asthmatic problems. Albuterol (Proventil) by MDI has been ordered as treatment. Which client response would indicate to the nurse practitioner that the client understands how to take his medication?

    1. "I will take one puff of the medication and then wait a minute before taking the second puff."

    2. "I will take two puffs of the medication every 4 hours, even if I am not short of breath."

    3. "It is important for me to take this medication on a regular cycle to prevent future attacks."

    4. "I will take two puffs, one right after the other, whenever I begin to get short of breath."

50. A client who was recently given a diagnosis of TB calls the clinic because her urine is reddish orange. She is taking isoniazid (INH; Laniazid), rifampin (Rifadin), and pyrazinamide. What would be an appropriate response for the nurse practitioner to make?

    1. "This is a urinary tract infection symptom; drink plenty of fluids."

    2. "This is a normal response to the rifampin."

    3. "Often, this is an indication of liver toxicity. Stop the medications."

    4. "This is probably bleeding and you should see a physician immediately."

51. A client with a history of bronchial asthma is seen in the clinic because of increased episodes of difficulty breathing. The client has been taking theophylline 100 mg PO tid. The client is a 40-year-old obese man with an 18–pack-year history of cigarette smoking and an excessive daily intake of coffee who eats a low-carbohydrate, high-protein diet. Which identified factors decrease the therapeutic effects of the theophylline?

    1. Age and gender.

    2. Coffee intake and weight.

    3. Age and weight.

    4. Smoking history and diet.

52. A 70-year-old man comes to the clinic with complaints that he has experienced increased difficulty breathing over the past few days. He has a history of chronic obstructive lung disease and coronary artery disease. He was recently given a diagnosis of hypertension. Examination reveals no jugular vein distention, slight increase in the AP diameter of the chest, and no productive cough; breath sounds are present, but expiratory wheezes are noted bilaterally, and he denies complaints of chest pain. His vital signs are pulse 72 bpm, respirations 34 breaths/min, and blood pressure 170/100 mm Hg. His current medications are ipratropium bromide (Atrovent) inhaler two puffs q6h, nitroglycerin transdermal patches, and propranolol (Inderal) 60 mg PO bid. What is the best treatment for this client?

    1. Discontinue the propranolol (Inderal) and begin administration of verapamil (Calan) 80 mg PO tid qd.

    2. Begin administration of theophylline (Theo-24; methylxanthine) 200 mg q12h PO.

    3. Discontinue the propranolol (Inderal) and begin administration of atenolol (Tenormin) 50 mg PO qd.

    4. Start using beclomethasone (Beclovent) inhaler, two puffs 3 to 4 times daily.

53. The recommended range for maintaining serum theophylline levels is:

    1. 0.05 to 2 μg/ml.

    2. 10 to 20 μg/ml.

    3. 20 to 25 μg/ml.

    4. 30 to 40 μg/ml.

54. A client in a long-term care facility whose roommate has been given a diagnosis of active TB should begin chemoprophylaxis:

    1. As soon as possible. Chemoprophylaxis should be initiated at the time of screening skin testing.

    2. Within 72 hours after PPD skin test results are obtained.

    3. Only if PPD skin test results are positive.

    4. In 3 months if the result of the repeated skin test is positive.

55. In adults with asthma, the most common reason that outpatient treatment fails, resulting in hospitalization, is:

    1. Exposure to allergens.

    2. Increased use of steroids.

    3. Improper inhaler technique.

    4. Use of cromolyn inhalers.

56. Which can elevate theophylline levels?

    1. Concomitant treatment with cimetidine (Tagamet).

    2. IV ampicillin therapy.

    3. Heavy smoking.

    4. History of seizure disorder.

57. A client with a long history of chronic airflow limitation has noticed a change in sputum over the past few days (increased amount of thick,

yellow-green mucus, congestion). What would be appropriate therapy?

1. Hismanal 10 mg PO qd.

2. Augmentin 500 mg PO tid × 10 days.

3. Tylenol with codeine.

4. Vancenase MDI 2 puffs prn.

58. Which medication is most effective in promoting a decrease in airway inflammation, as well as in providing long-term medication coverage in a client with asthma?

1. Montelukast (Singulair).

2. Beclomethasone diproprionate (Vanceril, Beclovent).

3. Albuterol (Proventil, Ventolin).

4. Salmeterol (Serevent).

59. The nurse practitioner is planning prophylactic treatment for a client with asthma. What is the best medication to use for the client with asthma who is not currently experiencing an exacerbation?

1. Antibiotics.

2. Inhaled glucocorticoids.

3. β_1-Agonist.

4. Methacholine challenge.

60. Clients with asthma need to be instructed to:

1. Begin using their inhaled steroids as soon as symptoms appear.

2. With the MDI, take two puffs of the β-agonist prn.

3. Use their inhaled steroids when they experience bronchospasm.

4. Start their antibiotic regimen when they experience bronchospasm.

61. The nurse practitioner understands that an appropriate medication regimen for a client with pulmonary TB that is drug-susceptible is:

1. Montelukast (Singulair) drug therapy with rifampin (Rifadin).

2. Combination therapy with streptomycin, pyrazinamide, and rimantadine (Flumadine).

3. Combination therapy with isoniazid (INH), pyrazinamide, and rifampin (Rifadin).

4. Single-agent therapy with pyrimethamine (Fansidar).

62. A client presents in the clinic with a dry, hacking, nonproductive cough that is interfering with her sleep. The nurse practitioner would encourage the client to purchase an over-the-counter preparation that contains:

1. Pseudoephedrine.

2. Diphenhydramine.

3. Guaifenesin.

4. Dextromethorphan.

63. A client with chronic asthma is seen in the clinic complaining of vomiting and stomach cramps. He is confused and is unsure what medications he is currently taking. His vital signs are blood pressure 158/92 mm Hg, pulse 152 bpm and irregular, and respirations 28 breaths/min and shallow. What STAT diagnostic study should be done?

1. Serum electrolytes.

2. Digoxin level.

3. Theophylline level.

4. ABGs.

64. A client is seen in the clinic complaining of increased difficulty breathing and an intermittent productive cough that worsens in the evening. The history revels that the client has a 20–pack-year history of smoking. Breath sounds are clear to auscultation. There is no evidence of fever, and no abnormalities are detected by means of chest radiography. The nurse practitioner instructs the client concerning the importance of smoking cessation and fluid therapy and prescribes:

1. Erythromycin 500 mg PO qid × 14 days.

2. Albuterol 2 mg PO tid.

3. Mucomyst inhalation 10 ml of 10% solution q4h prn.

4. Tetracycline 100 mg q12h × 14 days.

65. When initiating preventive care to decrease the incidence of pneumonia in clients in an extended care facility, the nurse practitioner would identify clients receiving immunosuppressive therapy, repeated courses of antibiotics, sedation, and:

1. β_1-Adrenergic blocking agents.

2. Calcium channel blockers.

3. Diuretics.

4. Histamine (H_2) antagonists.

66. An older adult client presents with complaints of dyspnea, cough, fatigue, and dependent edema that have been worsening over the past few days. In planning the treatment for this client, the nurse practitioner considers:

1. Streptokinase therapy.

2. Referral for hospitalization for evaluation of heart function.

3. Prescription for furosemide (Lasix) 40 mg PO qd.

4. Addition of a calcium channel blocker to the client's medications.

67. A client with a history of Parkinson's disease has a positive tuberculin skin test result, and INH is ordered as a prophylactic medication. Before beginning administration of INH, it is important for the nurse practitioner to determine:

1. Whether the client's Parkinson's disease is being treated with levodopa (Larodopa).

2. How long the client has had the diagnosis of Parkinson's disease.

3. How much respiratory compromise the client is currently experiencing.

4. The adequacy of urinary output and renal function.

68. A geriatric client with a history of COPD is seen because of an upper respiratory tract infection, and the nurse practitioner decides to prescribe erythromycin. On review of the client's history, what current medication would be a contraindication to the administration of erythromycin?

1. Theophylline (Theo-24).

2. Lisinopril (Zestril).

3. Moexipril (Univasc).

4. Atenolol (Tenormin).

69. A 50-year-old white man with a history of COPD presents to the clinic with increased dyspnea, elevated temperature of 39° C (102° F), pulse 104 bpm, respiratory rate of 44 breaths/min, O_2 saturation of 84%. On physical examination, the nurse practitioner notes diffuse rales and rhonchi bilaterally. The client's medication list includes Tenormin (Atenolol) 25 mg, PO, qd; prednisone (Deltasone) 10 mg, PO, qd; ipratropium bromide (Atrovent) 18 μg, 1-2 puffs, qid, prn; and fluticasone propionate (Advair) 100/50, 2 puffs, bid. The nurse practitioner makes the preliminary diagnosis of pneumonia, pending results of the chest x-ray examination. Which medication puts this patient at risk for immunocompromise?

1. Tenormin (Atenolol).

2. Prednisone (Deltasone).

3. Ipratropium bromide (Atrovent).

4. Fluticasone propionate (Advair).

5 Answers & Rationales

Physical Examination & Diagnostic Tests

1. **(2)** The sounds heard over normal lung tissue are called *vesicular breath sounds*. The inspiratory phase of the vesicular breath sound is heard better than the expiratory phase and is about 2.5 times longer for these low-pitched, soft sounds. Bronchial breath sounds are normally heard over the trachea. Bronchial breath sounds are high-pitched, loud sounds with a shortened inspiratory phase and a lengthened expiratory phase. Bronchovesicular breath sounds have an intermediate pitch and intensity with equal duration of expiratory and inspiratory sounds heard mainly over the second interspace anteriorly and between the scapulae posteriorly. Rhonchi are abnormal breath sounds that are low pitched with a snoring quality.

2. **(4)** Tactile fremitus is a palpable vibration of the thoracic wall that is produced when the client speaks. Bronchophony is the increase in loudness and clarity of vocal resonance. Whispered pectoriloquy is exaggerated bronchophony and is heard through a stethoscope when the client whispers words (e.g., "ninety-nine"). In egophony, the spoken voice has a nasal or bleating quality when heard through a stethoscope and the spoken "e-e-e" sounds like "a-a-a."

3. **(2)** Hyperresonance is an abnormal percussion tone in adults but occurs normally in a children's lungs. It is characterized by very loud intensity, very low pitch, long duration, and a booming quality.

4. **(3)** Both the anterior and posterior chest are to be percussed systematically and symmetrically, moving from left to right. Diaphragmatic excursion is usually only measured on the posterior chest.

5. **(1)** Pleural friction rubs are loud, dry, creaking or grating sounds produced by the rubbing together of inflamed and roughened pleural surfaces, which are heard best during the latter part of inspiration and the beginning of expiration and in the lower anterolateral chest. Option #3 is characteristic of sonorous rhonchi. Option #4 is characteristic of egophony.

6. **(1)** With aging, there is a decrease in the number of alveoli, and the alveoli become rigid and lose the ability to recoil. The loss of alveolar elasticity affects the ability of the client to exhale effectively, and there is an increase in the residual volume. There is also a decrease in basilar inflation and a decrease in the ability to expel foreign matter. The anteroposterior (AP) diameter of the chest increases, as it does in clients with kyphosis.

7. **(2)** The bifurcation of the trachea or bronchi on the posterior chest wall is the best area for assessment of tactile fremitus. Care should be taken to avoid the area over the scapula and sternum because bone dampens vibrations.

8. **(4)** Crepitation or crepitus (also called *subcutaneous emphysema*) is caused by air bubbles under the skin from a rupture somewhere in the respiratory system, or less commonly, from an infection by a gas-producing organism. Crepitation always requires attention.

9. **(2)** This landmark can be used to determine each of the second ribs and intercostal space and corresponding spaces below that level. It is a visible and palpable angle of the sternum at the point where the second rib attaches to the sternum.

10. **(2)** Fluid or a solid mass transmits the vibrations so that tactile fremitus may be felt on the exterior chest wall. Increased air trapping will cause a decreased or absent fremitus. A reactive airway results in wheezing caused by edema.

11. **(4)** The adult chest is somewhat asymmetric and the AP diameter is often half the transverse diameter. Pigeon chest (pectus carinatum) is a forward protrusion of the sternum with the ribs sloping back. Funnel chest (pectus excavatum) is a depression of the sternum. Barrel chest occurs when the AP diameter equals the transverse diameter.

12. **(2)** "Primary prevention is more effective than screening in reducing the lung cancer morbidity and mortality" (*Guide to Clinical Preventive Services*, 1996, p. 137). Current evidence-based research does not support routine screening for lung cancer. There is insufficient evidence that lung cancer screening by x-ray or sputum cytologic examination reduces mortality rates. Bronchoscopy with biopsy is a diagnostic test, not a screening test.

13. **(2)** The client should be initially evaluated for tuberculosis (TB). Pulmonary function studies, arterial blood gas (ABG) studies, and bronchoscopy are not indicated at this time. Complement fixation studies are done to diagnose atypical pneumonia.

14. **(2)** Hyperinflation caused by air trapping causes an increase in functional residual capacity (FRC), residual volume (RV), and total lung capacity (TLC) (which may be twice normal). Corresponding decreases in forced vital capacity (FVC) and forced expiratory volume in 1 second (FEV_1) occur. This causes a flattening of the diaphragm, decreased inspiratory efficiency, and increased work of breathing.

15. **(3)** Positive interpretation of PPD skin test results are as follows:

Induration	Positive in:
≥5 mm	Individuals with human immunodeficiency virus (HIV) infection
	Individuals with recent close contact with persons with active TB
	Individuals with chest x-ray film indicating healed TB
≥10 mm	Residents in long-term care facilities
	Health care workers
	Medically underserved individuals
	IV drug users
≥15 mm	All individuals

16. **(1)** The positive sputum smear for acid-fast bacillus is indicative of active TB. *P. carinii* is a common organism in healthy respiratory tracts; it becomes a problem if the client is immunocompromised. Hemolysis on a complement fixation test is a negative finding. When oxygen saturation is low and the leukocyte count is within the normal range, treatment is not as important as for TB.

Disorders

17. **(3)** The most common respiratory complication after a traumatic injury to the chest is pneumothorax caused by a fractured rib. Oximetry readings at 90% and increased pain are expected at this point and may not be indicative of a problem.

18. **(1)** Pneumococcal pneumonia caused by *S. pneumoniae* often presents abruptly with high fever, shaking chills (rigor), cough productive of purulent or rusty sputum, headache, and pleuritic chest pain. In acute bronchitis, cough is the primary symptom and is initially dry and nonproductive. Fever, dyspnea, wheezing, and possible mucoid sputum production are also characteristic of acute bronchitis.

19. **(1)** On discharge, a client must understand the importance of taking medications as prescribed. If doses are missed, it will increase the mutation of the tubercle bacillus and decrease the effectiveness of the medication. Respiratory isolation at home is not necessary, but if the child experiences problems of rash, nausea, and vomiting, the parent should contact the health care provider. Weekly sputum checks are not necessary.

20. **(2)** According to the American Heart Association, the protocol for cardiopulmonary resuscitation (CPR) (rescue breathing) in response to respiratory arrest would be to open the airway by tilting the head and lifting the chin.

21. **(1)** It is most important to determine what precipitates the dyspnea. Is it present during rest or does it occur with activity? What level of activity precipitates the problem? This information is necessary to determine the severity of the client's complaint.

22. **(1)** The most common area for a foreign body obstruction is the right bronchi; this will produce a unilateral retraction of the right chest wall. Retraction of the lower chest occurs with lower respiratory tract problems such as asthma. A pleural friction rub is heard when there is inflammation between the visceral and parietal pleura. Crepitation is present when air is leaking into the subcutaneous tissue.

23. **(1)** This is a normal finding because of the bulk of the liver. Atelectasis and consolidation will present with normal diaphragmatic movement but with dullness to percussion over the affected area. Obstructive lung disease will result in hyperresonance and limited diaphragmatic excursion, but it will be bilateral.

24. **(1)** Spontaneous pneumothorax occurs in healthy, thin young adults, especially after strenuous exercise; predominant symptoms include sudden pain and dyspnea. The clinical hallmark of asthma is wheezing; with pulmonary edema, predominant symptoms are coughing, frothy sputum, and crackles heard on auscultation. Bronchiectasis is most often chronic and is characterized by moist crackles and wheezing on auscultation; cough is usually present.

25. **(1)** The situation described is hyperventilation; if breathing is slowed by having the client breath into a paper bag, the carbon dioxide levels will be restored and the acid-base problem will be resolved. Albuterol, oxygen, ABGs, and IV fluids are not appropriate initial treatment.

26. **(1)** For the purpose of preventing dyspnea during activity, the bronchodilator should be used before walking or increased physical activity. The client should not stay in bed but should be encouraged to gradually increase activity. Fluid intake of 2 to 3 L/day should be encouraged, unless there are cardiac problems.

The flow rate of oxygen should not exceed 3 to 4 L.

27. **(3)** Elevated blood bicarbonate levels are expected in clients with chronic hypercapnia. Hypoventilation and acidemia can result when too much oxygen is delivered. Supplemental oxygen should not be discontinued because the PaO_2 levels decrease more quickly than the stimulus to breathe returns to eliminate the accumulated store of carbon dioxide. Discontinuing supplemental oxygen, even for a short period, could cause serious complications.

28. **(1)** Nutritional needs are meet by high-calorie, high-protein foods. High-carbohydrate foods need to be avoided in clients who retain carbon dioxide (CO_2) because carbohydrates metabolize into CO_2 as a waste product.

29. **(2)** Age-associated physiologic changes include:

   • Decreased compliance of the chest wall, making deep inspiration difficult.
   • The trachea and bronchi increase in diameter, increasing dead space and resulting in a decrease of volume of air reaching the alveoli. Increased small airway closure results in decreased vital capacity and increased residual volume.
   • The lung parenchyma become less elastic, which decreases the function of the alveoli.
   • Breathing becomes more shallow, and cough forcefulness decreases as a result of weakening of the respiratory muscles.

30. **(4)** The client is at risk for a pulmonary embolism as a result of hypercoagulation related to giving birth, smoking, and vascular injury (recent surgery). Assessment reveals common symptoms of pulmonary embolism: dyspnea, cough, and pleuritic pain. Diagnostic tests include ABGs, 12-lead electrocardiogram (ECG), chest x-ray examination, and echocardiogram.

31. **(3)** The flu or influenza is a highly contagious respiratory tract infection that occurs epidemically during the winter cold months. It is characterized by a sudden onset of chills, elevated temperature (101° F-104° F [38.3°C-40°C]), headache, fatigue, muscle pain, dry cough, laryngitis, rhinorrhea, and red eyes after an incubation period of 24 to 48 hours from time of exposure to respiratory droplets from an infected person or indirect exposure by drinking from a contaminated glass. Flu vaccines do not cause the flu; they are made with a killed virus.

32. **(2)** This client is considered to be in the "yellow" zone of personal best peak flow but is close to the "red" zone (50% or less of personal best). The client should use her bronchodilator immediately, and if she does not experience improvement, she may need emergency intervention by the nurse practitioner.

33. **(1)** The pneumococcal vaccine is recommended for elderly clients, since their immune systems are less efficient. The symptoms of fever, chest pain, and sputum production are suggestive of pneumonia.

34. **(2)** Confusion may be the first sign that the elderly client has pneumonia. The client may not have a fever or leukocytosis. The client may not experience any discomfort or a cough.

35. **(4)** *Streptococcus pneumoniae* is the most common cause of community-and nursing home-acquired pneumonia. *Haemophilus influenzae* is common in elderly clients with underlying chronic diseases (e.g., chronic obstructive pulmonary disease [COPD], diabetes). *Klebsiella pneumoniae* and other gram-negative bacteria are pathogens commonly found in alcoholics, immunocompromised hosts, and hospitalized clients. *Mycobacterium tuberculosis* is an infrequent cause of pneumonia.

36. **(2)** Pneumococcal vaccination and yearly influenza immunization will decrease complications and hospitalizations for the older client. The pneumococcal vaccination is not administered annually. Options #3 and #4 are not recommended. The purified protein derivative (PPD) test should be done annually for high-risk clients.

37. **(2)** *Klebsiella pneumoniae* and other gram-negative bacteria are important pathogens in alcoholics, immunocompromised hosts, and hospitalized clients. *Haemophilus influenzae* is common in elderly clients with underlying chronic diseases (e.g., chronic obstructive pulmonary disease [COPD], diabetes mellitus). *Staphylococcus aureus* generally affects elderly clients recovering from influenza; it is also frequent in hospitalized clients and clients with diabetes. *Streptococcus pneumoniae* is the most common bacterial pathogen (30%-40% of pneumonia cases) and the most common cause of community-and nursing home–acquired pneumonia.

38. **(2)** Up to 25% of elderly clients with newly diagnosed TB have a negative tuberculin skin test because of waning cellular immunity with senescence. If the result of the initial PPD test is negative, a repeat PPD test 1 week later is recommended for elderly clients. The repeat test is useful to stimulate a booster phenomenon in clients whose initial infection occurred many years ago. The other options contain incorrect information.

39. **(3)** Horner's syndrome—which is paralysis of the cervical sympathetic nerves resulting in ptosis, loss of sweating, constriction of the pupils, and sinking of the eyeball on one side—is very commonly associated with malignant tumors in the upper lung, leading to nerve compression.

40. **(4)** Superior vena cava obstruction is a complication of malignancy involving the mediastinum and rapidly progresses to an oncologic emergency.

41. **(3)** Hyponatremia results from an overproduction of antidiuretic hormone caused by ectopic production by the bronchogenic tumor. Ketoacidosis and trauma result in fluid loss, which causes hypernatremia, as does overuse of sodium-containing antacids.

42. **(3)** In older individuals, asthma is usually accompanied by infection. It is rarely allergic, and costal retraction and fever are not usually seen. Subcutaneous epinephrine is not standard treatment but is sometimes indicated in emergent situations.

43. **(1)** Late-phase asthma occurs 6 to 12 hours after the initial or acute bronchoconstrictive phase. The inflammatory response is the result of mast cell degranulation and release of histamine. Histamine acts on the lungs by causing bronchoconstriction, vascular permeability, and vasodilatation. In late-phase asthma, bronchoconstriction is refractory to most bronchodilator therapy.

44. **(3)** Nocturnal exacerbation of asthma is a common clinical sign. It is linked to variation in circulating catecholamines and vagal tone. Chronic hypoxemia and diffuse crackles are seen in the client with chronic bronchitis. Pruritus is often seen in contact allergic reactions.

45. **(2)** Asking the client about the consumption of wine with dinner is the most appropriate response. Many wines, especially white wines, contain sulfites that can trigger a mild allergic response.

46. **(2)** Desaturation and 10-second periods of apnea are diagnostic of sleep apnea. Loud snoring at night, frequent arousals during the night, and sleeping during the day are characteristic of the problem, but not diagnostic.

47. **(1)** Male gender, age greater than 55 to 60 years, obese, nasal allergies and polyps are common factors associated with obstructive sleep apnea. Snoring, daytime sleeping, and a general feeling of fatigue during the day are frequent symptoms the client may report.

48. **(1)** Ongoing daytime sleepiness is the hallmark of obstructive sleep apnea (OSA). Options #3 and #4 should be evaluated, but client has classic symptoms of OSA.

Pharmacology

49. **(1)** For the medication to be most effective, a 1-minute time lapse between the two puffs of medication is required. The first puff will open the upper airways. This will allow more effective penetration of the lower respiratory tract by the second puff of medication.

50. **(2)** The client would not stop taking the medications, because this is a common side effect of rifampin. (Rifampin may also cause soft contact lenses to become discolored).

51. **(4)** The use of tobacco increases the metabolism of theophylline, causing a need for greater dosage than required in nonsmokers. A high-protein, low-carbohydrate diet increases the metabolism of theophylline and decreases serum concentrations. Coffee (and other xanthine-containing beverages) may increase the central nervous system effects of xanthine derivatives.

52. **(1)** β-Blockers (Inderal and Tenormin) are known to cause exacerbation of chronic respiratory problems. Another antihypertensive agent, such as a calcium channel blocker, should be considered. The

client's pulse is 74 bpm and his blood pressure remains elevated, which indicates that the β-blocker is probably not effective in decreasing blood pressure in this client. Theophylline derivatives are not indicated unless other medications are not effective. Drug interactions and increased levels of toxicity cause problems for the elderly client.

53. **(2)** Therapeutic plasma levels range from 10 to 20 μg/ml. Drug levels of 20 μg/ml or greater are associated with toxic effects.

54. **(1)** Chemoprophylaxis should be initiated at the time of the screening skin testing. Skin testing should be repeated in 3 months if initial test results are negative. If the result of the second skin test is negative, chemoprophylaxis can be stopped.

55. **(3)** One of the most common causes of outpatient treatment failure is improper inhaler technique. Although exposure to allergens may trigger an asthma attack, the proper use of inhalers will control those attacks. Use of both steroids and cromolyn inhalers has decreased the severity of asthma attacks.

56. **(1)** Theophylline may be used in the treatment of chronic lung disease and can accumulate in toxic levels. Cimetidine decreases the hepatic clearance of theophylline. Nicotine and some antiseizure drugs may actually increase clearance, and ampicillin does not change the clearance.

57. **(2)** Antibiotic therapy is indicated when there is a change in color, consistency, or amount of sputum. Cough suppressants and antihistamines should be avoided.

58. **(2)** Beclomethasone diproprionate is a long-acting corticosteroid that stabilizes mast cells and greatly reduces mast cell degranulation on exposure to allergens. Albuterol is a short-acting bronchodilator that is used as a rescue medication. Serevent is a long-acting bronchodilator that is most useful in controlling nocturnal asthma symptoms. Singulair, a leukotriene receptor antagonist, inhibits bronchoconstriction and is used as an adjunct to bronchodilator and corticosteroids.

59. **(2)** Treatment of the client with asthma includes inhaled glucocorticoids because of their antiinflammatory effects. Antibiotics are

indicated if there is a concurrent infection such as acute bronchitis. β_2-Agonists are used for their bronchodilator effects and rapid onset of action. Methacholine challenge is used in the diagnosis of asthma.

60. **(2)** Clients with asthma should be instructed to keep their inhaled β_2-agonist with them at all times in case of bronchospasm and use them as needed. The β_2-agonists are effective in reversing bronchospasm. Inhaled steroids are long acting and will not provide immediate relief; therefore clients should be instructed to use them regularly as prescribed and use their inhaled β_2-agonist prn. Administration of antibiotics is not indicated for acute bronchospasm.

61. **(3)** These are the common drugs used for combination therapy for the treatment of TB in children. Rimantadine is an antiviral; Fansidar is an antimalarial. Single-agent therapy is not indicated because of the virulence of the tubercle bacillus.

62. **(4)** Dextromethorphan is specific for control of coughing. Guaifenesin is an expectorant, and Options #1 and #2 are decongestants to decrease nasal and upper respiratory tract congestion.

63. **(3)** The drug therapy regimen for chronic asthma may include theophylline. Toxic effects include anorexia, nausea, vomiting, confusion, restlessness, tachycardia, dysrhythmias, and seizures.

64. **(2)** The hallmark clinical presentation of acute bronchitis is a productive cough. The nurse practitioner should rule out pneumonia. Pneumonia was ruled out in this client by auscultation of clear breath sounds and a lack of abnormalities on the chest radiograph. Bronchodilators (Albuterol) have been found to eliminate the cough of acute bronchitis. Antibiotic therapy (erythromycin and tetracycline) is not recommended. Research has

demonstrated that antibiotic-susceptible organisms rarely cause acute bronchitis.

65. **(4)** H_2 receptor antagonists neutralize the normal gastric acid barrier, allowing for an increased colonization of gram-negative bacilli and *Staphylococcus aureus*.

66. **(2)** Worsening dyspnea and fatigue with increasing cough may be indicative of early pulmonary edema. Clients with pulmonary edema require hospitalization and oxygen therapy, IV furosemide (Lasix), and morphine. Clients who are believed to have pulmonary edema ***should not*** be treated on an outpatient basis. Calcium channel blockers are of little benefit in heart failure.

67. **(1)** Isoniazid (INH) requires concurrent administration of vitamin B_6 to prevent problems of optic neuritis. Vitamin B_6 will decrease the effectiveness of levodopa. If the client is to receive INH, his antiparkinson medication needs to be reevaluated.

68. **(1)** A combination of theophylline and erythromycin-based antibiotics may result in decreased metabolism of theophylline. Another antibiotic should be considered. *(Testing tip: three of the options are antihypertensive medications; only one is different and it is the correct answer.)*

69. **(2)** Prednisone (Deltasone) is a corticosteroid that suppresses immune response and puts the client in an immunocompromised state, making him more susceptible to infections. Clients who are taking prednisone (Deltasone) routinely should be taught that they are at risk for infections and to seek medical attention if they suspect they are becoming ill. Tenormin (Atenolol) is a β-blocker and is used an antihypertensive agent. Ipratropium bromide (Atrovent) is a bronchodilator used as a rescue inhaler. Fluticasone propionate (Advair) is also a bronchodilator used on a twice-daily basis.

Immune & Allergy

Physical Examination & Diagnostic Tests

1. When taking the history of a client with known allergies, what is the most important information to determine?

   1. Reaction associated with each allergen.

   2. Drug allergies.

   3. Food allergies.

   4. Environmental exposure.

2. Which test is used to determine the concentration of gamma globulins that contain most of the immunoglobulins?

   1. Immunofixation electrophoresis.

   2. Complement fixation test.

   3. Protein electrophoresis.

   4. Antinuclear antibody (ANA) test.

3. Which diagnostic studies are used in the differential diagnosis of systemic lupus erythematosus (SLE)?

   1. Complete blood count (CBC), SMA-12, and erythrocyte sedimentation rate (ESR).

   2. Chest radiograph and coagulation profile.

   3. ANA, ESR, and C-reactive protein test.

   4. CBC, urinalysis, and chest radiograph.

4. Which tests are appropriate for the nurse practitioner to order in an initial workup for asymptomatic clients at risk for human immunodeficiency virus (HIV) infection?

   1. CD4 count and HIV enzyme-linked immunosorbent assay (ELISA).

   2. Serology for cytomegalovirus, herpes simplex virus, and Epstein-Barr virus.

   3. HIV ELISA and Western blot.

   4. Hepatitis screen and Western blot.

5. The nurse practitioner would identify which laboratory finding as most significant in a client with joint pain, "butterfly rash," photosensitivity, weight loss, and fever?

   1. Presence of ANAs.

   2. Negative serum complement level.

   3. Decreased red blood cell (RBC) count.

   4. Glycosuria.

6. When assessing a client for angioedema, the nurse practitioner would examine the:

   1. Neck and ears.

   2. Heart sounds.

   3. Abdomen.

   4. Eyes and mouth.

7. Clients who believe they have been exposed to HIV should have an HIV antibody test how soon after the exposure?

   1. The next day and 2 months later.

   2. 6 months after exposure and again at 12 months.

   3. 6 to 12 weeks after exposure and again at 6 months.

   4. 4 weeks and 12 weeks.

8. The most reliable test for the presence of specific immunoglobulin E (IgE) antibody is:

   1. Skin testing.

   2. Radioallergosorbent test (RAST).

   3. Smears for eosinophils.

   4. CBC.

9. To make a diagnosis of allergic rhinitis in the primary care office setting, the nurse practitioner would consider performing:

   1. A nasal smear for eosinophils.

   2. A total serum IgE.

   3. Skin tests.

   4. RAST.

10. The nurse practitioner is evaluating the tuberculin skin test on an immunocompetent client who has no risk factors for tuberculosis. The purified protein derivative (PPD) test response is considered positive when it measures:

    1. 5 mm.

    2. 10 mm.

    3. 15 mm.

    4. 20 mm.

Disorders

11. A young adult presents to the clinic with a 10-day history of fever, myalgia, sore throat, and measles-like rash. The client is not taking any medications. Which of the following viral syndromes is characterized by a measles-like rash?

    1. Influenza.

    2. Varicella.

    3. HIV.

    4. Mononucleosis.

12. A young adult woman presents to the urgent care center reporting that the night before, a male "date" vaginally raped her. You will treat her for chlamydia, gonorrhea, and syphilis today in the clinic and start her on a month-long course of medications to prevent HIV (as well as pregnancy prevention medications). She wants to know why she needs to do this; no one she knows has "AIDS." Your counseling is based on the knowledge that:

    1. She could ask the "date" whether he has "AIDS."

    2. She probably doesn't really need to but it is a good idea to take the medications.

    3. More than 30% of the people infected with HIV do not know they are infected.

    4. HIV is not easily transmitted.

13. A client tells you that her husband's sister has HIV but now she is "cured." She takes medications and "her doctor cannot find the virus in her blood." Which response would be appropriate?

    1. Oh, I am so sorry; she must be mistaken. AIDS is not curable.

    2. That is wonderful news, but are you sure?

3. You must be very happy; I did not know that was possible.

4. I have heard that the new medications are very good and can make the virus counts go down very low.

14. A co-worker comes to you asking you for help and asks you not to tell the nurse manager that she has stuck herself with a needle while performing a phlebotomy. This has just happened. What would you do?

    1. Send her to the nurse manager.

    2. Sit with her and calm her down.

    3. Put on gloves, run water, and make her "bleed' the site under running water for several minutes.

    4. Put on gloves and pour Betadine on the area.

15. An adult client has presented to the clinic with fatigue, sore throat, and myalgia. On physical examination, lymphadenopathy and a slightly enlarged spleen are noted. Based on the history, acute HIV infection is added to the differential. What lab test result increases concern about HIV infection?

    1. Normochromic, normocytic anemia.

    2. Leukopenia and thrombocytopenia.

    3. Lymphocytosis.

    4. Proteinuria.

16. Client education regarding common antigens of anaphylaxis includes:

    1. Extreme weather.

    2. Egg albumin.

    3. Pungent odors.

    4. Animal dander.

17. The nurse practitioner understands that an HIV infection results in a reduction of:

    1. Helper T cells.

    2. Suppressor T cells.

    3. Killer T cells.

    4. Suppressor B cells.

18. Which finding is commonly associated with a diagnosis of SLE?

    1. Excitability, diarrhea, vomiting.

    2. High fever, measles-like rash on limbs, weight gain.

    3. Joint pain, malar rash, photosensitivity.

    4. Weight loss, diarrhea, epigastric pain.

19. After a repeat HIV antibody test, a client continues to have positive test results but is asymptomatic. What is important for the nurse to understand regarding the transmission of the virus by this client?

    1. The client is infectious when symptoms are active.

    2. The client is infectious for life.

    3. The dormant virus is not infectious while the client is asymptomatic and the T-cell count is high.

    4. Laboratory tests should be done monthly to identify the infectious periods of the disease process.

20. A young woman has just received news of a positive HIV test result. She does not want her sexual partner to be informed. What is the most appropriate response to her decision?

    1. Respect for her decision, since she is the client.

    2. Letting her know that you have a legal responsibility to inform her partner.

    3. Counseling her about your ethical responsibility to inform all sexual partners.

    4. Noting her decision in the record for future reference.

21. The nurse practitioner has been assigned a new client. The problem list indicates this client has CREST syndrome. What would the nurse practitioner be monitoring this client for?

    1. Scleroderma.

    2. Dental caries.

    3. SLE.

    4. Rheumatoid arthritis.

22. A client presenting with complaints of fatigue, malaise, arthralgias, oral ulcers, malar rash, and a positive ANA test result would most likely be given a diagnosis of:

    1. Rheumatoid arthritis.

    2. Fibromyalgia.

    3. Scleroderma.

    4. SLE.

23. What are the most common clinical manifestations of Sjögren's syndrome?

    1. Corneal dryness and lack of saliva.

    2. Increased urination and hunger.

    3. Abdominal discomfort and headaches.

    4. Joint destruction and alopecia.

24. An elderly female client presents to the nurse practitioner with a low-grade fever and a unilateral throbbing headache. She also reports scalp sensitivity and some visual disturbances. Lab results show a markedly elevated ESR and anemia. She has been relatively healthy except for a recent history of polymyalgia rheumatica (PMR). Symptoms indicate a clinical presentation of:

    1. Bacterial meningitis.

    2. Acute migraine headache.

    3. Temporal (giant cell) arteritis.

    4. Subdural hematoma.

25. A middle-aged female client presents with weight loss, heartburn, dysphagia, dry cough, pain, stiffness of the fingers and knees, and Raynaud's phenomenon. The nurse practitioner recognizes these as the symptoms of:

    1. Rheumatoid arthritis.

    2. Lupus erythematosus.

    3. Graft-versus-host disease (GVHD).

    4. Scleroderma.

26. The erythematous confluent macular eruption of the face known as *the butterfly rash* is characteristic of:

    1. Allergic drug eruption.

    2. SLE.

    3. Rosacea.

    4. Seborrheic dermatitis.

27. The nurse practitioner is discussing general health care with a female client with SLE who is in remission. What are important points to include in the teaching?

    1. Avoid getting pregnant.

    2. Decrease physical and psychological stress.

    3. Avoid isometric and aerobic exercise.

    4. Maintain diet low in fat and carbohydrates.

28. A 50-year-old male client presents with complaints of frequent sinus infections, a decrease in the ability to hear, and arthralgias. Laboratory findings are mild normochromic and normocytic anemia; elevated ESR; mild hypergammaglobulinemia (elevated immunoglobulin A); proteinuria; and hematuria with granular or cellular casts. Physical examination findings include mild conjunctivitis, vasculitic dermatitis, chronic cough, chest pain, dyspnea, paranasal sinus pain, occasional epistaxis, and imbalance of intake and output. What would be a tentative diagnosis?

    1. Connective tissue disease.

    2. Wegener's granulomatosis.

    3. Pulmonary neoplasm.

    4. Infectious granulomatous disease.

29. A client presents with sneezing, watery eyes, postnasal drip, and sore throat. What diagnosis do the symptoms suggest?

    1. Acute bronchitis.

    2. Allergic rhinitis.

    3. Asthma exacerbation.

    4. Influenza.

30. A 70-year-old woman presents with complaints of morning headache, malaise, and anorexia. What condition would the nurse practitioner suspect?

    1. Pneumonia.

    2. Temporal arteritis.

    3. Herpes zoster.

    4. Postmenopausal symptoms.

31. When teaching a client about risk factors for HIV and prevention of transmission, which statement is most appropriate?

    1. HIV can be transmitted by casual kissing.

    2. Unprotected oral sex with an infected partner is not advised.

    3. Sharing an office with an HIV-positive person increases the risk of exposure to HIV.

    4. Using the same bathroom as an infected family member puts you at risk of exposure to HIV.

32. Signs and symptoms that alert the nurse practitioner to identify a client who is at an increased risk for HIV infection include:

    1. Night sweats.

    2. Malaise and fatigue.

    3. Frequent sexually transmitted diseases.

    4. Swollen glands and diarrhea.

33. HIV is classified as a:

    1. Cytomegalovirus.

    2. Herpetic virus.

    3. Papillomavirus.

    4. Retrovirus.

34. What are the most frequently occurring symptoms of SLE?

    1. Splenomegaly and Raynaud's phenomenon.

    2. Pulmonary effusions and hepatomegaly.

    3. Butterfly rash on the face and lymphadenopathy.

    4. Fever, arthritis, arthralgia, and weight loss.

35. A systemic IgE-mediated antigen-antibody response resulting in a life-threatening massive release of mediators is:

    1. Generalized seizures.

    2. Allergic rhinitis.

    3. Anaphylaxis.

    4. Status asthmaticus.

36. The release of histamine results in:

    1. Bronchospasm, vasodilatation, and vascular permeability.

    2. Bronchodilatation, vasodilatation, and vascular permeability.

    3. Smooth muscle contraction, decreased vascular permeability, and vasoconstriction.

    4. Pain, increased vascular permeability, and bronchodilatation.

37. After bone marrow transplantation (BMT), the nurse practitioner can expect the onset of acute GVHD to occur:

    1. Between 10 and 15 days after BMT.

    2. Between 30 and 50 days after BMT.

    3. Between 1 and 5 days after BMT.

    4. At 100 days after BMT.

38. A client has recently undergone BMT. The nurse practitioner identifies signs and symptoms of GVHD to include:

    1. Fever, headache, and mental status changes.

    2. Chills, fever, and urticaria over flank area.

    3. Increased serum bilirubin; maculopapular rash; and green, watery diarrhea.

    4. Decreased RBC count and hematocrit and hemoglobin values; petechiae; and increased bleeding tendencies.

39. The pathogenesis of SLE is characterized by autoantibody development. This results in:

    1. Increased T suppressor cells.

    2. B-cell decrease.

    3. Polyclonal hypogammaglobulinemia.

    4. Decreased T suppressor cells and inhibited cell activity.

40. What cell is responsible for the activation of the immune response?

    1. Band neutrophil.

    2. T4 lymphocyte.

    3. Segmented neutrophil.

    4. B lymphocyte.

41. A 22-year-old man presents with breathlessness, weight loss, nonproductive cough, temperature of 38° C (100.4° F), pulse 124 bpm, respirations 36 breaths/min, blood pressure 120/78 mm Hg, and a history of a positive HIV serum test result. On the basis of this information, what is the most accurate diagnosis?

    1. *Klebsiella pneumoniae.*

    2. Kaposi's sarcoma.

    3. *Pneumocystis carinii* pneumonia.

    4. Lymphoma.

42. An adult is brought into the clinic, and the family states that he has a history of anaphylactic reactions. What signs and symptoms indicate to the nurse practitioner the client is experiencing another type of reaction?

    1. Cough, wheezing, and hives.

    2. Severe malaise, pallor, stridor, and dyspnea.

    3. Anxiety, nasal congestion, and tachycardia.

    4. Rhinorrhea, nausea, and gastrointestinal cramping.

43. A nurse at the clinic experiences a needle stick while caring for a client with known hepatitis. What immunoglobulin (Ig) should be administered to provide passive immunity?

    1. IgE.

    2. IgA.

    3. IgG.

    4. IgC.

44. Which sign and/or symptom is indicative of a type I hypersensitivity reaction?

    1. Contact dermatitis.

    2. Immediate wheal-and-flare reaction.

    3. Hematuria.

    4. High fever.

45. Which clients are at greatest risk for HIV infection and AIDS?

    1. Immunocompromised clients.

    2. Sexually active teenagers.

    3. Elderly adults.

    4. Marijuana users.

46. What are the cardiovascular effects of anaphylaxis?

    1. ST-segment and T-wave changes.

    2. Hypertension.

    3. Prolonged P-R intervals with elevated Q-T segment.

    4. Elevated serum enzyme levels.

47. When assessing a client for SLE, what ophthalmologic findings would the nurse practitioner determine to be consistent with this condition?

    1. Retinal hemorrhages.

    2. Conjunctivitis.

    3. Cotton-wool spots.

    4. Arteriovenous (AV) nicking.

48. What instruction does the nurse practitioner include in the education of the client with allergic rhinitis?

    1. Monitor air quality and the allergy index.

    2. Use a surgical-type mask when going outdoors.

    3. Remain inside during allergy season.

    4. Avoid working in the garden or yard.

49. A nurse from the operating room comes into the clinic with complaints of shortness of breath, itching, reddened hands, and wheezing. He indicates that when he is not working, he does not seem to have the symptoms. On the basis of the history and symptoms, what would the nurse practitioner evaluate for?

    1. Sick building syndrome.

    2. Bronchitis.

    3. Latex allergy.

    4. Contact dermatitis.

50. Which statement is true regarding latex allergy?

    1. It usually only produces symptoms of contact dermatitis and allergic rhinorrhea.

    2. It is a progressive disease that worsens with continued exposure.

    3. It affects <5% of the health care population.

    4. It is an autoimmune response.

Pharmacology

51. An adult patient comes to the urgent care center with nausea, vomiting, and acute abdominal pain. His history is significant for HIV disease and he takes the following HIV medications: Videx 400 mg ec once per day, Kaletra 3 pills twice per day, and Epivir 150 mg bid. He started taking these medications a month ago. After the examination, the nurse practitioner determines that Videx can cause pancreatitis and lactic acidosis. What lab tests would be ordered?

    1. CBC, CD4 count, viral load.

    2. CBC with differential, lipase, lactic acid, electrolytes, BUN, creatinine, and LFTs.

    3. Amylase, lipase, lactic acid.

    4. Lipase, amylase, LFTs.

52. Which drugs have been associated with a lupus-like syndrome?

    1. Sulfonamides (Septra DS), penicillin (Pen-Vee K, penicillin G).

    2. Progestin-estrogen combination oral contraceptives.

    3. Nonsteroidal antiinflammatory drugs (NSAIDs; Motrin).

    4. Procainamide (Pronestyl), hydralazine (Apresoline).

53. A client is given a diagnosis of temporal (giant cell) arteritis. What is the medication of choice?

    1. Prednisone (Deltasone).

    2. Ibuprofen (Motrin).

    3. Indomethacin (Indocin).

    4. Azathioprine (Imuran).

54. The clinic is notified that a college student is being brought in with a bee sting and is having difficulty breathing. Which medication should the nurse practitioner have available for the initial care?

    1. Lidocaine topical ointment.

    2. Epinephrine.

    3. Prednisone.

    4. Benadryl elixir.

55. What is the standard drug used for malaria prophylaxis?

    1. Ampicillin (Polycillin, Omnipen).

    2. Doxycycline (Vibramycin).

    3. Ceftriaxone (Rocephin).

    4. Chloroquine phosphate (Aralen).

56. Which medications are used in the treatment of allergic rhinitis?

    1. Antihistamines and corticosteroids.

    2. Antihistamines and analgesics.

    3. Cholinergic agents, antibiotics, and analgesics.

    4. Nasal saline, corticosteroids, and antibiotics.

57. Development of an adverse drug reaction is dependent on which factors?

    1. Client age, prior drug reactions, genetic factors, and degree of exposure.

    2. Client gender, route of administration, and history of atrophic disease.

    3. Client age, gender, and genetic factors.

    4. Genetic factors, prior drug reactions, and client gender.

58. A medication frequently used for the prophylaxis and initial treatment of *Pneumocystis carinii* pneumonia (PCP) is:

    1. Fluconazole (Diflucan).

    2. Amphotericin B (Fungizone).

    3. Trimethoprim-sulfamethoxazole (Septra, Bactrim).

    4. Acyclovir (Zovirax).

59. When instructing clients with allergic rhinitis about the use of nasal decongestants, it is important for the nurse practitioner to make sure they understand that:

    1. The condition is self-limiting and will resolve in a matter of weeks, regardless of whether clients are re-exposed to the allergen.

    2. A nasal decongestant used continuously for more than 3 days can result in a worsening of the symptoms.

    3. It is not necessary to avoid exposure to the allergen once therapy has been initiated.

    4. Allergic rhinitis is only seen in the spring and fall; the condition requires treatment during these seasons only.

60. What is the major advantage of using second-generation antihistamines, such as astemizole (Hismanal) and loratadine (Claritin)?

    1. Decreased cost.

    2. Increased anticholinergic activity.

    3. Delayed absorption.

    4. They do not cross the blood-brain barrier.

61. What is the desired action of sympathomimetics (adrenergics) in the treatment of allergic rhinitis?

    1. Promotion of vasoconstriction in nasal mucosa.

    2. Blocking of mast cell degranulation.

    3. Decrease in the effect of histamines.

    4. Increases in degranulation and end-organ response.

62. The nurse practitioner is prescribing astemizole (Hismanal) for a geriatric client's allergy problems. When considering the client's current medications, which medication would be a contraindication to the administration of astemizole?

    1. Erythromycin ethylsuccinate (EES).

    2. Verapamil (Calan).

    3. Propranolol (Inderal).

    4. Captopril (Capoten).

63. Cromolyn sodium (Intal) is used to:

    1. Reduce the histamine load.

    2. Antagonize the effects of histamine.

    3. Stabilize the mast cell membrane.

    4. Reduce antiemetic activity.

64. In the elderly client, histamine blocking agents may cause which side effects?

    1. Ataxia.

    2. Nausea.

    3. Diarrhea.

    4. Gastrointestinal upset.

65. What information is important for the nurse practitioner to include when teaching a client about the use of antihistamines?

    1. Use of topical antihistamines is safe and has relatively few side effects.

    2. Do not use over-the-counter (OTC) medications without consulting the health care provider.

    3. Constipation and urinary retention are expected side effects and do not need to be reported.

    4. Once the antihistamines have been taken for 3 days, avoidance of allergens is not necessary.

66. A primary advantage of using loratadine (Claritin) in treating a client with seasonal allergies is that it:

    1. Is supplied as an enteric-coated pill.

    2. May be prescribed for a once-a-day dosing.

    3. Costs considerably less than other medications.

    4. Effectively decreases nasal secretions.

67. What medications are drugs of choice in secondary therapy for the client with an anaphylactic reaction?

    1. Antibiotics and anticholinergics.

    2. NSAIDs.

    3. Decongestants and expectorants.

    4. Antihistamines and corticosteroids.

68. What is an appropriate antihistamine to recommend for a child with allergic rhinitis?

    1. Diphenhydramine (Benadryl).

    2. Dextromethorphan (Benylin).

    3. Guaifenesin (Robitussin).

    4. Brompheniramine (Dimetane).

69. Clients presenting with signs and symptoms of SLE would have their medication profiles reviewed to determine whether they are taking any medication that may have caused a drug-induced lupus-like syndrome. Which drug would be most likely to cause such a syndrome?

    1. Digoxin (Lanoxin).

    2. Procainamide (Pronestyl).

    3. Trimethoprim-sulfamethoxazole (Bactrim).

    4. Cimetidine (Tagamet).

Answers & Rationales

Physical Examination & Diagnostic Tests

1. **(1)** The reaction to each allergen is important to know. Often clients will indicate they have a reaction to a particular food or medication, such as nausea, stomach pain, or diarrhea, and consider it an allergy. The signs and symptoms of the reaction, speed of onset, how long it lasts, and what successful treatment has been used in the past are important information. It is important to distinguish between side effects of medication and true allergies to medication; therefore client statements of either drug and food allergies should be explored.

2. **(3)** In protein electrophoresis, proteins are electrically separated on a strip. It is a screening test to measure various proteins in body fluids, usually serum or urine. It assists in screening for diseases that are characterized by an increase or decrease in immunoglobulins. The complement fixation test and antinuclear antibody (ANA) test are diagnostic studies for rheumatoid problems. Serum protein electrophoresis can also be used to detect occult malignancy when a client's condition is deteriorating and no known cause can be found.

3. **(3)** Although all of the tests listed in the options may be included in a complete physical examination, laboratory tests specific to the diagnosis of systemic lupus erythematosus (SLE) include the ANA test, erythrocyte sedimentation rate (ESR), and C-reactive protein test. During flares, the ESR and C-reactive protein level are increased. The ANA titer in a client with SLE is positive at a 1:80 ratio.

4. **(3)** The initial screening test for human immunodeficiency virus (HIV) is the enzyme-linked immunosorbent assay (ELISA). If the test result is positive, confirmation of antibodies is done with a Western blot. Although serology and hepatitis screening along with a complete blood count (CBC) and tuberculin tine test are routinely performed, the initial workup starts with an ELISA. The CD4 count is performed during the active disease process.

5. **(1)** The majority of clients with SLE have ANAs in their blood. They also have leukopenia, thrombocytopenia, lymphopenia, and a positive lupus erythematosus (LE) cell prep. Proteinuria with cellular casts is often noted.

6. **(4)** Angioedema is most easily seen in the eyes and mouth. It is edema of the mucous membrane tissue. It can also be observed on the tongue, feet, hands, and genitalia. Diffuse erythema may be seen in the upper body parts. Gastrointestinal symptoms such as vomiting, cramping, and diarrhea may also be seen.

7. **(3)** The HIV antibody develops between 6 and 12 weeks after exposure. Because of the variability of antibody development, it is recommended that the test be repeated in 6 months to confirm the findings.

8. **(1)** The most reliable test for the presence of the specific IgE antibody is the skin test. The radioallergosorbent test (RAST) is less sensitive than skin testing and is difficult to

standardize. It is also difficult to reproduce results of the RAST. The smear for eosinophils and the CBC are not specific for IgE antibody.

9. **(1)** A nasal smear for eosinophils is a simple office procedure. Many clients who have uncomplicated allergic rhinitis have a normal serum IgE level. Skin testing should be performed by trained providers only. RASTs cost more and have lower sensitivity.

10. **(3)** A positive purified protein derivative (PPD) test result for an immunocompetent client is 15 mm. For a client who is HIV-positive or immunocompromised or who has been exposed to an active case of tuberculosis (TB), 5 mm is considered a positive result. For a client who has a chronic disease or has been exposed to HIV-positive people or people born in a foreign country, 10 mm is considered a positive result.

Disorders

11. **(3)** Neither influenza nor mononucleosis typically presents with a rash; varicella is characterized by a vesicular skin eruption. Acute HIV infection is characterized by a history of prolonged fever and a red, raised, discrete skin eruption, described as *morbilliform* or *measleslike*.

12. **(3)** Treating a woman who has been raped requires the time to provide patient education. It is not safe to ask the client to confront her attacker with a request for medical information. Evidence from studies of health care workers indicates that postexposure prophylaxis (PEP) does work. Traumatic sex increases the risk of transmission of diseases including HIV.

13. **(4)** You should repeat what the client has said to make you understand the client's statement. This would be a good time to add further information about HIV.

14. **(3)** Option #1 does not address the medical need; Option #2 is also necessary but not until after you have addressed the need to wash the site immediately and at length. Bleeding the site under water is more effective than use of topical antiseptics.

15. **(2)** Acute primary HIV infection causes a depletion of CD4 cells, which produces a leukopenia and also depletes the platelets. Normochromic normocytic anemia is more commonly present in advanced HIV; lymphocytosis is more consistent with mononucleosis.

16. **(2)** Egg albumin is just one of many identified common antigens that may cause an anaphylactic reaction. Others include vaccines, allergen extracts, sulfonamides, penicillins, hormones, legumes (especially peanuts), berries, nuts, seafood, and venom (bee, wasp, yellow jacket stings). Changes in weather and strong scents and odors are triggers that may precipitate an asthma attack resulting in bronchospasm and wheezing.

17. **(1)** HIV infection results in a severe, life-threatening reduction of helper T cells, along with an increase in suppressor T cells. The helper T cells help amplify or increase the production of antibody-forming cells from the B lymphocytes after an encounter with an antigen. Killer T cells are produced after mature helper T cells interact with an antigen. Suppressor T cells suppress the formation of antibody-forming cells from the B lymphocytes, which, when their numbers are increased, have a detrimental effect on the immunity and ability of the client with HIV to make antibody-forming cells.

18. **(3)** The symptoms most commonly experienced with SLE are joint pain, fatigue, Raynaud's phenomenon, chronic or low-grade or recurrent fever, sun sensitivity, hair loss, weakness, butterfly (malar) facial rash, and weight loss. Typically, the pulmonary, cardiac, renal, and central nervous systems are involved, which may cause multisystem failure and may contribute to mortality rates in clients with SLE.

19. **(2)** HIV infection creates a chronic infectious state in the body that is transmitted via blood or body fluids and transplacentally throughout the client's life span.

20. **(3)** An ethical response includes notification of all persons at risk.

21. **(1)** CREST (**C**alcinosis, **R**aynaud's phenomenon, **E**sophageal dysfunction, **S**clerodactyly, **T**elangiectasia) syndrome is associated with a slow progressive form of scleroderma.

22. **(4)** This client has 4 of the 11 criteria necessary for a diagnosis of SLE. There is no single test for SLE, but the presence of these characteristics plus results of other lab tests (ANA test, ESR, and C-reactive protein test) can establish the diagnosis.

23. **(1)** Corneal dryness and lack of saliva are the most common clinical manifestations of Sjögren's syndrome. Clients may also have joint inflammation, but this rarely leads to joint destruction.

24. **(3)** About 40% of clients with temporal (giant cell) arteritis have a history of polymyalgia rheumatica (PMR). The other diagnoses may have some of these symptoms, but only arteritis has all the symptoms listed in the situation. It is especially critical to note visual disturbances, because these clients can experience sudden blindness. Definitive diagnosis is made by means of biopsy. Treatment normally consists of increasing the client's prednisone (Deltasone) dosage to 60 mg daily in divided doses for 4 weeks, then beginning a gradual decrease in monitoring the ESR.

25. **(4)** The symptom of Raynaud's phenomenon distinguishes this as scleroderma. The esophageal dysfunction is often an initial symptom in this disease, which is four times more common in females.

26. **(2)** The butterfly rash is one of the characteristic symptoms of SLE.

27. **(2)** Since SLE is considered an autoimmune disorder, psychological and physical stress can cause an exacerbation. A balanced diet helps to limit the side effects of some of the medications, while regular exercise helps to reduce arthralgia and myalgia associated with SLE. Barrier contraception is recommended for women with SLE. Pregnancy is usually allowed during periods of remission; however, the stress of pregnancy could cause an acute exacerbation of SLE. The pregnant client would have to be closely monitored by both her rheumatologist and gynecologist.

28. **(2)** Wegener's granulomatosis is a multisystem disorder that occurs equally in both sexes. Peak occurrence is between 40 and 60 years of age. The disease usually targets the upper respiratory tract and the kidneys. Connective tissue disease, pulmonary neoplasm, and infectious granulomatous disease would be considered in the differential diagnoses.

29. **(2)** The signs and symptoms presented are classic for allergic rhinitis. Acute bronchitis would present with cough and yellow or green sputum production. An asthma exacerbation would present with wheezing, chest tightness, decreased forced vital capacity, and history of exposure to an allergen. Influenza has an acute onset with fever, chills, and general malaise.

30. **(2)** The nurse practitioner should rule out temporal arteritis, an inflammatory disorder of unknown etiology affecting large-and medium-sized arteries. It occurs two times more frequently in women, most frequently in the elderly, and rarely in the African American population. The clinical findings would reveal temporal tenderness and temporal bruits. About 40% of the clients who have PMR also have temporal arteritis, and the elderly client may be attributing some of her arthralgia and myalgias to normal changes of aging rather PMR. The nurse practitioner should also check an ESR and consider a referral to a rheumatologist.

31. **(2)** Unprotected oral sex with an HIV-positive person puts one at risk for infection with the virus. Contact such as casual kissing or sharing an office or bathroom does not transmit the virus. The virus is transmitted in bodily fluids and secretions.

32. **(3)** Frequent sexually transmitted diseases would alert the nurse practitioner to the client's lack of protected sex and the possibility of multiple partners. Night sweats, malaise, fatigue, swollen glands, and diarrhea can be associated with many other illnesses.

33. **(4)** HIV is a retrovirus. It contains an enzyme, reverse transcriptase, that copies RNA into DNA. When the virus binds to a CD4 receptor, it inserts its RNA and enzymes into the cell, where a copy of the virus's RNA is made and enters the nucleus of the cell. As the infected host cell reproduces, the HIV DNA is duplicated and passed on.

34. **(4)** Although any of the clinical symptoms mentioned in the options can be present in clients with SLE, fever, weight loss, arthritis, and arthralgias occur most often. Butterfly rash of the face and lymphadenopathy occur

<50% of the time. Pulmonary effusion, hepatomegaly, splenomegaly, and Raynaud's phenomenon occur in less than a third of the cases.

35. **(3)** The massive release of mediators triggers a series of events in target organs. Prior sensitization to the antigen must have occurred for an anaphylactic reaction to be triggered. Anaphylaxis may result from injection of an antigen, ingestion of food or drugs, or inhalation of antigens.

36. **(1)** The release of histamine results in bronchospasm, vasodilatation, and vascular permeability, leading to wheezing, increased mucus production in the lungs, and edema of the airway.

37. **(2)** The onset of acute graft-versus-host disease (GVHD) occurs between 30 and 50 days after bone marrow transplantation (BMT). It results from immunocompetent donor T lymphocytes attacking the host tissues.

38. **(3)** The signs and symptoms of GVHD include maculopapular rash; generalized erythroderma with desquamation; increased bilirubin, serum glutamic-oxaloacetic transaminase (SGOT), and/or alkaline phosphatase levels; abdominal cramping; and diarrhea. Infection is characterized by fever, mental status changes, and headaches. Decreased red blood cell (RBC) count, decreased hematocrit and hemoglobin values, and petechiae are signs of anemia. Fever, chills, and urticaria are indications of a reaction to white cells in the marrow.

39. **(4)** T lymphocytes are the white cells responsible for control of the immune response. In SLE, T suppressor cells are decreased and cell activity is inhibited. This results in hypergammaglobulinemia and B-cell proliferation.

40. **(2)** The T4 lymphocyte is known as *the T helper cell*. T helper cells are responsible for the proliferation of lymphocytes and macrophages, causing activation of the cells in response to an antigen. The B lymphocytes are effector cells that mediate humoral responses by production of antibodies. Band neutrophils and segmented neutrophils are slightly mature and fully mature neutrophils, respectively. Neutrophils are the most abundant cells in the bone marrow and blood.

41. **(3)** According to the history of an HIV-positive test result and the symptoms presented, the client is at risk for development of *Pneumocystis carinii* pneumonia. Further examination would include obtaining a chest radiograph and pulse oximetry to determine oxygen saturation. The lack of purplish lesions is considered in ruling out Kaposi's sarcoma. *Klebsiella pneumoniae* is a nosocomial, rather than a community acquired, infection. Lymphoma in HIV usually occurs as non-Hodgkin's lymphoma with the primary site in the brain.

42. **(2)** Severe malaise, pallor, stridor, and dyspnea are signs and symptoms associated with a severe anaphylactic reaction. Symptoms may occur immediately or up to 2 hours after exposure to the allergen. Severe reactions require immediate intervention.

43. **(3)** The nurse should be given IgG because IgG is the major antibody against viruses and bacteria. IgG is the principal mediator of the secondary immune response and requires repeated exposure to the same antigen to increase the immune response. There is no IgC antibody. IgA is the secretory immunoglobulin found in tears, saliva, and mucous secretions of the lungs and gastrointestinal tract. IgE mediates allergic reactions.

44. **(2)** A type I hypersensitivity reaction causes an immediate wheal-and-flare reaction. Contact dermatitis is seen in a type IV (delayed) reaction. Hematuria is seen in a type II reaction caused by the presence of preformed circulating cytotoxic antibodies, as in a blood transfusion reaction or autoimmune hemolytic anemia. High fever can be seen in the type III hypersensitivity reaction when large quantities of antigen-antibody complexes are released in the body.

45. **(2)** Sexually active teenagers are the fastest growing group of HIV-positive clients because of unprotected sexual activity. Immunocompromised clients and elderly adults are at no greater risk for infection with HIV than any other group. However, it must be noted that elderly men constitute an increasing number of HIV-positive clients because of their use of prostitutes after the loss of their life partners. Risk factors for HIV infection include unprotected sexual contact with someone of unknown HIV status, multiple sexual partners, IV drug use, hemophilia, and blood transfusions received before 1985.

46. **(1)** Changes in the electrocardiogram (ECG) are associated with coronary and myocardial ischemia. Although the electrocardiographic changes suggest myocardial injury, there is no change in the serum enzyme levels. Other signs and symptoms include hypotension and tachycardia.

47. **(3)** Cotton-wool spots are the most common ophthalmologic problem associated with SLE. Retinal hemorrhages and arteriovenous (AV) nicking can be seen in the client with hypertension. Conjunctivitis is an infection of the conjunctiva.

48. **(1)** Clients with allergic rhinitis should monitor the air quality and allergy index in their area. A surgical-type mask will not filter out small allergens. Remaining inside during allergy season is an unrealistic expectation and can lead to decreased socialization and increased depression for the client. Clients can enjoy a summer garden if they are careful about the types of plants and flowers they include. For example, the client with an allergy to ragweed should avoid daisies, dahlias, and chrysanthemums.

49. **(3)** The operating room nurse likely has a latex allergy. The incidence of latex allergies has increased dramatically since the onset of standard precautions and increased use of latex gloves. In an effort to keep up with the increased demand for gloves, changes have been made in the manufacturing process, which have resulted in a higher protein count in the gloves. The increased exposure to the protein has led to the development of latex allergy in a large number of health care workers.

50. **(2)** Latex allergy is a progressive disease that worsens with continual exposure. The symptoms range from contact dermatitis to anaphylaxis. Currently, latex allergy affects 17% of health care workers and 39% of dental professionals. Latex allergy is an acquired immune response to the latex protein allergen. There is no vaccine, and the only defense is to avoid contact with latex.

Pharmacology

51. **(2)** There is no need to assess the patient's immune function at this point, and it is not going to change the course of management of the acute illness. Options #3 and #4 would get at the diagnosis of pancreatitis but would provide information on the patient's hydration status, the rest of his biliary tree, or the presence of acute infection.

52. **(4)** Procainamide (Pronestyl), hydralazine (Apresoline), and isoniazid (INH) have been shown to induce a lupus-like syndrome. Discontinuation of the medication results in disappearance of the clinical signs and symptoms. Antibiotics such as sulfonamides (Septra DS) and penicillin (Pen-Vee K, penicillin G) have been associated with anaphylactic reactions in some clients. Oral contraceptives may cause increased blood pressure and increase the risk for development of thromboemboli. Nonsteroidal antiinflammatory drugs (NSAIDs) such as Motrin have been associated with gastrointestinal upset and gastric pain, especially when taken on an empty stomach, and are contraindicated in patients with renal disease.

53. **(1)** Temporal arteritis, seen primarily in the elderly, can lead to blindness if not treated immediately with a corticosteroid such as prednisone. The usual daily dose of prednisone (Deltasone) is 60 mg, in divided doses initially, then in a single morning dose (steroids should never be used on an every-other-day basis). A *slow taper* can be started after 4 weeks, if the client is asymptomatic and the ESR is decreased. Tapering of the dose is very individualized, and the client may be receiving medications for several months to years. Average time for disease remission is 3 to 4 years (range, 1-10 years).

54. **(2)** Epinephrine would be the first-line drug to be injected for the treatment of the respiratory distress associated with an anaphylactic reaction. The dosage for epinephrine (1:1000, SC) is 0.3 to 0.5 ml/kg for an adult. Benadryl's onset of action is not fast enough. Lidocaine would only topically treat the pain and not the respiratory problem. Antiinflammatory medications would not be given initially but could be given later if needed for relief of generalized discomfort and/or pain at the site of the sting.

55. **(4)** Chloroquine phosphate is the standard drug used for malaria prophylaxis. The dosage is 5 mg/kg body weight (up to 300 mg for an

adult). Doxycycline (Vibramycin) is often used to treat diarrhea associated with traveling to areas where diarrhea is commonly caused by drinking water; it is also used to treat chlamydia and pelvic inflammatory disease. Ceftriaxone (Rocephin) is used to treat bacterial septicemia or infections caused by gram-negative bacilli in the respiratory and urinary tracts. Ampicillin (Polycillin, Omnipen) is used to treat a variety of infections and as prophylaxis for bacterial endocarditis.

56. **(1)** Unless there is a secondary bacterial infection, antibiotics are contraindicated. Antihistamines and reduction of exposure to the allergen will help to reduce the symptoms. For continued control and stabilization of mast cells, corticosteroids are indicated.

57. **(1)** Adults are at greater risk for adverse drug reactions, probably because of the increased number of medications they have used, the amount of exposure, and the effects of aging on the immune system. Clients with prior drug reactions are more likely to have reactions to new drugs. The risk of an adverse drug reaction occurs in the first 2 to 3 weeks of therapy. Prolonged course of drug use, high dosage, and intermittent therapy increase the risk of an adverse reaction. Genetic factors may contribute to an increased number of mediators and may influence metabolic pathways. Gender has no effect except that when muscle relaxants and chymopapain are used, women are at greater risk of having an adverse drug reaction. Route of drug administration contributes to the risk; IV is associated with the greatest risk, followed (in order) by IM, SC, PO, and topical.

58. **(3)** Trimethoprim-sulfamethoxazole (Septra, Bactrim) is used to treat and prevent *Pneumocystis carinii* pneumonia. Usually a 21-day course of the drug is indicated. It may take 7 to 10 days to see a clinical response. Fluconazole (Diflucan) and amphotericin B are antifungal drugs, and acyclovir (Zovirax) is an antiviral agent used primarily to treat herpes simplex virus types 1 and 2 and herpes zoster (shingles).

59. **(2)** The use of nasal decongestants for more than 3 days can result in a rebound effect when use is discontinued. This will lead to increased nasal congestion as a result of reflex vasodilatation. The condition may take as long as 2 to 3 weeks to resolve. Allergic rhinitis is not a self-limiting illness associated only with the spring and fall. Even though therapy is initiated, the client should be instructed to avoid exposure to the allergen as much as possible.

60. **(4)** The major advantage of the second-generation antihistamines is that they do not cross the blood-brain barrier; therefore they do not cause sedation or psychomotor dysfunction. There is little anticholinergic activity and less dry mouth and constipation. The cost of these antihistamines is 15 to 30 times greater than that of first-generation antihistamines. The medications are rapidly absorbed within 1 to 2 hours of oral administration on an empty stomach.

61. **(1)** Sympathomimetics (adrenergics) cause vasoconstriction, thereby reducing edema and secretions. Inhaled corticosteroids stabilize mast cells and block degranulation.

62. **(1)** Erythromycin ethylsuccinate (EES) and astemizole (Hismanal) should not be administered concurrently. Fatal dysrhythmias may be precipitated by this combination.

63. **(3)** Cromolyn sodium is used to stabilize the mast cell membrane to prevent release of histamine when the cell comes in contact with an antigen. It does not affect the amount of histamine released from the cell, exacerbate the effects of histamine, or reduce antiemetic activity.

64. **(1)** The use of histamine blocking agents can cause paradoxical central nervous system stimulation resulting in ataxia in the elderly. Antihistamines can cause many simultaneous side effects in the elderly, such as impaired vision and gait, which can lead to falls. Antihistamines may cause impaired thinking in some older adults, which may interfere with their functional skills (cognition) and could necessitate an unexpected hospitalization or nursing home stay. Additionally, antihistamines may interact with their numerous medications, as well as exacerbate their side effects, such as dry mouth and constipation.

65. **(2)** The client should be instructed not to use over-the-counter (OTC) medications without consulting the nurse practitioner or pharmacist. The nurse practitioner should explain to the client that OTC medications and

herbal supplements are considered drugs and have possible interactions with prescribed medications. The client should be advised to inform the nurse practitioner of all OTC medications and herbal supplements that he or she is taking to avoid possible interactions. The client should be cautioned about the extended use of topical antihistamines. Antihistamines do not affect circulating histamine; therefore it is important for the client to avoid exposure to a known allergen. Constipation and urinary retention are adverse effects that should be reported to the nurse practitioner.

66. **(2)** An advantage of using loratadine (Claritin) is the once-a-day dosing, which helps with client compliance. The cost is greater than that of some of the other first-generation antihistamines. Loratadine/pseudoephedrine (Claritin D) is available as an antihistamine/decongestant with twice-a-day dosing, and loratadine/pseudoephedrine extended release (Claritin D 24 Hour) is available for once-a-day dosing.

67. **(4)** Medications such as antihistamines and corticosteroids are used to counter mediator release and block release of additional mediators. Nonsteroidal antiinflammatory drugs (NSAIDs), antibiotics, and decongestants are contraindicated in the treatment of an anaphylactic reaction.

68. **(4)** Both diphenhydramine (Benadryl) and brompheniramine (Dimetane) are antihistamines and could be prescribed. The brompheniramine (Dimetane) would have less central nervous system sedating effects than the diphenhydramine (Benadryl). Dextromethorphan (Benylin) is an antitussive, and guaifenesin (Robitussin) is an expectorant.

69. **(2)** Procainamide (Pronestyl) is one of the most common offenders. Twenty percent of clients receiving this drug experience clinical drug–induced SLE. The other drugs listed have not been associated with SLE.

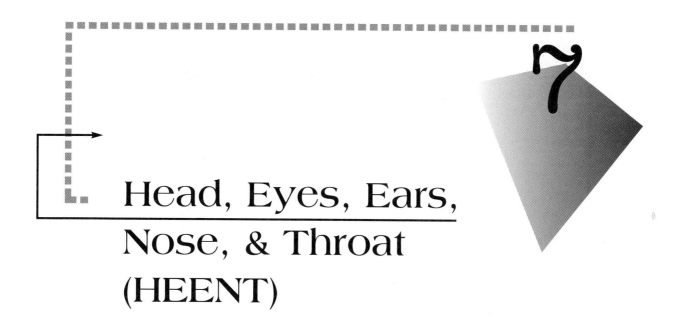

Head, Eyes, Ears, Nose, & Throat (HEENT)

Physical Examination & Diagnostic Tests

Head

1. The nurse practitioner is examining lymph nodes in the neck. What is palpated in the anterior triangle of the neck?

   1. Posterior cervical chain.
   2. Anterior superficial chain.
   3. Periauricular lymph nodes.
   4. Supraclavicular lymph nodes.

Eyes

2. When using an ophthalmoscope, the nurse practitioner:

   1. Holds the ophthalmoscope in the right hand (uses right eye) while examining the client's left eye.
   2. Starts the examination with the lens set at zero.
   3. Begins in a position 1 inch from the eye to check the red reflex.
   4. Examines the anterior chamber in a well-lighted room and asks the client to focus on an object.

3. The nurse practitioner checking for strabismus would use which test?

   1. Cover-uncover test.
   2. Bruckner's test.
   3. Ishihara's test.
   4. Snellen's test.

4. The nurse practitioner observes lid lag in a client with:

   1. Myasthenia gravis.

   2. Hyperthyroidism.

   3. Hordeolum.

   4. Chalazion.

5. The nurse practitioner is examining an elderly woman. There is a glossy white circle around the pupil of one of her eyes, and the pupil has a decreased reaction to the direct light reflex. There is a history of presbyopia. Correct interpretation of these findings is:

   1. Beginning development of cataracts with a significant decrease in visual acuity.

   2. Normal changes in the eyes as a result of the aging process.

   3. A decrease in depth perception and the early eye changes associated with glaucoma.

   4. Visual changes caused by long-term treatment with digitoxin and corticosteroids.

6. The nurse practitioner is preparing to examine the eyes of an adult client. To examine the optic disc and retinal vessels, the practitioner uses what aperture on the ophthalmoscope?

   1. Small aperture.

   2. Red-free filter.

   3. Slit.

   4. Grid.

7. When testing the eyes for the presence of a normal consensual response, the nurse practitioner will:

   1. Shine the light into the client's pupil and observe the rate of pupillary constriction.

   2. Direct the light into one pupil and observe for the constriction or response of the other pupil.

   3. Hold a card in front of one eye and have the client focus on a fixed object, remove the card, and observe movement of the newly uncovered eye.

   4. Ask the client to focus on an object, then direct a light source to the bridge of the nose while observing for symmetrical reflection in both eyes.

8. On ophthalmic examination, there appears to be a narrowing or blocking of the vein at the point where an arteriole crosses over it. The significance of this finding is:

   1. The client needs to be evaluated for chronic hypertension.

   2. This may be indicative of increased ocular pressure associated with glaucoma.

   3. The finding is associated with papilledema causing decreased venous drainage.

   4. This may represent a small embolus in the retinal vessels.

9. When examining the eyes, the nurse practitioner determines that the pupils change in size when the client focuses from a close object to a distant object. This is interpreted as:

   1. Normal visual accommodation.

   2. Intact extraocular motor nerves.

   3. Appropriate consensual response.

   4. Visual acuity within normal limits.

Ears

10. When examining the ears of an adult client, the nurse practitioner determines that the tympanic membrane is gray and translucent. This is interpreted as:

    1. Scarring from previous infections.

    2. Decreased circulation to the membrane.

    3. Presence of serous fluid behind the membrane.

    4. Normal characteristics of the adult ear.

11. The purpose of conducting the Rinne test is to determine conduction of sound through the bone and through the auditory canal. A normal Rinne test result is described as:

    1. Equal conduction through the mastoid bone and the ear canal.

    2. Air conduction twice as long as bone conduction.

    3. Bone conduction twice as long as air conduction.

    4. Sound is clearer with bone conduction than with air conduction.

12. When the tympanic membrane is assessed, specific landmarks are determined and described according to the face of a clock. Where are the normal landmarks for the right tympanic membrane located?

    1. Direct light reflex at 5- to 6-o'clock position, malleus at 1- to 2-o'clock position with umbo in center.

    2. Manubrium slanted to the left with malleus at 10-o'clock position.

    3. Direct light reflex in center of membrane with malleus at 9-o'clock position.

    4. Umbo to the left with anterior malleolar folds at 10-o'clock position.

Nose

13. The nurse practitioner understands that nasal mucosa:

    1. Is redder than oral mucosa.

    2. Is pale and translucent in appearance.

    3. Appears pink and boggy, without exudate.

    4. Appears dark pink with watery secretion.

Throat

14. Throat cultures are indicated for the following suspected causes of pharyngitis:

    1. Rhinovirus and coronavirus infection.

    2. Group A β-hemolytic streptococci.

    3. Mononucleosis.

    4. *Candida albicans.*

15. A young adult arrives at the nurse practitioner's clinic with complaints of low-grade fever, sore throat, a slight headache, and fatigue. On physical examination, the nurse practitioner finds exudative tonsils bilaterally, red pharynx with white patches, and enlarged posterior cervical neck nodes. The nurse practitioner would expect to find:

    1. Positive rapid strep test result.

    2. Positive Monospot test result.

    3. Decreased white blood cell (WBC) count.

    4. Positive viral throat cultures.

Disorders

Head

16. An adult client presents to the nurse practitioner's office with a white plaque near the base of the tongue. The nurse practitioner notes that the plaque does not wipe off and assesses it as:

    1. Hemangioma.

    2. Leukoplakia.

    3. Papilloma.

    4. Erythroplasia.

17. Which of the following are predominant risk factors for oral carcinoma?

    1. History of dental infections, age <40 years.

    2. Tobacco use, alcohol use.

    3. Herpes simplex virus type 1, tobacco use.

    4. Alcohol use, history of dental abscess.

18. The hallmark of early oral cancer is:

    1. Tissue retraction.

    2. Thickening oral tissues.

    3. Persistent (>14 days) local inflammation.

    4. Halitosis and cough.

19. An adult male client is being evaluated for a complaint of a sore throat. He states that he has difficulty swallowing and has some mouth pain. On exam, the nurse practitioner finds that the client's mouth, tongue, and pharynx are coated with white curd-like plaques that are difficult to remove and leave a red surface when scraped with a tongue blade. What would be the best action for the nurse practitioner to take at this time?

    1. Refer him to an ear, nose, and throat specialist for evaluation.

    2. Prescribe Amoxicillin 500 mg PO tid × 10 days.

    3. Encourage the client to have human immunodeficiency virus (HIV) screening.

    4. Recommend clear liquids only for the next few days.

20. The nurse practitioner knows that the most common site for head and neck cancer to occur is the:

    1. Sinuses.
    2. Oral cavity.
    3. Larynx.
    4. Nasal cavity.

Eyes

21. A client who is a sheet metal worker complains that he has had something in his right eye since this morning. Before beginning treatment, the nurse practitioner should:

    1. Instill local anesthetic.
    2. Check the visual acuity.
    3. Flush the eye with tap water for 30 minutes.
    4. Stain the eye with fluorescein.

22. A client is being prepared for cataract surgery. What information is important for the nurse practitioner to provide to the client?

    1. The procedure is short, and the client usually goes home the morning after the surgery.
    2. Both eyes will be patched for the first 24 hours, and it is important for the client to stay in bed.
    3. There may be problems with headache and eye pain for the first 24 hours; take the pain medication provided.
    4. Clients usually go home in 2 to 3 hours after the surgery; there will be increased tearing, but it should not be painful.

23. A client works as a welder. He finished work about 8 hours ago and discovered the protective glass on his welding hood was cracked. He is complaining of agonizing pain and photophobia. The correct diagnosis and action are:

    1. Chemical keratitis; dilate with atropine twice daily.
    2. Viral conjunctivitis; sulfonamide drops four times daily.
    3. Corneal abrasion; binocular patching with polymyxin ointment.
    4. Ultraviolet keratitis; antibiotic drops, non-steroidal antiinflammatory drug (NSAID) topical drops, patching optional.

24. A geriatric client presents to the clinic with a complaint of blurred vision that has been getting increasingly worse over the past 2 years. The client also has also a problem with glare but no problems with pain. The nurse practitioner would first check for the presence of:

    1. Glaucoma.
    2. Retinal detachment.
    3. Macular degeneration.
    4. Cataracts.

25. An adult client presents to the nurse practitioner for evaluation of an eye that has been red and itchy for 1 day. The client states that when he awoke, the eye was matted shut. The client can recall no trauma to the eye. The pupils are equal and reactive, and the client denies any pain in the eye. The nurse practitioner treats this client for:

    1. Conjunctivitis.
    2. Corneal abrasion.
    3. Glaucoma.
    4. Iritis.

26. Which assessment of the eye is a deviation from the commonly occurring age-related changes?

    1. Arcus senilis.
    2. Presbyopia.
    3. Sensitivity to glare.
    4. Sustained nystagmus.

27. During a routine physical examination of a 30-year-old client, the nurse practitioner identifies arcus senilis. The significance of this disorder is:

    1. High potential for future blindness.
    2. None, normal variant of aging process.
    3. Abnormal lipid metabolism requiring medical management.
    4. Hereditary variant of no consequence.

28. A 70-year-old client comes to the clinic complaining of an increased sensitivity to glare, difficulty adapting to darkness, and altered depth perception. The nurse practitioner should suspect:

    1. Cataract.
    2. Macular degeneration.

3. Glaucoma.

4. Normal age-related changes.

Ears

29. In teaching clients how to avoid acoustic trauma caused by noise in the very loud range, the nurse practitioner knows that noise is loudest from a:

1. Vacuum cleaner.

2. Power mower.

3. Clothes washer.

4. Food blender.

30. A geriatric client is complaining of difficulty hearing. He relates that the problem seems to have gotten worse over the past few years. What finding would support a diagnosis of presbycusis?

1. Complain that they can hear voices, but everyone mumbles.

2. Rinne test indicates air conduction greater than bone conduction.

3. History of long-term use of tetracycline antibiotics for chronic infections.

4. Family history of chronic hearing loss.

31. Which of the following organisms is least likely to cause otitis media?

1. *Moraxella catarrhalis.*

2. *Streptococcus pneumoniae.*

3. *Chlamydia trachomatis.*

4. *Haemophilus influenzae.*

32. Which finding in the ear would indicate a deviation from the normal aging process?

1. Dull, retracted, white tympanic membrane.

2. An elongated lobule.

3. A sensorineural hearing loss.

4. Bulging tympanic membrane with a distorted cone of light.

33. Which statement by the nurse practitioner indicates an understanding of conductive hearing loss in the older client?

1. "This has occurred because of damage of the eighth cranial nerve from gentamycin."

2. "This is a result of an inner ear infection."

3. "This is a normal part of aging and is referred to as presbycusis."

4. "This may be reversible after the cerumen is removed from the ear canal."

34. Sensory hearing loss is common in industrial settings and preventable with the use of adequate hearing protection. This type of hearing loss is usually first noted with changes at what level?

1. 500 Hz.

2. 200 Hz.

3. 3000 to 4000 Hz.

4. Above 4000 Hz.

Nose

35. An adult client presents to the nurse practitioner's office with fever and complaints of right facial pain, copious yellow nasal discharge, and acute pain and headache when bending over. The symptoms have been occurring for about 5 days. There is no transillumination of the right maxillary sinus and that area is very tender to palpation. The client's diagnosis is:

1. Chronic sinusitis.

2. Acute sinusitis.

3. Dental abscess.

4. Temporal arteritis.

36. The nurse practitioner teaches a young adult client the following as the most effective measure to prevent the common cold:

1. Judicious use of vitamin C during cold season.

2. Ensuring adequate sleep and fluids.

3. Meticulous handwashing, preferably with an antibacterial soap and warm water.

4. Avoiding contact with children and adults who have a runny nose, cough, and sore throat.

Throat

37. A 20-year-old client presents to the nurse practitioner's office with the chief complaint of "severe sore throat" for 3 days. The client states that he also had a fever but does not know how high it got, and he has been very tired with the sore throat. The physical exam revealed enlarged tonsils with large patchy exudate, inflamed pharynx, and nontender posterior cervical lymphadenopathy. The rest of the findings were unremarkable. The nurse practitioner would make the diagnosis of:

   1. Infectious mononucleosis.
   2. Leukemia.
   3. Scarlet fever.
   4. Oral candidiasis.

38. Which of the following clinical findings is associated with bacterial streptococcal pharyngitis?

   1. Rhinorrhea.
   2. Cough.
   3. Enlarged tonsils with exudate.
   4. Small oral vesicles.

Pharmacology

39. The antibiotic(s) of choice for mild cases of acute sinusitis in the adult is (are):

   1. Amoxicillin (Amoxil) 500 mg PO tid × 14 days; trimethoprim-sulfamethoxazole (Bactrim) DS PO 1 q12h × 14 days; penicillin V potassium (Pen-Vee K) 500 mg bid PO × 14 days.
   2. Trimethoprim-sulfamethoxazole DS PO 1 q12h × 14 days; penicillin V potassium (Pen-Vee K) 500 mg PO bid × 14 days.
   3. Penicillin G 150,000 U IM × 1 day; Amoxicillin 500 mg PO tid × 14 days.
   4. Amoxicillin 500 mg PO tid × 14 days; trimethoprim-sulfamethoxazole DS 1 q12h PO × 14 days.

40. A geriatric client is given a diagnosis of chronic open-angle glaucoma. She has a history of bradycardia and first-degree atrioventricular block. In consideration of her treatment, what medication should be avoided?

   1. Pilocarpine (Isopto Carpine).
   2. Timolol (Timoptic).
   3. Hydrochlorothiazide (Diuril).
   4. Acetazolamide (Diamox).

41. Which antibiotic would be appropriate for the nurse practitioner to prescribe for β-lactamase production by strains of *Haemophilus influenzae* and *Moraxella catarrhalis* in a client with acute otitis media (AOM)?

   1. Amoxicillin (Amoxil).
   2. Erythromycin-sulfisoxazole (Pediazole).
   3. Penicillin V potassium (Pen-Vee K).
   4. Amoxicillin with clavulanate potassium (Augmentin)

42. The treatment plan for a client given a diagnosis of infectious mononucleosis includes which of the following?

   1. Rest during acute phase.
   2. Avoid exercise during acute phase.
   3. Corticosteroids during acute phase.
   4. Ampicillin orally for 10 days.

43. A client has had yellowish green nasal discharge and frontal headache for a week. The client's temperature has gone up to 101.2° F (38.4° C)on most afternoons. She has a cough that worsens when she lies down. The findings on physical exam are within normal limits except for the drainage and a slightly erythematous pharynx. She does not have any drug allergies and has not been taking any medications in the last few months. Which medication would be best to prescribe for her?

   1. Diphenhydramine hydrochloride (Benadryl).
   2. Erythromycin (E-Mycin).
   3. Pseudoephedrine hydrochloride (Sudafed).
   4. Amoxicillin with clavulanate potassium.

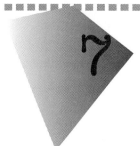

Answers & Rationales

Physical Examination & Diagnostic Tests

Head

1. **(2)** The conceptualization of triangles is useful in determining the location of palpable lymph nodes in the neck. The sternocleidomastoid muscle is the division between the anterior (containing the anterior superficial cervical chain) and the posterior (containing the posterior cervical chain) triangles. The trapezius muscle marks the posterior border of the posterior triangle. The supraclavicular or scale nodes are palpated in the angle formed by the clavicle and the sternocleidomastoid muscle.

Eyes

2. **(2)** The correct use of the ophthalmoscope involves using the right hand and right eye to examine the client's right eye. The room should be semidarkened for best visualization. The examiner initially inspects the lens and vitreous body from a distance of about 12 inches (at zero setting) and moves closer to the eye, usually rotating the lenses to the positive numbers (+15 to +20), which assists in focusing on near objects.

3. **(1)** The cover-uncover test is used to detect strabismus; Bruckner's test is used to check for the red reflex; Ishihara's test is used to determine color perception; and Snellen's test is used to evaluate far vision.

4. **(2)** If the lid margin falls above the limbus (junction line where the sclera and cornea meet) so that some sclera is visible, hyperthyroidism may be present. The lid may lag behind the limbus as the gaze moves from an upward to a downward position. Ptosis is a drooping lid margin that falls at the pupil or below and may indicate an oculomotor lesion or myasthenia gravis. A chalazion is an inflammation or cyst of the meibomian glands, which lie within the posterior portion of the eyelid. A localized infection of the small glands around the eyelashes in the hair follicle at the lid margin is called *a hordeolum*.

5. **(2)** With cataracts, there is a clouding of the lens, not a circle around the pupil. The circle around the pupil is arcus senilis, which is normal in the geriatric client. The visual acuity of the client cannot be determined from the information provided. There are no observable pupillary changes in the beginning stages of glaucoma, which is identified by checking the intraocular pressure.

6. **(2)** The red-free filter is used to examine the optic disc for pallor and vascular changes, as well as to detect retinal hemorrhages. The small aperture is used for small pupils, the slit is for the anterior eye, and the grid is for estimating the size of lesions found in the fundal area.

7. **(2)** Consensual response is pupillary constriction of one eye when there is a direct light stimulus to the pupil of the other eye.

8. **(1)** Arteriovenous nicking is associated with longstanding hypertension. Intraocular pressure cannot be determined from an

ophthalmic examination. Papilledema is associated with swelling around the optic disc, and small emboli are represented by an abrupt impediment in or severe narrowing of an arteriole not associated with the point at which the retinal veins and arteries cross.

9. **(1)** Changes in pupil size in focusing from near to distant objects is normal accommodation. Extraocular eye movements refer to the ability to move the eye. Consensual response is constriction of the eye in response to light being shined in the opposite eye. The Snellen eye chart is used to determine visual acuity.

Ears

10. **(4)** This describes the normal characteristics of the tympanic membrane. There is no evidence of scarring or fluid.

11. **(2)** The normal Rinne test result is air conduction (AC) that is twice as long as bone conduction (BC) (AC > BC).

12. **(1)** This describes the correct position for these landmarks on the right ear. In Option #2, the manubrium slants to the right with the malleus at the 1- to 2-o'clock position for the right ear. Option #3 describes the correct position for the left ear. In Option #4, the umbo is in the center with anterior folds at the 1- to 2-o'clock position for the right ear.

Nose

13. **(1)** Nasal mucosa is redder than oral mucosa. Increased redness of the nasal mucosa usually indicates infection. Pale, boggy turbinates along with watery secretion often occur with allergic rhinitis. The normal secretion is mucoid. Purulent, crusty, or bloody secretions are abnormal.

Throat

14. **(2)** Rapid screening for strep throat can be done with a throat swab and an antigen agglutination kit, but there is a 5% to 10% false-negative rate; therefore it is suggested that a culture be performed. The heterophile antibody test (Monospot test), which rapidly detects heterophile antibodies, has sensitivity and specificity (95% specific and 90% sensitive) comparable to those of older heterophile antibody tests for the diagnosis of mononucleosis. *Candida albicans* and

rhinovirus are not diagnosed by means of bacterial cultures. Oral candidiasis can be diagnosed by means of a potassium hydroxide smear.

15. **(2)** The client in this situation has risk factors (age) and symptoms of mononucleosis; therefore the Monospot or heterophile antibody test should be done. The classical triad of mononucleosis symptoms is sore throat, fever, and posterior cervical lymphadenopathy with or without mild tenderness. Rapid screening for strep throat can be done with a throat swab and an antigen agglutination kits and would be done first; however, the result would probably be negative. A white blood cell (WBC) count would be ordered if the nurse suspected bacterial pharyngitis, because an increase in WBC count is found with bacterial infection and a decrease is associated with viral agents.

Disorders

Head

16. **(2)** Leukoplakia is a white patch present on the oral mucosa that cannot be rubbed off. Hemangiomas are benign blood vessel proliferations of the lips, tongue, or buccal mucosa. Erythroplasia is an asymptomatic, red, velvety lesion of the mouth, which sometimes indicates malignancy. Papillomas are benign verrucous lesions that are manifestations of human papillomavirus infection.

17. **(2)** The predominant risk factors for oral cancer are tobacco and alcohol use. The risk increases with the number of cigarettes smoked per day. The disease is age related, occurring in those older 40 years and increasing with age. The male/female ratio is 3:1. Other risk factors are use of cigars, pipes, and smokeless tobacco. Human papillomavirus has been considered in the etiology of squamous cell carcinoma in the upper head and neck.

18. **(3)** Erythroplasia is accompanied by an inflammatory reaction in a client with suspected oral cancer. If the erythematous lesion persists over 14 days, early oral cancer should be suspected. Tissue retraction and thickening of the oral tissues are later signs of oral cancer. Halitosis (odor) may be associated with dysfunction within the oral cavity, nasal cavity,

or sinuses or with esophageal disorders. Cough is the primary symptom of respiratory disorders such as acute bronchitis or pneumonia.

19. **(3)** Adults who present with thrush (oral candidiasis) may be immunologically impaired. It is important to make the diagnosis of human immunodeficiency virus (HIV) early to so that treatment can be started. Treatment with amoxicillin may actually worsen the condition.

20. **(2)** The nurse practitioner knows that the risk factors for head and neck cancer include tobacco and alcohol use. Poor oral hygiene and occupational exposure to asbestos, coke, nickel, wood, or leather are also risk factors. Therefore the most common site is the oral cavity, accounting for 48% of the head and neck cancer diagnoses.

Eyes

21. **(2)** The nurse practitioner should check the visual acuity before treatment as a basis for comparison in the event of complications. Local anesthetic will be helpful for a detailed exam, after the initial inspection and during removal, if indicated. Flushing with normal saline solution may be helpful in removing an object that is visualized. Staining the eye should come later when the nurse is preparing to examine the eye for abrasion under ultraviolet light.

22. **(4)** Clients go home almost immediately after the procedure. Eye patches may be worn for the first 24 hours. Care should be taken to protect the eye on which surgery was performed from injury. There is some discomfort, but pain should not be a problem. The client can be up and around as tolerated.

23. **(4)** Exposure to a welding arc can cause ultraviolet burns to the cornea. Treatment with ophthalmic antibiotic drops and topical ophthalmic nonsteroidal antiinflammatory drug (NSAID) drops, such as diclofenac (Voltaren), can be done at home, with recovery expected in 2 to 3 days. Patching is controversial and generally reserved for severe cases during the first 24 hours after injury only.

24. **(4)** Cataracts are characterized by painless loss of visual acuity over time. Retinal detachment most often occurs suddenly, with partial loss of the field of vision. Glaucoma results in the loss of peripheral vision, and macular degeneration primarily involves the central vision field.

25. **(1)** In clients with corneal abrasion, glaucoma, and iritis, the chief complaint is pain. Conjunctivitis presents with no pain and with a history of purulent discharge.

26. **(4)** Sustained nystagmus is indicative of a neurologic complication. The other options include normal age-related changes.

27. **(3)** Arcus senilis is caused by the deposit of lipids at the junction of the cornea and sclera or hyaline degeneration and is present in many people older than 50 years. When it is identified in younger individuals, it points to a disorder of lipid metabolism.

28. **(4)** These findings are normal age-related changes. Signs and symptoms of cataracts include reduced visual acuity; painless, progressive loss of vision; and sensitivity to light, especially during night driving. Reduced color discrimination and double vision may also be seen. Macular degeneration will present with a loss of central vision. Primary open-angle glaucoma will present with occasional headaches, and occasionally, halos around lights and may be asymptomatic in early stages. Primary angle-closure glaucoma will present with episodes of blurred vision, halos around lights at night, and redness.

Ears

29. **(2)** Although all of these household appliances are noisy, the client should wear ear plugs or muffs when using a power lawn mower regularly for long periods.

30. **(1)** In presbycusis, the ability to hear high-frequency sounds is diminished. Patients with presbycusis have difficulty distinguishing consonant sounds, so words such as "shoe" and "true" are heard as "oo." The Rinne test result will indicate that bone conduction is two times greater than air conduction. Tetracyclines are not ototoxic, and the family history may or may not contribute to the problem.

31. **(3)** The bacteria that most frequently infect the middle ear are similar to those that frequently infect the nasopharynx: *S. pneumoniae, H. influenzae,* and *M. catarrhalis. Escherichia coli* and *Klebsiella* species. Viruses may also cause AOM. *Chlamydia trachomatis* is not a frequent causative agent.

32. **(4)** This would be indicative of an inflammation of the middle ear (AOM). The other options are normal changes that occur with aging.

33. **(4)** Conductive hearing loss may result from AOM, perforation of the eardrum, and obstruction of the ear canal, as by cerumen. The other options describe causes of sensorineural hearing loss.

34. **(4)** Sensory hearing loss presents with high-frequency loss, above the 4000-Hz level, and then progresses into voice frequencies at 2000 to 3000 Hz.

Nose

35. **(2)** The client is experiencing the classic symptoms of acute sinusitis. Symptoms of chronic sinusitis are nasal discharge, congestion, headache, or cough for more than 30 days. Symptoms of a dental abscess are a constant, severe tooth-associated pain and jaw tenderness. Temporal arteritis causes pain in the jaw, tongue, and face but no nasal discharge.

36. **(3)** Transmission of cold viruses is indirect (e.g., self-inoculation from virus on surfaces of inanimate objects to mucous membranes of the nose and mouth). It is less likely to be spread by the aerosol route. Thus the client should avoid touching the nose and mouth unless the hands have been thoroughly washed. It is impractical to avoid contact, because cold viruses are found everywhere. Although many individuals believe vitamin C prevents colds, there is little evidence to support the claim.

Throat

37. **(1)** Mononucleosis is commonly seen in adolescents and young adults. It often presents with fever, exudate on the tonsils, generalized lymphadenopathy, malaise, posterior cervical adenopathy, and palatine petechiae. Leukemia presents with anorexia, irritability, lethargy, and bone pain. The peak incidence is in 3- to 5-year-olds. Scarlet fever presents in children 2 to 10 years old with fever, abdominal pain, headache, sore throat, and strawberry tongue. Oral candidiasis presents with white curd-like plaques on erythematous mucosa. The tongue is red with a white coat.

38. **(3)** Characteristics of bacterial pharyngitis include headache, mild to severe erythema of tonsils with white or yellow exudate, dysphagia, positive anterior cervical nodes, sore throat with dysphagia, fever >101° F (38.3° C) to 102.5° F (39.1° C), and nausea. Viral organisms that cause herpangina present with small oral vesicles. Cough is the primary symptom of acute bronchitis. Rhinorrhea is associated with allergic rhinitis.

Pharmacology

39. **(4)** Amoxicillin (Amoxil) is the first-line antibiotic for mild cases of acute uncomplicated sinusitis in the adult because of cost-effectiveness, efficacy, and cure rates ranging from 67% to 100%. For cases of moderate severity and in geographic areas with high rates of resistance to β-lactam antibiotics, amoxicillin/clavulanate is the next choice. Additional choices include trimethoprim-sulfamethoxazole (Bactrim), cefuroxime (Ceftin), azithromycin (Zithromax), and clarithromycin (Biaxin).

40. **(2)** β-Adrenergic blockers cause problems with bradycardia; timolol (Timoptic) can be absorbed systemically from the eye and should not be used.

41. **(2)** Amoxicillin with clavulanate potassium (Augmentin) is effective against β-lactamase production. Amoxicillin is ineffective against β-lactamase production. Erythromycin-sulfisoxazole and trimethoprim-sulfamethoxazole have recently been deemed less effective. Cephalosporins are effective against β-lactamase production by strains of *H. influenzae* and *M. catarrhalis*. Penicillin V potassium (Pen-Vee K) is not effective against this group of organisms. Cephalexin, cefuroxime, or cefixime can be used as an alternative.

42. **(1)** The treatment of mononucleosis includes bed rest while the client has fever and myalgia (10-14 days), administration of acetaminophen or ibuprofen, warm saline solution gargles, and use of throat lozenges or spray. The client must avoid strenuous exercise and contact sports for 2 months because of the risk of splenic rupture even if no splenomegaly is detected. Corticosteroids are recommended only in

clients with impending airway obstruction. Ampicillin is not recommended because of the possibility of an allergic reaction. About 95% of clients with mononucleosis recover uneventfully with supportive treatment.

43. **(4)** The client is experiencing symptoms of moderately severe acute sinusitis as indicated by her symptoms of facial pressure, headache, and postnasal discharge. The first-line antibiotic to prescribe for this condition is amoxicillin/clavulanate because of its safety and efficacy. Oral antihistamines such as diphenhydramine should not be used unless the client has allergies. Oral decongestants (pseudoephedrine hydrochloride) are not as effective as topical agents (e.g., nasal spray) for clients with sinusitis. Erythromycin is not a first-line antibiotic for sinusitis.

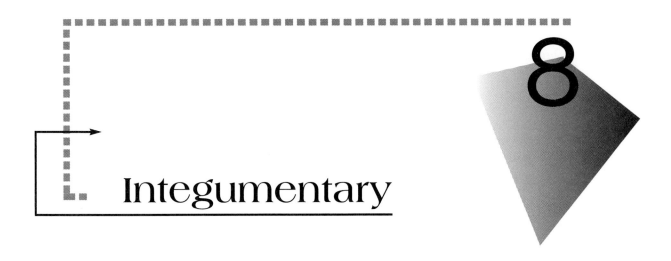

Integumentary

Physical Examination & Diagnostic Tests

1. The nurse practitioner describes an annular skin lesion as usually arranged in:

   1. Groups of vesicles erupting unilaterally.

   2. A line.

   3. A pattern of merging together, not discrete.

   4. A circle or ring.

2. A client has pitting of the nails. The nurse practitioner understands this is associated with:

   1. Psoriasis.

   2. Iron deficiency anemia.

   3. Malnutrition.

   4. Hyperthyroidism.

3. The nurse practitioner is inspecting a dark-skinned individual for signs of jaundice. The best place to observe is:

   1. Sclera of the opened eye.

   2. Palms and soles of the hands and feet.

   3. Oral mucosa.

   4. Nail beds.

4. In assessment of the hydration status of a client, the best place to evaluate skin turgor on an adult is:

   1. Just below the clavicle.

   2. Below the scapula on the back.

   3. On the inside of the forearm.

   4. On the back of the hand.

5. The Wood's lamp is used to evaluate skin lesions. When the light is shone on the client's skin, a green-yellow fluorescence indicates:

   1. Presence of fungi.

   2. Lichenification.

   3. Keratinized cells.

   4. Bacterial colonies.

6. On examination of a client's skin, the nurse practitioner finds a lesion that is about 0.75 cm in diameter, brown, circumscribed, flat, and nonpalpable. What is the correct term for this lesion?

   1. Macule.

   2. Papule.

   3. Nodule.

   4. Wheal.

7. The history and findings on physical examination of a client indicate past occurrences of lichenification. The nurse practitioner identifies the characteristics of this lesion as:

   1. Dried, crusty exudate, slightly elevated.

   2. Rough thickened epidermis, accentuated skin markings.

   3. Keratinized cells shaped in an irregular pattern with exfoliation.

   4. Loss of epidermis with hollowed-out area and dermis exposed.

8. Clubbing of the nails occurs in clients with chronic respiratory conditions. The nurse practitioner assesses for this condition by:

   1. Evaluating the nail for transverse depressions and ridges.

   2. Placing both of the client's hands together with palms inward and index fingers aligned.

   3. Placing nail beds of each index finger together to determine angle of nail plate.

   4. Determining whether there is diffuse discoloration of the nail bed from decreased oxygenation.

9. A circumscribed, elevated lesion >1 cm in diameter and containing clear serous fluid is best described as a:

   1. Papule.

   2. Vesicle.

   3. Bulla.

   4. Pustule.

10. In performing a skin assessment, the nurse practitioner understands that the following appearance would necessitate immediate intervention:

    1. A 5-mm, symmetrical, uniformly brown mole on the thigh that has been present and has not changed in appearance for more than 5 years.

    2. Multiple small (1-3 mm), flat moles across the upper back that are dark brown in color, round, and have smooth edges.

    3. A 3-cm waxy papule, with a "stuck-on" appearance, noted on the face.

    4. A new 2-mm mole that is brown with a red, irregular border, and is occasionally pruritic.

11. Dermatophyte skin infections can be diagnosed from skin scrapings prepared with which solution for microscopic exam?

    1. Hydrochloric acid.

    2. 20% potassium hydroxide (KOH) solution.

    3. Gram's stain.

    4. Distilled water.

12. When administering skin tests to an immunocompromised client, the nurse practitioner must consider:

    1. The importance of not applying more than one skin test at a time.

    2. That the skin test may react more aggressively than expected.

    3. Identification and use of a known allergen as a control.

    4. That the immunocompromised client should not be skin tested.

Disorders

13. A client complains of intolerable itching in the pubic area. On examination, the nurse practitioner notes erythematous papules and tiny white specks in the pubic hair. The differential diagnosis includes all **except:**

    1. Pediculosis pubis.

    2. Scabies.

    3. Impetigo.

    4. Atopic dermatitis.

14. An elderly lady has an area of vesicles in clusters with an erythematous base extending from her spine, around and under her arm and

breast, to the sternum on her left side. She says the area was very tender last week and the vesicles started erupting yesterday. She is complaining of severe pain in the area. What is the probable diagnosis for this condition?

1. Psoriasis.
2. Herpes zoster.
3. Contact dermatitis.
4. Cellulitis.

15. What is a chronic skin condition that is sometimes associated with arthritis?
    1. Eczema.
    2. Psoriasis.
    3. Neurodermatitis.
    4. Pityriasis rosea.

16. Which is a true statement about psoriasis?
    1. It is usually worse in the summer.
    2. It is highly contagious.
    3. It can be exacerbated by stress.
    4. All clients have accompanying pruritus.

17. What should a client with actinic keratosis be told?
    1. These are a normal part of aging and are benign.
    2. These lesions can develop into squamous cell carcinomas.
    3. This is part of an allergic reaction and the offending allergen needs to be identified.
    4. This skin condition responds well to sunlight, which will help alleviate the symptoms.

18. The following are all true statements regarding urticaria **except:**
    1. Most cases of acute urticaria are mediated by immunoglobulin E mast cell degranulation.
    2. Chronic urticaria may be related to occult infections.
    3. Urticaria is characterized by itchy, red swellings of a few millimeters to a few centimeters in size.
    4. Laboratory studies are necessary to identify the causative agent.

19. A client who is known to be human immunodeficiency virus (HIV)–positive presents with several painless, persistent, raised purple lesions on the face. What is the most likely diagnosis of the lesions?
    1. Seborrheic dermatitis.
    2. Molluscum contagiosum.
    3. Kaposi's sarcoma.
    4. Fungal infection.

20. In differentiating between nummular eczema (dermatitis) and dyshidrotic eczematous dermatitis, the nurse practitioner knows that:
    1. Nummular eczema is characterized by flushing and clusters of papulopustules on the cheek and forehead.
    2. Dyshidrotic eczematous dermatitis is a chronic vesicular type of hand and foot eczema characterized by vesicles (tapioca-like), scaling, lichenification, and pruritus.
    3. Nummular eczema is a hereditary disorder characterized by chronic scaling plaques that usually appear bilaterally on exposed areas (knees, elbows).
    4. Dyshidrotic eczematous dermatitis primarily affects young adults, is contagious, and is characterized by firm papules with a clefted surface and multiple conical vegetations.

21. A middle-aged male client presents to the clinic with a complaint of being bitten last night by another individual during a fight. He has a bite mark on his forearm and the skin has been broken. He reports that he had a tetanus shot about 8 years ago. Management recommended by the family nurse practitioner should include all **except:**
    1. Administration of 0.5 ml of tetanus toxoid IM.
    2. Instructing client to watch for signs of infection.
    3. Administration of penicillin plus a penicillinase-resistant penicillin.
    4. Closure of wound with sutures or Steri-strips.

22. Nail involvement secondary to primary foot and hand tinea, which is characterized by accumulation of subungual keratin that produces thickened, distorted, crumbling nails, is termed:

    1. Hippocratic nails.

    2. Onychomycosis.

    3. Koilonychia.

    4. Anonychia.

23. A middle-aged client presents for an office visit with a complaint of a measles-like rash on his trunk and spreading to his extremities. He was seen several days ago for bronchitis and began taking trimethoprim-sulfamethoxazole (Bactrim DS) 1 tablet PO bid. What is the recommended action for the family nurse practitioner?

    1. Instruct client to continue taking Bactrim and see whether any change in the rash occurs.

    2. Discontinue Bactrim.

    3. Discontinue Bactrim for 3 days and restart the medication.

    4. Decrease Bactrim to half the original dose.

24. A client complaining of hyperhidrosis should be counseled that:

    1. This is a normal occurrence.

    2. There are no therapies for this complaint.

    3. Bathing in a 20% alcohol solution of aluminum chloride hexahydrate (Drysol) may be beneficial.

    4. A history and physical exam need to be completed so that any medical etiologies can be ruled out.

25. During the physical examination, the nurse practitioner observes a macular-papular skin lesion on a client's back that is warty, scaly, greasy in appearance, and light tan in color. What would be the probable diagnosis?

    1. Actinic keratosis.

    2. Basal cell carcinoma.

    3. Seborrheic keratosis.

    4. Senile lentigines.

26. The nurse practitioner is assessing an older client who has herpes zoster (shingles) in the prodromal stage. What would the practitioner expect to find in the assessment of this client?

    1. Erythematous lesions present over 4 different parts of the body.

    2. A red, pinpoint, painless rash.

    3. A burning pain in a line on only half of the client's chest that does not cross the midline.

    4. Painless purulent lesions for 2 days, followed by complaints of itching, burning, and nausea.

27. What would be the appropriate treatment for a client with herpes zoster (shingles)?

    1. Acyclovir (Zovirax).

    2. Miconazole (Monistat-Derm).

    3. Clotrimazole (Lotrimin).

    4. Corticosteroid (prednisone).

28. An elderly retired farmer presents with a dome-shaped, pearly, firm nodule with telangiectasia on his nose. In making a diagnosis, the nurse practitioner recognizes this to be:

    1. Compound nevus.

    2. Melanoma.

    3. Bullous pemphigoid.

    4. Basal cell carcinoma.

29. An adult female presents with an irregular variegated nevus on her lower left back that has doubled in size in the past 3 months. What would be an appropriate action for the nurse practitioner?

    1. Do a punch biopsy to confirm the diagnosis.

    2. Take a photograph of the lesion and recheck it in 1 month.

    3. Refer client to a dermatologist immediately.

    4. Reassure the client that these are normal changes related to hormone variations.

30. A client complains of pain in his right chest wall that has been present for the past 48 hours. On examination, the nurse practitioner notices a vesicular eruption along the dermatome and

identifies this as herpes zoster. The nurse practitioner informs the client that:

1. All symptoms will disappear in 3 days.

2. Oral medication can dramatically reduce the duration and intensity of symptoms.

3. He has chickenpox and can be contagious to his grandchildren.

4. The eruptions will recur at regular intervals.

31. A young adult female presents to the nurse practitioner's office, stating that she has a red rash over her trunk that itches and has been present for 2 weeks. She has tried over-the-counter lotions and creams, with no relief of symptoms. She states that it started as a small, round red patch on her chest and has since spread across her chest, back, arms, and legs. Physical exam reveals a generalized distribution of erythematous, scaly macular lesions that run parallel to each other, creating a "Christmas tree" pattern. The nurse practitioner should:

1. Obtain a thorough medication history, investigate any potential allergens, and send the client to an allergy specialist.

2. Prescribe triamcinolone acetonide 0.025% (Aristocort A) cream to be applied bid for 2 weeks.

3. Teach the client that this viral disease is self-limiting and to avoid prolonged or excessive exposure to sunlight.

4. Refer the client to a dermatologist for a biopsy.

32. An adult male client presents to the nurse practitioner's office complaining of flu-like symptoms, a large red spot in the right groin, headaches, and generalized muscle pain. These symptoms have persisted for approximately 4 to 5 weeks. In taking the client's history, it would be most important to determine whether the client:

1. Was using new skin care products, detergents, etc.

2. Was taking any new medications, vitamins, herbal therapies, etc.

3. Has had a recent insect bite or has been potentially exposed to insects such as ticks.

4. Has been exposed to anyone who has tuberculosis.

33. A nurse practitioner is teaching a client how to use permethrin 1% creme rinse (Nix) for treatment of pediculosis capitis. What is the most important information the nurse practitioner should give to the client?

1. Shampoo hair daily for 1 week with permethrin 1% (Nix).

2. After hair is shampooed and towel-dried, apply permethrin 1% (Nix) creme rinse to scalp and hair, and leave this on for 10 minutes before rinsing.

3. The shampoo should not be used again, because it is toxic and may be absorbed systemically and cause acute respiratory problems.

4. It is not necessary to treat other members of the family or launder bedding or clothing.

34. A client seen at the clinic gives a history of an insect bite the previous evening. What presenting symptom would be associated with the bite of a brown recluse spider?

1. Paresthesias in all extremities.

2. Edematous, erythematous area with coalescing macules.

3. Tissue sloughing in the bite area within 8 to 10 hours.

4. Development of a central black eschar of "sinking infarct" within 6 to 12 hours.

35. The nurse practitioner understands that cat bites become infected more often than dog bites because:

1. Dogs have a "cleaner mouth" than cats.

2. Cat bites are often deep puncture wounds.

3. Dog bites are usually on the face, which makes them less susceptible to infection.

4. Cat bites are usually associated with clawing and spreading of microorganisms.

36. When do bites from insects, spiders, snakes, and bees most commonly occur?

1. Fall.

2. Spring to fall.

3. Winter.

4. Any time of the year.

37. A client was bitten by a neighbor's dog 3 days ago. An infection has developed in a large wound on his lower leg. What would be appropriate treatment for this client?

    1. Prescribe amoxicillin/clavulanate potassium (Augmentin) 250 mg PO tid × 14 days.

    2. Approximate the edges of the wound together with sutures.

    3. Prescribe cephalexin (Keflex) 500 mg PO tid × 7 days.

    4. Have the client return to the clinic for follow-up in 2 weeks.

38. Medical management for a brown recluse spider bite includes:

    1. Warm, moist soaks of the area.

    2. Ice pack and elevation of the area.

    3. Active and passive range of motion (ROM) to area.

    4. Avoidance of antihistamines.

39. A young adult has been bitten by a black widow spider while doing yard work. He is having a severe reaction; the nurse practitioner expects:

    1. Hypotension and shock.

    2. Localized pain, erythema, and edema in the area.

    3. Black eschar of sloughing tissue within 4 hours of the bite.

    4. Abdominal rigidity, nausea, and headache.

40. An outdoor guide is explaining about snakes and snake bites and relates the following to his group about the coral snake: "Red on yellow, kill a fellow; red on black, venom lack." Later on, one of the group members is bitten by a snake described as having broad rings of red and black separated by narrow rings of yellow. The nurse practitioner understands that this client will probably experience all **except:**

    1. Numbness and change in sensation.

    2. Local swelling at the fang mark site.

    3. Dizziness and diplopia.

    4. No symptoms, because the snake was not poisonous.

Pharmacology

41. An obese woman presents to the clinic with complaints of tenderness and irritation under both of her breasts. The examination reveals a very irritated, moist, inflamed area with macules and papules present. What is the best treatment for this woman?

    1. Application of nystatin cream 2 to 3 times a day for 10 days; thorough drying of the area and exposure to light and air.

    2. Systemic antistaphylococcal antibiotics (dicloxacillin) and soaking with pads moistened with normal saline solution 3 times a day.

    3. Gentle washing of the area and removal of crusts, then application of antibiotic ointment.

    4. Antiviral treatment (acyclovir) and application of topical ointment to prevent secondary infection.

42. Which classification of drugs has the potential to exacerbate psoriasis?

    1. β-Blockers.

    2. Thiazide diuretics.

    3. Vasodilators.

    4. Tricyclic antidepressants.

43. In treatment of severe inflammatory acne in a young adult female client, the nurse practitioner understands that:

    1. Isotretinoin (Accutane) provides an effective first-line therapy.

    2. The benefits of treatment will be noted in 5 to 7 days.

    3. Counseling on stringent dietary changes is important.

    4. Systemic antibiotics are effective treatments.

44. All of the following are true of postherpetic neuralgia **except:**

    1. Capsaicin (Zostrix) cream may alleviate some of the discomfort.

    2. In the majority of clients, postherpetic pain decreases gradually over several weeks.

3. Acyclovir (Zovirax) 200 mg, 5 capsules a day PO in divided doses, is an effective therapy.

4. It is more common in clients older than 60 years.

45. When treating genital warts with topical podophyllin, it is important for the family nurse practitioner to:

1. Apply preparation directly to the wart and approximately 5 mm around base of wart.

2. Cover with a dressing so the solution remains moist and caution client not to remove the dressing for 24 hours.

3. Instruct client to wash off medication in 4 to 6 hours.

4. Treat with liquid nitrogen before applying podophyllin.

46. What is the recommended treatment for rosacea?

1. Oral hydrocortisone.

2. Oral ketoconazole.

3. Low-dose tetracycline.

4. Topical 5-fluorouracil.

47. When lidocaine is used with 1% to 2% epinephrine as a local anesthetic in the repair of an injury, it is essential to keep in mind that the maximum allowable dose is:

1. 7 mg/kg.

2. 2 mg/kg.

3. 10 mg/kg.

4. 5 mg/kg.

48. An elderly client presents to the nurse practitioner complaining of a painful, tingling rash across the right side of his abdomen. Exam reveals vesicles with erythematous bases; some of the vesicles are draining cloudy fluid, while others are crusted. The nurse practitioner makes the diagnosis of herpes zoster infection and initiates antiviral therapy for the patient. The patient states that the painful rash has kept him from sleeping for the past 4 nights. What would be appropriate therapy for this client's pain?

1. Amitriptyline (Elavil) 10 mg PO qhs, nonsteroidal antiinflammatory drugs (NSAIDs) prn as directed.

2. High-dose corticosteroid therapy.

3. Application of heat directly to the area involved.

4. No appropriate therapy is currently available to treat neuropathic pain.

49. On a return visit to the clinic, a client who is receiving sulfonamide therapy exhibits the following symptoms: generalized rash, mucous membrane lesions, sloughing of the skin of the palms and feet, high fever, and generalized malaise. These findings would alert the nurse practitioner to consider:

1. Hepatitis B.

2. Stevens-Johnson syndrome.

3. HIV infection/acquired immunodeficiency syndrome (AIDS).

4. *Pneumocystis carinii* pneumonia.

50. A young adult female presents to the nurse practitioner's office with a prolonged history of facial acne. She has been seen by several dermatologists and has been treated over the past 3 years with multiple therapies, including topical antibiotics, drying agents, intralesional injections of corticosteroids, and multiple systemic antibiotics, without success. After consulting with the collaborating physician, the nurse practitioner prescribes isotretinoin (Accutane). Teaching/counseling related to the use of this medication includes:

1. No dietary/alcohol restrictions.

2. Exposure to sunlight without burning can be helpful in hastening the healing process.

3. Elimination of all fat from the client's diet.

4. Emphasis on the importance of using effective contraception if the client is sexually active.

Answers & Rationales

Physical Examination & Diagnostic Tests

1. **(4)** Annular skin lesions may be arranged in a circular manner or in an arciform (arc-shaped) pattern (e.g., tinea corporis). Multiple groups of vesicles erupting unilaterally that follow the course of cutaneous nerves are herpetiform or zosteriform (e.g., herpes zoster). Linear lesions are arranged in a line (e.g., allergic contact dermatitis in response to poison ivy). Confluent lesions merge and are not discrete (e.g., scarlet fever rash).

2. **(1)** Psoriasis, peripheral vascular disease, diabetes, tuberculosis, and other infectious diseases such as syphilis are associated with pitting deformities of the nail that may vary from pinpoint to pinhead size and may be linear or irregular in distribution. Iron deficiency anemia, eczema, malnutrition, and pellagra are associated with koilonychia (spoon nails). Hyperthyroidism and hypothyroidism are associated with onycholysis, which is a separation of the nail from the nail bed, originating at the free edge and progressing proximally.

3. **(1)** The place to inspect is that portion of the sclera that is observed when the eye is open. If jaundice is suspected, the posterior portion of the hard palate should be examined for a yellowish cast. Pallor and cyanosis can be noted in the nail beds, palms, and soles.

4. **(1)** The best place is just below the clavicle or on the abdomen for an adult. The best place to evaluate skin turgor for hydration status on children is the fleshy part of arms or legs because a child with a distended abdomen may have a tight abdomen, which appears to have adequate turgor, even though the child may actually be dehydrated.

5. **(1)** Fungal lesions will be visualized as a green-yellow fluorescence when viewed with the Wood's lamp in a dim room.

6. **(1)** A macule is <1 cm in diameter; nonpalpable; and brown, red, purple, or tan (freckles, flat moles, rubella). A papule is elevated and palpable (warts, pigmented nevi). A nodule is 1 to 2 cm in diameter, elevated, and deeper (lipoma). A wheal is elevated and irregular and has a variable diameter (insect bites, urticaria).

7. **(2)** Lichenification occurs with chronic irritation, often of an exposed extremity (chronic dermatitis). Crusts are dried exudate; scales are heaps of keratinized cells from exfoliation (psoriasis); and loss of epidermis is excoriation, as seen in an abrasion.

8. **(3)** The angle of the nail beds should form a diamond when the nail beds are approximated. Transverse ridges and grooves may occur as a result of trauma. Placing the palms together provides no assessment data, and diffuse discoloration may be caused by a fungal infection or an injury.

9. **(3)** Bulla is the correct term. A papule is solid, a vesicle is <1 cm in diameter, and a pustule contains a purulent exudate.

10. **(4)** The appearance of a new mole with high-risk features including irregular border, color changes, and changes in sensation (e.g., pruritus) would necessitate immediate biopsy

to rule out melanoma and/or referral to a dermatologist. Uniform moles, those that are symmetrical and have smooth borders, and those that are not showing signs of change are those that can be followed up with annual skin assessments. Seborrheic keratosis is a benign skin growth that usually presents on sun-exposed areas and appears waxy or "stuck-on"; it requires no treatment.

11. **(2)** On microscopic examination, fungal scrapings in potassium hydroxide (KOH) solution will appear as thread-like hyphae crossing cell walls. The other solutions are not indicated for use in identification of dermatophytes.

12. **(3)** It is important to remember to apply controls when skin testing the immunocompromised client. Ask clients what diseases they believe they have immunity to, such as measles. Apply the "known" allergen and the reagent to be tested. If the client is unable to mount an immune response at all, the known allergen will not react. By not applying the controls, the nurse practitioner may assume a skin test response is negative, when in fact, the client's immune system is unable to respond.

Disorders

13. **(3)** Intense itching is characteristic of pediculosis pubis, scabies, and atopic dermatitis. Impetigo starts out as a tender, erythematous papule and progresses from a vesicular stage to a honey-crusted stage with no itching.

14. **(2)** Herpes zoster typically presents with a history of tenderness, followed by eruptions and vesicles that follow a dermatome on one side of the body. This is very painful. Other symptoms may include fever, headaches, and malaise.

15. **(2)** Approximately 10% to 30% of people with psoriasis have an accompanying form of arthritis called *psoriatic arthritis*. The other options are dermatologic conditions but are not directly associated with arthritis.

16. **(3)** Stress can exacerbate psoriasis. Sunlight helps psoriasis, so it is usually better in the summer. It is not contagious, and only about 30% of clients with psoriasis experience itching.

17. **(2)** Actinic keratoses are potentially precancerous lesions and are found in areas of skin exposed to sunlight. Because of the increasing popularity of sunbathing, they have even been seen in persons 30 to 50 years old.

18. **(4)** Laboratory studies are not likely to be helpful in evaluation of urticaria. Identification of causes is usually based on history and physical findings. The other statements are true of urticaria.

19. **(3)** Although any one of these conditions can affect the skin, particularly that of a human immunodeficiency virus (HIV)–positive client, the description relates most closely to Kaposi's sarcoma and warrants a biopsy.

20. **(2)** Despite the name, *dyshidrotic eczematous dermatitis* (bullous form called *pompholyx*), there is no evidence of sweating. Most clients have an atopic history, and emotional stress is often a precipitating factor in the appearance of the vesicles. Nummular (discoid) eczema is a chronic, pruritic, inflammatory dermatitis that occurs in the form of coin-shaped plaques composed of small papules and vesicles grouped on an erythematous base. Option #1 describes rosacea. Option #3 describes psoriasis. Option #4 describes a verruca or common wart.

21. **(4)** Wound closure should be delayed for approximately 24 to 48 hours until absence of infection can be confirmed. Mouth flora of humans is abundant, and with a bite, there is the possibility of heavy bacterial inoculum and potential severe infection. Tetanus toxoid is indicated, since there has been no booster in the last 5 years.

22. **(2)** Onychomycosis is the correct term. Hippocratic nails are clubbed nails and fingers associated with chronic heart and lung disorders; koilonychia is a concavity of the nail plate often associated with iron deficiency anemia; and anonychia is a total congenital absence of the nail.

23. **(2)** In cases of suspected drug reactions, it is recommended that the drug be discontinued and documented as the cause of the reaction in the client's record so it is not reintroduced.

24. **(4)** Excessive sweating can be normal, but the client needs to provide a history and have a physical exam performed to rule out any underlying causes. Therapies for hyperhidrosis are available. The Drysol is only for use on the feet and axilla. Full bathing is not recommended with this solution.

25. **(3)** The appearance indicates seborrheic keratosis. Actinic keratosis is an irregular, rough, scaly, white to erythematous macular lesion found most commonly on the dorsal surface of the hands, arms, neck, and face. It has malignant potential. Basal cell carcinoma is a smooth, round nodule with a pearly gray border and central induration. Senile lentigines are gray-brown, irregular, macular lesions on sun-exposed areas of the face, arms, and hands.

26. **(3)** Herpes zoster (shingles) is a vesicular dermatomal eruption related to a reactivation of latent varicella virus. It increases with advanced age and is characterized by burning pain and paresthesia along one or two dermatomes. This will not cross the midline. This discomfort may be accompanied by fever, malaise, or headache. The vesicular stage lasts 2 to 3 weeks. The vesicles are initially clear or blood-filled and become purulent. The area along the dermatome is erythematous, and the vesicles crust and then scab, which may leave hypopigmented scars. The other options describe painless lesions and are not specific to this prodromal stage.

27. **(1)** Antiviral therapy with acyclovir 800 mg 5 times per day for 7 days may speed healing if started within 2 to 3 days of onset, especially in immunocompromised individuals. Miconazole and clotrimazole are antifungal creams, and the prednisone would only be used to decrease the incidence of postherpetic neuralgia. Prednisone may increase the incidence of disseminated infection.

28. **(4)** These are classic signs of a basal cell carcinoma, also supported by the employment history of the client. Melanoma would be pigmented, compound nevus would not be firm or have telangiectasia, and bullous pemphigoid results in bullous lesions.

29. **(3)** The nurse should refer the client to a dermatologist immediately, since these findings are highly suggestive of a melanoma. Biopsy should never be done on a melanoma, and any delay could be detrimental to the outcome.

30. **(2)** Oral acyclovir is very effective in reducing intensity and duration of symptoms if administration is started early in the course of the disease. Herpes zoster does not usually recur at regular intervals but frequently lasts for several weeks.

31. **(3)** This client presents with a classic case of pityriasis rosea, a benign, self-limiting skin eruption of unknown etiology. Although a medication/allergen history would be warranted, referral to an allergy specialist or dermatologist would not be necessary. Triamcinolone would not be indicated, because the treatment is mainly symptomatic. Sunlight in moderate amounts has been shown to hasten healing in some cases.

32. **(3)** The signs and symptoms presented are classic for Lyme disease, which is transmitted by ticks. Therefore it would be important to inquire about potential exposure to ticks during the period before the development of signs and symptoms. Exposure to new skin care products would be important if the practitioner suspected an allergic reaction, which is not consistent with the signs and symptoms presented. Although a thorough medication history should always be obtained, it is most likely not going to reveal the cause of the signs and symptoms in this case. Tuberculosis does not present in this manner.

33. **(2)** This is the correct procedure for the shampoo; that is, after hair is shampooed and towel-dried, permethrin 1% (Nix) creme rinse should be applied to scalp and hair and left on for 10 minutes before rinsing. After the rinse, nits are removed with a nit comb. Shampoo treatment is repeated after 7 days, if living lice are still observed. Clothing and bedding should be washed or dry-cleaned. Family members should also be treated.

34. **(4)** Brown recluse spiders produce sharp pain at the instant of the bite, with subsequent minor swelling and erythema. Tissue necrosis may occur within 4 hours. A blue-gray to black macular halo may surround the bite, with eventual widening and sinking of the center of the lesion, leading to a "sinking infarct." This leaves a deep ulcer that takes weeks or months to heal.

35. **(2)** Deep puncture wounds are more likely to become infected with anaerobic organisms. The narrow, sharp feline incisors deeply puncture

tissue and may easily penetrate a bone or joint. Bites on the hand have the highest infection rate, whereas bites on the face have the lowest infection rate.

36. **(2)** Insects are more active, reproduce, and are present in greater numbers in the warm months (i.e., spring to early fall).

37. **(1)** Amoxicillin clavulanate potassium (Augmentin) is an excellent choice for the empiric treatment of animal bites. Keflex is not indicated because there are resistant strains of *Pasteurella multocida*, an organism present in 25% of dog bites and 50% of cat bites. An infected bite should be followed up on a daily basis until the infection clears. Open-wound management is indicated, not suturing.

38. **(2)** Heat application is contraindicated; ice packs are preferred, as is elevation, to decrease the edema. The area should be immobilized. Tetanus toxoid may be given along with antihistamines to reduce swelling and relieve itching.

39. **(4)** In addition to these symptoms, bronchospasm, hypertension, seizures, and altered mental status may occur. Black eschar is associated with a brown recluse spider bite.

40. **(4)** This was a poisonous coral snake bite. The typical symptoms are those listed plus the following: nausea, vomiting, and muscle fasciculations.

Pharmacology

41. **(1)** The description is consistent with candidiasis intertriginous, which is treated with an antifungal ointment or oral medication. It is not a staphylococcal infection; the area does not need to be kept moist but needs to be kept dry. An antibiotic ointment will not relieve the problem. Herpes zoster is treated with antiviral medications; this is not described as particularly painful, and it is bilateral.

42. **(1)** β-Blockers can exacerbate psoriasis. They are believed to decrease cyclic adenosine monophosphate–dependent protein kinase (an inhibitor of cell proliferation). Drugs in the other stated classifications have no known effect on psoriasis.

43. **(4)** Systemic antibiotics (such as tetracycline) offer the most effective treatment for inflammatory acne. Accutane is also very effective, but because of serious teratogenic side effects, it is not first-line treatment. Improvement in acne will not be noted for 4 to 8 weeks, and dietary changes have not been demonstrated to have any beneficial effect.

44. **(3)** Acyclovir offers no benefit for postherpetic pain, since this is a treatment for the acute phase during initial eruption of vesicular lesions.

45. **(3)** Clients need to be instructed to wash off podophyllin. It is to be applied sparingly, only to the wart, while avoiding normal skin, and allowed to dry thoroughly before the client dresses. There is no rationale for treatment with both liquid nitrogen and podophyllin.

46. **(3)** Systemic treatment with low-dose tetracycline is very effective for rosacea; topical treatment with metronidazole or low-dose hydrocortisone may also be useful. Oral cortisone and antifungal agents are not known to be effective. Topical 5-fluorouracil is used in the treatment of actinic keratosis, a precancerous skin condition.

47. **(1)** The maximum allowable dose for adults is 7 mg/kg lidocaine with epinephrine and 5 mg/kg lidocaine without epinephrine. Although local anesthetics are commonly used, the maximum allowable doses are rarely emphasized, and overdose can result in anaphylactic shock.

48. **(1)** Amitriptyline in low doses has been shown to be effective in treating neuropathic pain. Nonsteroidal antiinflammatory drugs (NSAIDs) can also be effective in treating the inflammatory component of herpes zoster pain. The most effective nonpharmacologic method of treating pain from shingles is the application of cool compresses. Heat has been shown to exacerbate neuropathic pain in some cases. Antidepressants and anticonvulsants have been shown to be effective adjuvant therapy in the treatment of neuropathic pain.

49. **(2)** Stevens-Johnson syndrome is a severe form of erythema multiforme that can be fatal. The clinical picture of this syndrome is mucous membrane lesions, conjunctival and corneal lesions, fever, malaise, arthralgia, and sloughing of the skin of the hands and feet. The distinguishing characteristics that

differentiate this condition are the eruption of vesicles, ulcerations of the mucosa, and the sloughing skin.

50. **(4)** Isotretinoin is extremely teratogenic; therefore a sexual assessment, along with a pregnancy test in women with child-bearing capacity, and contraceptive counseling should be done for all clients. The combination of alcohol and isotretinoin can cause a disulfiram-like reaction; therefore the use of alcohol should be avoided. Isotretinoin can cause photosensitivity, so the nurse practitioner should counsel the client to avoid sunlight, wear protective clothing and sunglasses, and apply sunscreen to all sun-exposed areas without acne. No conclusive relationship between diet and acne has been established.

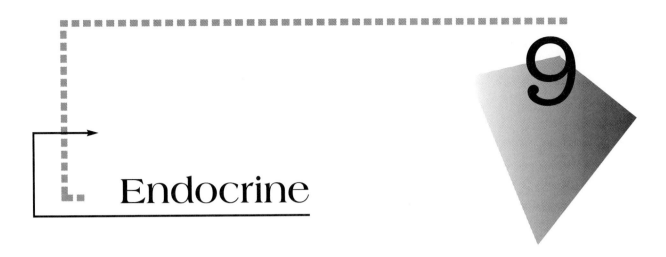

Endocrine

Physical Examination & Diagnostic Tests

1. What is the correct procedure for palpation of a client's thyroid gland?

   1. Stand behind the client, hyperextend the head, and palpate both sides simultaneously.

   2. Have the client lower his chin and lean his head slightly toward the side being evaluated.

   3. Hyperextend the head and have the client lean away from the side being evaluated.

   4. Have the client lean away from the side being examined and take a swallow of water.

2. When a client sips water and swallows, the thyroid gland:

   1. Moves downward and slightly posterior and feels smooth on palpation.

   2. Elongates and enlarges during the swallow and immediately returns to a resting position.

   3. Moves slightly out during the sipping and backward during the swallowing.

   4. Moves upward during the swallow and feels symmetrical and smooth to palpation.

3. Which question is **not** part of the Carville Diabetic Foot Screen?

   1. Has there been a change in the foot since the last evaluation?

   2. Does your foot hurt when you walk?

   3. Does the foot have an abnormal shape?

   4. Are the nails thick, too long, or overgrown?

4. While conducting the interview for a physical examination, the nurse practitioner identifies what finding in the client's history as being commonly associated with thyroid carcinoma?

   1. Family history of thyroid cancer.

   2. History of hyperthyroidism.

   3. Irradiation of the neck.

   4. Smoking for 15 years.

5. When doing a physical examination on a client with hyperthyroidism, a common neurologic finding is:

   1. Memory, attention, and problem-solving deficits.

   2. Diminished deep tendon reflexes.

   3. Severe cognitive impairment.

   4. Delusions and psychosis.

6. The treatment goal for glycemic control in a person with type 2 diabetes is to achieve and maintain a hemoglobin A_{1c} (HgbA$_{1c}$) level of:

   1. <10%.

   2. Between 6% and 9%.

   3. <7%.

   4. >8%.

7. Which findings would alert the nurse practitioner that a client might be experiencing a problem with the endocrine system?

   1. Coagulation abnormalities and fatigue.

   2. Growth abnormalities and glucose intolerance.

   3. Hypoxia and jaundice.

   4. Steatorrhea and abdominal distention.

8. The nurse practitioner finds a solitary nodule on a client's thyroid gland during a routine physical examination. The diagnostic test of choice is:

   1. Thyroid scan and antibody level.

   2. Thyroid-stimulating hormone (TSH) level and sonogram.

   3. X-ray examination of the thyroid.

   4. Fine-needle aspiration (FNA) biopsy.

9. An adult female client presents to the nurse practitioner's office, complaining of fatigue, weakness, and weight gain over the past 4 months. Physical examination reveals an elevated blood pressure, facial and supraclavicular fullness, hirsutism noted on the face, proximal muscle weakness, and facial and truncal distribution of acne. Appropriate laboratory tests the nurse practitioner should order include:

   1. Antinuclear antibody test (ANA) and a rheumatoid factor (RF) test.

   2. Three-hour glucose tolerance test and lipid profile.

   3. Red blood cell count and a calcium level.

   4. Dexamethasone suppression test, a urine free cortisol level, and TSH/thyroxine (T_4) test.

10. The nurse practitioner would anticipate what laboratory values in the client with Graves' disease?

    1. TSH levels to be increased.

    2. TSH levels to be decreased.

    3. TSH levels to be within normal limits (WNL).

    4. T_4 levels to be decreased.

11. What information is correct regarding foot screening with a nylon filament (5.07 Semmes-Weinstein)?

    1. Use a 25-g filament and apply along perimeter of any scar or ulcer tissue.

    2. Apply the filament at a 45-degree angle to the skin surface.

    3. Apply sufficient force for approximately 1.5 seconds to cause the filament to bend.

    4. Slide the filament across the skin and make repetitive contact to each of the 10 sites.

12. For a diagnosis of diabetes to be made, the client must have 2 fasting plasma glucose levels documented on 2 different occasions greater than or equal to:

    1. 200 mg/dl

    2. 140 mg/dl

    3. 126 mg/dl

    4. 110 mg/dl

Disorders

13. Which statement best describes type 1 diabetes?

    1. It is an autosomal dominant genetic disorder.

    2. It is caused by an autoimmune destruction of the β cells.

3. Overnutrition and resulting obesity are major risk factors.

4. It may be prevented by exercise, which increases the concentration of insulin receptors.

14. A client has had diabetes for more than 5 years. With whom should the nurse practitioner maintain an annual referral for this client?

    1. A cardiologist.

    2. A dietitian.

    3. A vascular surgeon.

    4. An ophthalmologist.

15. Hirsutism in a female with normal menstruation and normal plasma androgens is most likely:

    1. Caused by an ovarian tumor.

    2. A symptom of Cushing's syndrome.

    3. Idiopathic.

    4. Associated with polycystic ovary disease.

16. Pathophysiologic changes responsible for decreased testosterone levels develop in the:

    1. Hypothalamus.

    2. Anterior pituitary.

    3. Testes.

    4. All of the above.

17. The most common cause of poor control of type 1 diabetes during the adolescent period is:

    1. Too frequent evaluation of blood sugar.

    2. Increased intake of protein.

    3. Too much exercise.

    4. Denial of the severity of the condition.

18. When counseling a client with diabetes about foot care, it is important to emphasize:

    1. Daily foot soaks in warm, soapy water.

    2. Careful daily foot inspections.

    3. Trimming corns and calluses regularly.

    4. Trimming toenails close to the bed of the nail.

19. An adult client presents to the nurse practitioner for evaluation of polyuria, polydipsia, and weight loss. Which lab test result would require immediate intervention by the nurse practitioner?

    1. An $HgbA_{1c}$ level of 14%.

    2. A serum glucose level of 150 mg/dl.

    3. An $HgbA_{1c}$ level of 6.0%.

    4. A serum glucose level of 65 mg/dl.

20. An adult client is being evaluated for hypoglycemia caused by a blood sugar of 58 mg/dl. The nurse practitioner would begin formulating the differential diagnosis by:

    1. Determining whether the hypoglycemia is fasting or postprandial.

    2. Ascertaining whether it is related to alcohol use.

    3. Determining whether the client has other medical problems.

    4. Reassuring the client that it is a benign problem.

21. An older adult male client complains of lethargy, cold intolerance, weight gain, and yellowing of the palms. The most important laboratory study ordered by the nurse practitioner in diagnosing this condition is:

    1. Complete blood count.

    2. Liver enzymes.

    3. Thyroid panel.

    4. Cardiac enzymes.

22. A middle-aged, normally healthy female presents for evaluation of intermittent palpitations. She also reports mood variability, tremulousness, difficulty falling asleep, and a 10-lb weight loss despite a normal appetite. She feels warm most of the time and wonders whether she is perimenopausal. She has no history of heart disease. The objective data that would yield the most useful information would be results of:

    1. Electrocardiogram (ECG).

    2. TSH and free T_4 tests.

    3. Electrolyte panel.

    4. Holter monitoring.

23. An adult client presents to the clinic complaining of fatigue, weakness, weight gain in spite of lack of appetite, and feelings of depression. Physical examination reveals an obese, alert female with thinning hair, bilateral chest puffiness, increased facial hair, supraclavicular fat pad, thin arms and legs, purple striae on the abdomen, and multiple ecchymotic areas on extremities. Her vital signs are blood pressure (BP) 158/96 mm Hg, pulse 88 bpm, respirations 22 breaths/min. Laboratory tests reveal a fasting blood sugar (FBS) level of 200 mg/dl, electrolyte panel WNL except for potassium 3.0 mEq/L, hemoglobin 11.8 g, and hematocrit 34%. This assessment information would support the nurse practitioner's diagnosis of:

    1. Addison's disease.

    2. Pheochromocytoma.

    3. Cushing's syndrome.

    4. Hypoaldosteronism.

24. Which of the following is the best alternative for treating hyperthyroidism diagnosed during the first trimester of pregnancy?

    1. Radioactive iodine in smaller than usual dose during the first trimester.

    2. Propylthiouracil during the first trimester, subtotal thyroidectomy during the second trimester, no thyroid replacement.

    3. Propylthiouracil during the first trimester, subtotal thyroidectomy during the second trimester, thyroid replacement.

    4. No treatment until after delivery.

25. Clinical findings in a client with hypothyroidism include:

    1. Hyperactive bowel sounds.

    2. Oily skin and acne.

    3. Postural tremors of the hands.

    4. Edema of the face and eyelids.

26. A young adult male reports anxiety, tremulousness, headaches, palpitations, and sweating 2 to 4 hours after eating. Findings on physical examination are normal. No lab test results are currently available. No history of any medical conditions is reported. What is the most likely diagnosis?

    1. Dumping syndrome.

    2. Hypoglycemia.

    3. Alcohol abuse.

    4. Hyperthyroidism.

27. Which of the following is the most likely cause of hypercalcemia in the medically well asymptomatic adult?

    1. Hyperthyroidism.

    2. Hyperparathyroidism.

    3. Hyperpituitarism.

    4. Hypothyroidism.

28. A middle-aged male with no previous medical history presents with a 30-lb weight gain in 2.5 months. He denies any medication use or allergies. He was recently laid off of a very active job and has been sedentary. Physical exam reveals BP 172/ 111 mm Hg, central obesity, and FBS level 200 mg/dl. What is the most likely cause of this client's weight gain?

    1. Cushing's disease.

    2. Hypothyroidism.

    3. Depression.

    4. Diabetes.

29. A middle-aged female presents with agitation, confusion, fever, tachycardia, and diaphoresis. Her daughter states that these symptoms were preceded by nausea, vomiting, and abdominal pain. There is no history of cardiac disease, diabetes, or substance abuse. She began receiving some "anti drug" 2 weeks ago and is scheduled for some kind of throat surgery next week (per daughter). On the basis of this history, the nurse practitioner immediately orders:

    1. TSH and T_4 tests.

    2. Urinalysis.

    3. Spinal tap.

    4. Computed tomography of the head.

30. A 45-year-old female client presents to the nurse practitioner's office, complaining of a 6-month history of fatigue, 15-lb weight gain, lethargy, an inability to tolerate cold temperatures, forgetfulness, hair loss, and constipation. Physical findings include dry coarse skin, periorbital edema and puffy facies, bradycardia, hyporeflexia and muscle weakness, and a smooth goitrous thyroid. The nurse practitioner would make the diagnosis of:

1. Congestive heart failure (CHF).

2. Diabetes mellitus (DM).

3. Hypothyroidism.

4. Thyroid cancer.

31. A client with diabetes has been taking 6 U of regular insulin and 12 U of Lente insulin in the morning. In the evening she has been taking 3 U of regular insulin and 8 U of Lente insulin. The client has been monitoring her blood glucose levels and she shows the nurse practitioner the following chart.

	7 AM	Noon	5 PM	Bedtime
Monday	100	76	98	109
Tuesday	119	75	88	110
Wednesday	119	66	86	100
Thursday	123	70	111	122
Friday	128	60	99	110

The nurse practitioner adjusts the client's insulin level by:

1. Increasing the dose of regular insulin.

2. Decreasing the dose of regular insulin.

3. Decreasing the dose of Lente insulin.

4. Increasing both insulin doses.

32. The role of the nurse practitioner in the initial management of a client with a thyroid nodule involves:

1. Referring the client to an endocrinologist for further evaluation.

2. Obtaining a biopsy specimen by FNA of the nodule and sending it to the cytology department.

3. Ordering a sonogram and a thyroid scan.

4. Ordering levothyroxine (Synthroid) to reduce the size of the nodule.

33. When teaching a client with diabetes about "sick day" guidelines, the nurse practitioner explains that the client should:

1. Stop measuring blood glucose and only check urine for ketones.

2. Not take your usual dose of insulin at the usual time.

3. Be sure to take metformin (Glucophage) and acarbose (Precose), even if nausea and vomiting are present.

4. Administer extra doses of regular insulin according to instructions for blood glucose levels above 240 mg/dl.

34. A young adult female client presents to the clinic with complaints of nervousness, tremulousness, palpitations, heat intolerance, fatigue, weight loss, and polyphagia. After obtaining a complete history and performing a physical examination, along with thyroid function tests, the nurse practitioner makes the diagnosis of hyperthyroidism, recognizing that the most common cause of this condition is:

1. Thyroid cancer.

2. Graves' disease.

3. Pituitary adenoma.

4. Postpartum thyroiditis.

35. A young adult male client presents to the nurse practitioner's office, stating that he found a lump in his neck while shaving. Physical examination reveals a firm, 2-cm nodule that is fixed and nontender located on the right lobe of the thyroid gland. Right posterior cervical lymphadenopathy is also noted. The nurse practitioner should:

1. Order a TSH level to determine thyroid function, and refer the client to a surgeon for a fine-needle biopsy of the nodule.

2. No intervention is necessary at this time; schedule a follow-up visit in 6 months.

3. Prescribe levothyroxine (Synthroid) 0.1 mg PO daily and schedule a 6-week follow-up visit.

4. The client's thyroid should immediately be ablated with radioactive iodine, and the patient should be referred to an endocrinologist.

36. A client with Graves' disease is to have radioactive I^{131} therapy. When teaching about this treatment, what information should the nurse practitioner include?

    1. Clients are highly radioactive for approximately 7 days after treatment and need to be isolated.

    2. Clients should not become pregnant during or after receiving this therapy because of the potential for teratogenic effects.

    3. Clients may experience hypothyroidism after this treatment and will therefore need to have regular TSH and T_4 levels determined and may require thyroid hormone replacement therapy.

    4. This therapy is contraindicated in clients with cardiac disease.

37. During an evaluation of a client with prediabetes, the nurse practitioner identifies what finding in the client's objective data as being associated with the dysmetabolic syndrome (insulin resistance syndrome)?

    1. Triglycerides >150 mg/dl.

    2. High-density lipoprotein (HDL) cholesterol level >40 mg/dl in men and >50 mg/dl in women.

    3. BP <130/85 mm Hg.

    4. Fasting glucose level <110 mg/dl.

38. While taking a history from a client, the nurse practitioner identifies what finding that may be associated with osteopenia/osteoporosis?

    1. High calcium intake.

    2. Minimal alcohol intake.

    3. Smoking 1 pack of cigarettes per day for 20 years.

    4. Walking 30 minutes 4 days a week.

39. Of the following risk factors for osteoporosis, which would the nurse practitioner see primarily in men?

    1. Smoking 2 packs of cigarettes per day.

    2. Excessive use of alcohol.

    3. Low testosterone level.

    4. Minimal exercise.

40. When prescribing a meal plan for a client with type 2 diabetes, the nurse practitioner educates the client that the macronutrient with the most influence on the postprandial glucose levels is

    1. Fiber.

    2. Fat.

    3. Protein.

    4. Carbohydrate.

Pharmacology

41. When prescribing oral medications for an overweight person with type 2 diabetes who also has a voracious appetite, the nurse practitioner is likely to select which of the following medications to encourage weight loss and reduce appetite?

    1. Nateglinide (Starlix).

    2. Pioglitazone (Actos).

    3. Metformin (Glucophage).

    4. Glyburide (Micronase).

42. Glargine (Lantus) is an insulin analog that essentially has no peak and is usually administered:

    1. Before meals.

    2. With Humalog (Lispro).

    3. Before breakfast and dinner.

    4. Once a day.

43. An adult male client with type 2 diabetes has a creatinine level of 1.8 mg/dl. Which of the following drugs is contraindicated?

    1. Pioglitazone (Actos).

    2. Metformin (Glucophage).

    3. Repaglinide (Prandin).

    4. Acarbose (Precose).

44. Clients who begin receiving metformin (Glucophage) need to be monitored closely for what potential side effect?

    1. Significant increase in weight.

    2. Elevation of low-density lipoprotein (LDL) cholesterol level.

    3. Lactic acidosis.

    4. Increase in insulin requirements.

45. The nurse practitioner has written an order for a client with type 2 diabetes to take glipizide (Glucotrol) 10 mg PO bid. This medication is believed to reduce the blood glucose level by:

    1. Delaying the cellular uptake of potassium and insulin.

    2. Stimulating insulin release from the pancreas.

    3. Decreasing the body's need for and utilization of insulin at the cellular level.

    4. Interfering with the absorption and metabolism of fats and carbohydrates.

46. The nurse practitioner would expect which symptom to be a side effect of metformin (Glucophage)?

    1. Gastrointestinal upset.

    2. Photophobia.

    3. Hyperglycemia.

    4. Skin eruptions.

47. A client is receiving antithyroid medication. The nurse practitioner understands that:

    1. Lifelong daily treatment is necessary to keep TSH levels within the normal range.

    2. Antithyroid medications do not cross the placenta.

    3. The medications are somewhat expensive and have serious cardiac and hematologic side effects.

    4. Clients remain on the medications for 1 to 2 years and then the medication is gradually withdrawn.

48. When prescribing an antihypertensive medication for a client with type 2 diabetes, the nurse practitioner is aware that the drug classifications that would tend to reduce insulin sensitivity are:

    1. Diuretics and calcium channel blockers.

    2. Diuretics and β-blockers.

    3. Calcium channel blockers and angiotensin-converting enzyme (ACE) inhibitors.

    4. α-Blockers and ACE inhibitors.

49. A 35-year-old female sees the nurse practitioner with a complaint of cold intolerance, fatigue, dry skin, weight gain, and heavy menstrual periods. On physical exam, she is found to have a pulse of 58 bpm; a "waxy," sallow complexion; and a firm goiter. Her TSH level is checked and found to be 176 mU/L. The best treatment choice for this client is:

    1. Begin administration of levothyroxine (Synthroid) at 0.025 mg PO qd and repeat TSH test in 2 weeks.

    2. Administer a "loading dose" of oral levothyroxine (Synthroid) and prescribe a full replacement dose of levothyroxine (Synthroid).

    3. Administer a "loading dose" of IV levothyroxine (Synthroid) and prescribe a half replacement dose of levothyroxine (Synthroid).

    4. Begin administration of levothyroxine (Synthroid) at a dose of 0.1 mg PO qd and recheck TSH level in 6 weeks.

50. The nurse practitioner is seeing a man for a preoperative evaluation and exam. He is scheduled to undergo coronary artery bypass grafting. Physical exam reveals the client to have mild facial puffiness, hoarse voice, and dry skin. Thyroid function tests were done and the client was found to have a TSH level of 34 mU/L. The recommended treatment for this client is:

    1. Give a loading IV bolus of levothyroxine (Synthroid) 0.5 mg and proceed with surgery.

    2. Cancel surgery and send him home to begin treatment with a daily dose of oral levothyroxine (Synthroid) 0.1 mg and reschedule surgery.

    3. Begin treatment with oral levothyroxine (Synthroid) and monitor client in the hospital until the euthyroidism is achieved.

    4. Proceed with surgery and treat hypothyroidism postoperatively.

51. The nurse practitioner is seeing an obese, middle-aged female client for a follow-up visit. She was given a diagnosis of type 2 diabetes 3 months ago and started a regimen of diet and exercise. Today her fasting plasma glucose level is 200 mg/dl and HgbA$_{1c}$ level is 10%. She has lost 2 lb. She reports that her home glucose level has ranged from 180 to 300 mg/dl. The rest of the results of the chemistry profile are WNL. The best treatment choice for this client is:

    1. Review her diet and exercise plan, increase exercise regimen, and reduce caloric intake. Schedule her for another follow-up visit in 3 months.

    2. Begin administration of sliding-scale insulin and instruct her on recording glucose and insulin requirements. Schedule her to return in 1 week for reevaluation.

    3. Initiate treatment with metformin (glucophage).

    4. Initiate treatment with an oral sulfonylurea agent (e.g., glyburide).

52. What is associated with long-term overtreatment with levothyroxine (Synthroid)?

    1. Tachycardia.

    2. Severe osteoporosis.

    3. Insomnia.

    4. Sweating.

53. A middle-aged male presents for a diabetes follow-up exam. He has been in good health without identified complications of diabetes. His FBS is 100 and his personal records indicate that he is taking insulin in the prescribed amounts and times. Vital signs are BP 142/98 mm Hg, pulse 80 bpm, respirations 20 breaths/min. Today's plan would include:

    1. Beginning treatment with diuretics and a β-blocker.

    2. Beginning administration of an ACE inhibitor and considering addition of a diuretic.

    3. Obtaining an ECG and a chest x-ray film.

    4. Having him return for BP check in 5 to 7 days.

54. An adult male has recently began taking insulin. His regimen is two daily injections, with two thirds of the total daily insulin in the morning and one third in the evening. He is using the 70/30 mixture of intermediate- and short-acting insulin in both injections. He presents for a follow-up visit with his log of blood glucose levels. The nurse practitioner notes that his recorded glucose levels before the evening meal have been in the 60 to 70 mg/dl range. Other checks during the day are in the 100 to 120 mg/dl range. What adjustments need to be made?

    1. Intermediate insulin, change 70/30 combination to self-mix and reduce AM intermediate dose.

    2. Regular insulin, reduce AM dose of 70/30.

    3. Intermediate insulin, reduce AM dose of 70/30.

    4. Regular insulin, change 70/30 to self-mix and reduce AM regular dose.

55. A client receiving antithyroid drug therapy for hyperthyroidism presents with complaints of palpitations and dry mouth for the past 2 days. He has had a cough and cold symptoms for the past 3 days, which he has been treating with over-the-counter medications. Which medication would the nurse practitioner encourage the client to avoid?

    1. Benzocaine (Chloraseptic) lozenge.

    2. Guaifenesin (Robitussin).

    3. Ibuprofen (Advil).

    4. Pseudoephedrine (Sudafed).

56. What is the most frequent complaint of clients who use insulin pumps?

    1. Problems with elevated glucose after changing the catheter-type (nonneedle) infusion set.

    2. Skin and site problems with dressing adhesive not sticking and redness and pain at infusion site.

    3. Mechanical problems with the pump's digital readout.

    4. Understanding "sick day" management modifications.

57. The nurse practitioner understands that pioglitazone (Actos) or rosiglitazone (Avandia) is indicated for:

    1. Clients with gestational diabetes.

    2. Clients with brittle (type 1) diabetes.

3. Clients with type 2 diabetes who require insulin who have poor glycemic control and insulin resistance.

4. Clients with type 2 diabetes to prevent the rapid postprandial blood glucose surges by delaying carbohydrate absorption.

58. An older client with a history of hypertension and coronary bypass surgery has been given a diagnosis of hypothyroidism. Appropriate medication management is:

1. Levothyroxine (Synthroid) 0.1 mg daily and return in 6 weeks for follow-up.

2. Desiccated thyroid extract 2 grains daily and return in 6 weeks for follow-up.

3. Levothyroxine (Synthroid) 0.025 mg daily for 6 weeks with slow gradual increase in dosage every 4 to 6 weeks until therapeutic level is achieved.

4. Methimazole (Tapazole) 15 mg daily in three divided doses, gradually increasing dose every 4 weeks until a therapeutic level is achieved.

59. A client is given a new diagnosis of hypothyroidism and begins receiving levothyroxine (Synthroid) 0.1 mg PO daily. Which of the following statements describes appropriate follow up by the nurse practitioner?

1. No follow-up visits are necessary.

2. The client should return to the clinic in 4 to 6 weeks for TSH level to determine whether there has been symptomatic improvement.

3. The client should have blood drawn weekly for determination of levothyroxine levels.

4. The client should have monthly CBCs while taking levothyroxine (Synthroid), because the medication has been found to be myelosuppressive.

60. Classes of medications commonly used to treat hyperthyroid conditions include:

1. Antibiotics and corticosteroids.

2. ACE inhibitors, anxiolytics, and antithyroid medications.

3. β-Blockers, nonsteroidal antiinflammatory drugs (NSAIDs), and antithyroid medications.

4. Calcium channel blockers and corticosteroids.

61. A client with hypothyroidism has been receiving daily levothyroxine (Synthroid) for 3 weeks. The client now presents with complaints of chest pain. The nurse practitioner should:

1. Discontinue the levothyroxine (Synthroid), because this is a contraindication to continuing this medication.

2. Schedule the client for a stress test.

3. Decrease the dose of levothyroxine (Synthroid), order an ECG, and consult with a collaborating physician.

4. Prescribe an anxiolytic agent for the client.

62. A young adult is discharged home with a prescription for DDAVP (desmopressin acetate) for diabetes insipidus after removal of a pituitary tumor. On examination, it is noted that the client is lethargic but has 4+ deep tendon reflexes. The nurse practitioner suspects:

1. Noncompliance with therapy.

2. Water intoxication

3. Increased vasopressor effect.

4. Interaction with over-the counter (OTC) cough medicine products.

63. When monitoring a client's insulin therapy regimen, the nurse practitioner is aware that the NPH to regular insulin proportions are:

1. 2:1 in the AM and 1:1 in the PM.

2. 1:1 in the AM and 1:2 in the PM.

3. 1:2 in the AM and 2:1 in the PM.

4. 1:1 in the AM and PM.

64. The nurse practitioner understands that lispro insulin (Humalog):

1. Can be injected just before eating.

2. Is less costly than regular insulin.

3. Increases the likelihood of late postprandial hypoglycemia because of its length of action.

4. Has a long-term safety profile and does not cause any teratogenic effects.

65. When prescribing sulfonylureas, the nurse practitioner educates the client that the most common side effect of therapy is:

    1. Upset stomach.

    2. Diarrhea.

    3. Angina.

    4. Hypoglycemia.

66. The primary action of pioglitazone (Actos) and rosiglitazone (Avandia) is to

    1. Decrease hepatic glucose output.

    2. Increase secretion of insulin from the pancreas.

    3. Increase glucose uptake into the muscle and fat.

    4. Increase the postprandial uptake of glucose into the intestine.

9 Answers & Rationales

Physical Examination & Diagnostic Tests

1. **(2)** During examination of the thyroid, it is important to have the client relax the sternocleidomastoid muscles. This can be done by having the client lean toward the side being evaluated.

2. **(4)** The thyroid gland is fixed to the trachea and thus ascends during swallowing. This assists the nurse practitioner in distinguishing thyroid structures from other neck masses. The gland's size, degree of enlargement, consistency, and surface characteristics and the presence of nodules or bruits are noted during the examination.

3. **(2)** There are five questions in the Carville Diabetic Foot Screen. They are as follows: Has there been a change in the foot since the last evaluation? Is there a foot ulcer now or history of foot ulcer? Does the foot have an abnormal shape? Is there weakness in the ankle or foot? Are the nails thick, too long, or overgrown? There is no reference to pain in this screening.

4. **(3)** Papillary carcinoma is the most common form of thyroid cancer. It is associated with a history of exposure to radiation. Family history, history of hyperthyroidism, and smoking are not considered significant risk factors for this malignancy.

5. **(1)** The high level of thyroid hormone affects the nervous system, causing sympathomimetic symptoms such as brisk deep tendon reflexes, fine rapid tremor of the hands, restlessness, irritability, insomnia, dreams, and nightmares but rarely severe cognitive impairment and psychosis.

6. **(3)** The American Diabetes Association (ADA) recommends a hemoglobin A_{1c} (HgbA$_{1c}$) level of <7% as an important treatment goal to decrease the risk of long-term complications. An HgbA$_{1c}$ level of >8% is an indication that action needs to be taken, either by making a change in medication or reinforcing education.

7. **(2)** Growth abnormalities are associated with anterior pituitary dysfunction, and glucose intolerance is associated with diabetes related to pancreas dysfunction. Coagulation abnormalities and fatigue would be associated with hematologic dysfunction. Hypoxia would be associated with oxygenation problems, and jaundice, with liver or biliary problems. Steatorrhea is associated with malabsorption syndrome and cystic fibrosis.

8. **(4)** Although the primary care provider may obtain thyroid-stimulating hormone (TSH) and antibody levels, the preferred diagnostic tool for the endocrinologist is the fine-needle aspiration (FNA) biopsy. Scans, sonography, and x-ray films can be used in initial screening; they do not assist in the determination of whether the nodule is malignant. The aspirate is sent out for cytologic examination and interpretation.

9. **(4)** The dexamethasone suppression test is the best screening test for Cushing's disease, and a 24-hour urine collection for measurement of free cortisol is the best confirmatory test for Cushing's disease. Measurement of TSH/thyroxine (T$_4$) levels may also be appropriate to rule out a thyroid condition, since some of the client's signs and symptoms

are consistent with thyroid dysfunction. Antinuclear antibody (ANA) and rheumatoid factor (RF) tests are ordered when rheumatoid arthritis or systemic lupus erythematosus (SLE) is suspected; this client's clinical picture is not consistent with these conditions. A red blood cell count would be done to rule out anemia, a potential problem for this client because of the history of fatigue, but the rest of the clinical picture points to something other than anemia. There are no clinical findings to suggest that a calcium level should be determined.

10. **(2)** TSH levels should be decreased in a client with Graves' disease, because thyroid-stimulating immunoglobulins bind to TSH receptors, which increase T_4 synthesis and release, subsequently suppressing TSH levels.

11. **(3)** Correct procedure is to use a 10-g (5.07 Semmes-Weinstein) filament and apply it to 10 sites on the foot (1 on the top of the foot and 9 on the heel, sole, and toes). The filament is to be applied perpendicularly (at a 90-degree angle) to the skin surface and sufficient force is to be applied for 1.5 seconds to cause the filament to bend. The filament should not be allowed to slide across the skin or make repetitive contact with each test site. Randomizing the selection of test sites (start with big toe → heel → instep area → little toe → etc.) and the time between successive tests to reduce client guessing and having the client close his or her eyes also helps.

12. **(3)** In 1997, the ADA revised the classification and diagnostic criteria for diabetes to include any 1 of the 3 following findings, which must be confirmed on a subsequent day:

- Random plasma glucose level greater than or equal to 200 mg/dl and acute symptoms of diabetes (polyuria, polydipsia, or polyphagia).
- Fasting plasma glucose level greater than or equal to 126 mg/dl.
- Two-hour plasma glucose level greater than or equal to 200 mg/dl.

Disorders

13. **(2)** Type (1) diabetes is caused by destruction of the β cells mediated through the immune system. The other three choices refer to type 2 diabetes.

14. **(4)** An annual eye exam with the pupils dilated should be done by a specialist who can recognize subtle abnormalities. Although the other health care providers can offer important contributions to diabetic care, referrals to them would be done on an as-needed basis rather than annually.

15. **(3)** Because of the normal menstrual periods and androgen plasma level, this hirsutism would be considered idiopathic. Diseases related to the ovaries would cause changes in the menstrual cycle, and a client with Cushing's syndrome would have adrenal androgen overproduction.

16. **(4)** Testosterone production is regulated by the hypothalamic-pituitary-testicular (HPT) axis. Thus abnormalities in any one of these areas can affect the production of testosterone.

17. **(4)** All of these contribute significantly to difficulty controlling diabetes in the teen years. Hormonal changes and the desire to become independent increase emotional conflicts. Teens have a great desire to be like their peers and do not want to be regimented in following a specific diet and adhering to a treatment plan.

18. **(2)** It is important for clients with diabetes to have their feet inspected daily, either per self-exam or by a family member. Feet should be washed daily but never soaked. Corns and calluses should be cared for by a professional. Nails should be trimmed straight across to avoid injury to the nail beds.

19. **(1)** The normal serum glucose level for adults ranges from 70 to 120 mg/dl. Diabetic acidosis is not of concern until the glucose level is >300 mg/dl. A hemoglobin A_{1c} (HgbA$_{1c}$) level of >8.0% indicates poor glucose control over the past few months.

20. **(1)** True hypoglycemia can be categorized as to whether it is fasting or postprandial. Postprandial hypoglycemia may be caused by early adult-onset diabetes or postgastrectomy syndrome. Fasting hypoglycemia is most commonly caused by excessive doses of insulin or by sulfonylureas alone or in combination with biguanides and/or thiazolidinediones.

21. **(3)** The symptoms are suggestive of hypothyroidism, and thyroid studies (TSH level) would be the most important.

22. **(2)** This middle-aged female client presents with many of the classic symptoms of early hyperthyroidism. A suppressed TSH level with an elevated free T_4 level establishes the diagnosis of hyperthyroidism.

23. **(3)** The client's physical findings and habitus, along with hypertension and hypokalemia, are associated with Cushing's syndrome, which is a state of excessive cortisol production caused by a pituitary tumor. A Cushing's-like syndrome is often associated with prolonged glucocorticoid administration. Obesity is the primary finding in Cushing's syndrome, along with the "moon face," "dowager" or "buffalo hump," truncal obesity, hirsutism in women, and impotence and loss of body hair in men. Addison's disease is characterized by hyperkalemia, hyponatremia, hypoglycemia, anemia, and hypercalcemia. Clients with hypoaldosteronism (impaired renin secretion) have hyperkalemia. Pheochromocytoma would be included in the differential diagnosis for this client because of the hypertension; the other findings are not consistent with this diagnosis.

24. **(3)** Administration of low-dose antithyroid drugs is considered a good alternative to prevent the ill effects of hyperthyroidism on the mother and developing fetus until surgery can be performed. It is noted that some opt to use an antithyroid drug until after delivery and then have surgery. Removal of the thyroid during the second trimester can be performed safely and is the usual recommendation. Thyroid hormone replacement is essential after removal of the gland.

25. **(4)** Accumulation of hyaluronic acid in interstitial tissues increases capillary permeability to albumin and accounts for the interstitial edema that is noted in the face and eyelids of individuals with hypothyroidism.

26. **(2)** Although alcohol abuse may be a cause of hypoglycemia, this client is presenting with classic symptoms of postprandial hypoglycemia. It would be a good idea to assess for alcohol abuse as the cause of hypoglycemia.

27. **(2)** Hyperparathyroidism accounts for more than 60% of cases of hypercalcemia and is likely to be the explanation for elevated serum calcium levels.

28. **(1)** Although Option #3 may explain the weight gain, Cushing's disease is correct because of the constellation of symptoms of rapid weight gain, hypertension, and elevated blood sugar level. These symptoms suggest adrenal dysfunction. Serum cortisol and corticotropin levels should be checked.

29. **(1)** This woman is likely experiencing the life-threatening syndrome that can occur in decompensated hyperthyroidism. The clues are her symptom presentation and progression, the new "anti drug," and the upcoming throat surgery.

30. **(3)** The symptoms describe the classic presentation of a client with hypothyroidism. A client with congestive heart failure (CHF) would exhibit jugular venous distention and have rales and peripheral edema. The criteria for diagnosing diabetes mellitus (DM) are polydipsia, polyphagia, polyuria, and weight loss. Thyroid cancer commonly presents without physical symptoms, and often the only physical finding is a hard, fixed nodule on the thyroid gland.

31. **(2)** The client's blood sugar level is low around lunch time, which is when the level of regular insulin is peaking (3 to 4 hours), so a reduction in the dose of regular insulin would be beneficial.

32. **(1)** The nurse practitioner's role in primary care for a client with a thyroid nodule initially involves the early identification of the thyroid nodule on physical examination, referral of the client to an endocrinologist for further evaluation, and possibly doing some preliminary TSH and antibody testing. The endocrinologist performs the FNA biopsy. Levothyroxine may or may not be used to diminish the size of the nodule on the basis of the findings from the FNA biopsy and the endocrinologist's chosen treatment plan.

33. **(4)** It is important for clients with diabetes to understand that when they are sick, their blood glucose levels will probably increase, even when they are not eating. It is most important for them to monitor blood glucose levels every 2 to 4 hours and check urine for ketones if the glucose level is >240 mg/dl. The medications in Option #3 *should not* be given

until the client's nausea and vomiting have subsided and he or she has resumed a normal diet (blood glucose monitoring is important during this period).

34. **(2)** Graves' disease, an autoimmune condition also known as *diffuse toxic goiter*, is the most common cause of hyperthyroidism in this age group. Much less common causes include cancer of the thyroid, adenoma of the pituitary gland, and postpartum (or silent) thyroiditis.

35. **(1)** The TSH level should be ordered to determine whether the client's condition is euthyroid, hypothyroid, or hyperthyroid. The client should also be sent to an endocrinologist/surgeon because biopsies should be performed on all nodules of the thyroid to rule out malignancy. Watching and waiting is inappropriate without having a biopsy performed. Thyroid hormone replacement therapy would only be indicated in clients with hypothyroidism in whom thyroid cancer has been ruled out. Thyroid ablation may be indicated in clients whose FNA biopsy results are positive for thyroid cancer, but this cannot be determined without a surgeon's intervention.

36. **(3)** Hypothyroidism often follows this treatment, with 50% of clients requiring replacement therapy in the first year and nearly 100% requiring replacement therapy within 10 years. For this reason, regular monitoring of TSH/T$_4$ levels should be done. Clients emit a small amount of radioactivity after receiving the dose used to treat this condition but do not require isolation for 7 days. Radioactive iodine is very safe without an increased risk of gonad chromosomal abnormalities; therefore there is no contraindication to becoming pregnant after therapy. Clients are counseled to avoid becoming pregnant while receiving treatment and to avoid children and pregnant women after receiving the oral ablation dose. This therapy is recommended for clients who have cardiac disease associated with their thyroid condition.

37. **(1)** The National Cholesterol Education Program (NCEP) Adult Treatment Panel (ATP) III states that the metabolic syndrome exists when a client has met three of the following criteria:

- Triglyceride level >150 mg/dl.
- High-density lipoprotein (HDL) cholesterol level <40 mg/dl in men and <50 mg/dl in women.

- Waist circumference >102 cm (>40 inches) in men and >88 cm (>35 inches) in women.
- Blood pressure 130/85 mm Hg.
- Fasting glucose level >110 mg/dl.

38. **(3)** Smoking has been shown to cause thinning of the bones and lead to the development of osteopenia/osteoporosis. Options #1, #2, and #4 are all self-care practices that may prevent or delay the onset of osteopenia/osteoporosis.

39. **(3)** Low testosterone levels can occur as a result of treatment for prostate cancer and can also occur with longstanding liver disease. Options #1, #2, and #4 are risk factors for osteoporosis that can occur in men and women alike.

40. **(4)** Carbohydrate is the macronutrient with the greatest impact on postprandial glucose levels. Ingested protein has minimal effect on the blood glucose levels. A diet high in fat may be associated with cardiovascular disease. Fiber has little effect on the plasma glucose response, but it may result in a decrease in low-density lipoprotein (LDL) cholesterol.

Pharmacology

41. **(3)** Metformin (Glucophage) is associated with weight loss and appetite suppression, although the actual cause of weight loss is unknown. Nateglinide (Starlix) and glyburide (Micronase) are considered insulin secretagogues, which tend to stimulate insulin secretion from the pancreas, thus causing a slight weight gain. Pioglitazone (Actos) is an insulin sensitizer and increases glucose uptake by muscle and fat. Common side effects include fluid retention and increase in central adiposity.

42. **(4)** Glargine (Lantuss) is considered a long-acting (background) insulin that is usually given once a day. It was introduced to the market in 2001 and is thought to last 24 hours without a peak. It is a clear insulin that must be given alone and not mixed with any other insulin. Humalog (Lispro) or Nova log (Aspart) is usually given 3 times a day with meals.

43. **(2)** Metformin (Glucophage) should not be given to men with a serum creatinine level greater than or equal to 1.5 mg/dl and women with a serum creatinine level greater than or equal to

1.4 mg/dl because it can predispose these clients to lactic acidosis. Pioglitazone (Actos) and Repaglinide (Prandin) are primarily metabolized in the liver and require monitoring of liver function studies. Acarbose (Precose) is primarily metabolized in the gastrointestinal tract.

44. **(3)** Lactic acidosis is a potentially severe and fatal reaction to metformin. Metformin does not contribute to weight gain; it often helps with weight loss and decreases low-density lipoprotein (LDL) cholesterol and triglyceride levels and insulin requirements.

45. **(2)** The sulfonylureas reduce blood glucose levels by stimulating insulin release from the pancreas. Also, over a long period, they may actually increase insulin effects at the cellular level and decrease glucose production by the liver. This is the reason that sulfonylureas are used for clients with type 2 diabetes who still have a functioning pancreas.

46. **(1)** Anorexia, nausea, and a metallic taste in the mouth are common side effects. Over time, the gastrointestinal symptoms subside and can be relieved by taking the medication with food or by starting administration at a lower dose.

47. **(4)** Antithyroid medications (propylthiouracil or methimazole) are relatively inexpensive and do cross the placenta. The client continues to take the medications for 1 to 2 years with the hope for a permanent remission of symptoms when medications are withdrawn.

48. **(2)** Both of these drug classifications tend to reduce insulin sensitivity and can cause hyperglycemia. Angiotensin-converting enzyme (ACE) inhibitors, calcium channel blockers, and selective α-blockers are metabolically neutral; some may actually have a beneficial effect.

49. **(4)** The client's symptoms indicate hypothyroidism along with the elevated TSH level; the normal range for TSH is 0.5 to 4.7 mU/L. A full replacement dose of levothyroxine (Synthroid) should be started based on client's age, and TSH level should be checked in 6 weeks, since it can take that long for a given dose to become effective. Loading doses should never be given except in cases of coma, which is treated with IV medication in the hospital.

50. **(4)** Clients with coronary artery disease and mild to moderate hypothyroidism can safely undergo urgent surgery (including bypass

procedures) without prior replacement. The rate of complications is no greater than that for clients without hypothyroidism, and the cardiac risks are lessened compared with initiating replacement therapy preoperatively.

51. **(3)** Metformin is a better option for an obese client, because metformin is frequently associated with weight loss, whereas sulfonylureas may actually cause a weight gain. Insulin is not a good choice, because it is an overly aggressive approach to a mildly elevated glucose level and clients tend to be less receptive to treatment requiring injections. Diet and exercise were unsuccessful, and the longer her blood sugar level remains elevated, the greater is the risk for end-organ damage.

52. **(2)** All but osteoporosis are related to acute overdosage of levothyroxine and can be relieved by omitting the dose for 3 days and then starting with a lower dose.

53. **(4)** Before treatment for elevated blood pressure (BP) is initiated, it is recommended that three elevated readings be recorded on three separate occasions. There is no evidence to suggest that this gentleman had an elevated BP on prior visits.

54. **(1)** This is the best answer, because the AM intermediate dose affects the glucose level before dinner. Altering the dose of regular insulin will affect levels before lunch and before bedtime; however, these levels are okay. To reduce the dose of intermediate-acting insulin while maintaining the level of regular insulin, the client will need to self-mix the intermediate-acting and regular insulin, using less of the intermediate-acting insulin.

55. **(4)** Pseudoephedrine (Sudafed) and other decongestant medications that contain sympathomimetics lead to adverse reactions of central nervous system (CNS) overstimulation, palpitations, headache, hypertension, nervousness, etc. Robitussin in combination (i.e., Robitussin-CF [dextromethorphan, phenylpropanolamine, guaifenesin] or Robitussin-PE [pseudoephedrine, guaifenesin]) can also cause palpitations and CNS overstimulation. Robitussin-DM (dextromethorphan, guaifenesin) is predominantly associated with gastrointestinal upset, drowsiness, headache, and rash as adverse effects.

56. **(2)** Infusion site problems and skin irritation are by far the most frequent complaints of a client who uses an insulin pump. Often, it is a major reason for the client's decision to discontinue using the pump. Clients also find it is more time-consuming and costly. However, in 1993 the Diabetes Control and Complications Trial (DCCT) demonstrated a reduced risk of microvascular complications when insulin pumps and multiple daily injections were used.

57. **(3)** Clients with gestational diabetes are treated with insulin, not an insulin sensitizer. Pioglitazone (Actos) and rosiglitazone (Avandia) act by decreasing peripheral insulin resistance in skeletal muscle and adipose tissue without enhancing insulin secretion. They improve glucose tolerance and decrease insulin resistance in clients with insulin-requiring type 2 diabetes. Option #4 refers to the action of α-glucosidase inhibitors (e.g., acarbose [Precose] and miglitol [Glyset]).

58. **(3)** Older clients, especially those with heart disease, need to begin receiving the smallest amount of thyroid medication replacement (0.025 mg, not 0.1 mg) and gradually have the amount increased until a therapeutic level is achieved. If thyroid replacement occurs too quickly, the heart may decompensate. Two grains of thyroid extract is too much. Methimazole (Tapazole) is an antithyroid medication and is indicated for treatment of hyperthyroidism.

59. **(2)** The response to therapy is based on clinical symptomatology and results of a TSH assay approximately 4 to 6 weeks after initiation of therapy. This is continued until a stable dose is obtained. The TSH assay and a free T_4 level are the two standard tests that can be used to monitor the status of the thyroid; a levothyroxine level cannot be measured. Levothyroxine (Synthroid) is not a myelosuppressive agent.

60. **(3)** β-Blockers are initially prescribed to reduce the signs and symptoms of the condition and to reduce the peripheral conversion of T_4 to triiodothyronine (T_3); nonsteroidal antiinflammatory drugs (NSAIDs) are indicated for reducing inflammation associated with thyroiditis; and antithyroid medications, such as propylthiouracil (PTU) or methimazole (Tapazole), are used to treat severe hyperthyroidism. Corticosteroids are sometimes used in the treatment of thyroiditis, but the remaining classes of medications (namely, antibiotics, ACE inhibitors, calcium channel blockers, and anxiolytics) are not routinely used in the management of hyperthyroidism.

61. **(3)** Decreasing the dose of levothyroxine and evaluating the cardiac status of the patient are the appropriate interventions in this situation, in addition to involving the collaborating physician regarding further workup. Discontinuing the thyroid replacement would be inappropriate because the client's hypothyroidism remains and requires therapy to continue for life. An anxiolytic may be a helpful adjunct, but it is certainly not appropriate as the sole intervention, because it does not address the cardiac symptoms.

62. **(2)** DDAVP (desmopressin acetate) promotes reabsorption of water in the renal tubules, which can lead to water intoxication. The signs of water intoxication are lethargy, behavioral changes, disorientation, and neuromuscular excitability.

63. **(1)** Insulin injections for the child/adolescent are 2:1 proportion NPH/regular in the AM and 1:1 in the PM. Changes are made on the basis of blood sugar level, which is determined 4 times a day. The proportion is based on the periods of insulin activity.

64. **(1)** Lispro (Humalog) is the first analog of human insulin that has several advantages over regular insulin, including a more rapid onset and shorter duration of action. It reaches peak activity within 1 to 2 hours and has a 4-hour duration, as compared with 6 to 8 hours for regular insulin. It is convenient for many clients, because it can be injected immediately before eating (10 to 15 minutes). Because it has been on the market only since June 1996, there is no long-term safety profile established and the teratogenicity is unknown. In addition, it is more expensive than insulin and some third-party payers may not reimburse clients.

65. **(4)** Hypoglycemia and weight gain are the most common side effects of sulfonylurea therapy.

66. **(3)** Pioglitazone (Actos) and rosiglitazone (Avandia) are insulin sensitizers, which increase the glucose uptake by muscle and fat. Metformin (Glucophage) decreases hepatic glucose output. Oral sulfonylureas increase the secretion of insulin in the pancreas. α-Glucosidase inhibitors increase the postprandial glucose uptake in the intestine.

10 Musculoskeletal

Physical Examination & Diagnostic Tests

1. A goniometer is a measuring device used during physical examination of the musculoskeletal client. The nurse practitioner uses this tool to determine:

   1. Strength of the muscles in the extremities.

   2. The degree of joint flexion and extension.

   3. Range of motion of the extremities.

   4. Point of joint flexion that is painful.

2. The nurse practitioner places a client in the prone position with the knee flexed to 90 degrees. The tibia is firmly opposed to the femur by exerting downward pressure on the foot. The leg is rotated externally and internally. If locking of the knee occurs, this is accurately called a positive:

   1. Drawer sign.

   2. McMurray's test.

   3. Apley's sign.

   4. Bulge sign.

3. A client has numbness and tingling in the thumb and first two fingers when pressing the backs of the hands together (flexes wrists at 90 degrees) for 60 seconds. This is a positive:

   1. Tinel's sign.

   2. Drawer sign.

   3. McMurray's test.

   4. Phalen's maneuver.

4. What is the name of the sign that occurs when compressing the suprapatellar pouch back against the femur and feeling for fluid entering the spaces?

   1. Drawer sign.

   2. Kernig's sign.

   3. Balloon sign.

   4. Bulge sign.

5. De Quervain's disease can be diagnosed in part by a positive:

   1. Finkelstein's sign.

   2. Tinel's sign.

   3. Phalen's sign.

   4. Lachman's sign.

6. The primary examination techniques to use for assessing the musculoskeletal system are:

   1. Inspection and percussion.

   2. Auscultation and palpation.

   3. Inspection and palpation.

   4. Palpation and percussion.

7. What can the nurse practitioner use to confirm a diagnosis of polymyalgia rheumatica (PMR)?

   1. Chest radiograph.

   2. Serum protein electrophoresis.

   3. Corticosteroid challenge.

   4. Erythrocyte sedimentation rate (ESR).

8. When performing an assessment, the nurse practitioner understands that the metacarpophalangeal (MCP) joints are frequently involved in:

   1. Gout.

   2. Rheumatic fever.

   3. Rheumatoid arthritis (RA).

   4. Osteoarthritis (OA).

9. In the evaluation of polyneuropathy, which study *would not* be recommended?

   1. Sedimentation rate.

   2. Complete blood count (CBC).

   3. Hemoglobin A_{1c} (HbA_{1c}) level.

   4. Electromyography (EMG).

10. During assessment of a client who reports back injury, it is critical to ask about:

    1. Family history of back problems.

    2. Previous injury.

    3. Personal history of chronic illness.

    4. Mechanism of injury.

11. Tinel's sign and Phalen's maneuver are used in identifying a common work-related disorder that the nurse practitioner recognizes as:

    1. Lateral epicondylitis.

    2. Carpel tunnel syndrome.

    3. Dupuytren's contracture.

    4. Thoracic outlet syndrome.

12. An elderly client complains of fatigue, weakness, lightheadedness, and anorexia. He also complains of hot, swollen proximal interphalangeal (PIP) and metacarpophalangeal (MCP) joints. These symptoms occurred 5 months ago and reoccurred a few days ago. Which lab findings would be most conclusive of these assessments?

    1. Mean corpuscular volume (MCV) 104 femtoliters, low serum ferritin level.

    2. MCV 92 femtoliters, high serum ferritin level.

    3. Elevation in the uric acid level.

    4. Elevation in the white blood cell (WBC) count.

13. How is the talar tilt test conducted?

    1. The tibia is grasped with one hand and backward pressure is applied to the heel.

    2. The ankle is gently inverted and laxity of the ligament is graded.

    3. The examiner passively inverts, everts, dorsiflexes, and plantar flexes the ankle.

    4. The client actively inverts, everts, dorsiflexes, and plantar flexes the ankle.

14. Varus pressure on a knee that is slightly flexed (30 degrees) tests:

    1. Medial collateral ligament stability.

    2. Lateral collateral ligament stability.

    3. Medial cruciate ligament stability.

    4. For the presence of a lateral meniscus tear.

Disorders

15. The nurse practitioner realizes that the most common cause of shoulder pain is:

    1. Frozen shoulder.

    2. Thoracic outlet syndrome.

    3. Impingement syndrome.

    4. Osteoarthritis.

16. A 45-year-old female complains of knee pain when kneeling and a "clicking" noise when walking up steps. On exam, there is a slight knee effusion and tenderness when the patella is palpated against the condyles. The diagnosis for this client is:

    1. Anterior cruciate tear.

    2. Dislocated patella.

    3. Chondromalacia patella.

    4. Tendinitis.

17. A client has been given a diagnosis of a complete rotator cuff tear of the left shoulder. The nurse would expect the client to have difficulty in:

    1. Abducting the left arm.

    2. Supinating the left forearm.

    3. Shrugging the shoulders.

    4. Touching the left hand to the right shoulder.

18. A client has been diagnosed with PMR. The nurse practitioner understands that this disorder is:

    1. An autoimmune, multisystem problem wherein the body makes antibodies to its own proteins.

    2. A degenerative disorder with no inflammatory changes and in which joint cartilage wears away with age and eventually causes bone spurs.

    3. An inflammatory disorder involving the axial skeleton and large peripheral joints.

    4. An inflammatory connective tissue disorder that primarily affects older women and is associated with giant cell (temporal) arteritis.

19. In teaching a client about fibromyalgia, the nurse practitioner includes what information?

    1. Diagnostic studies such as ESR and CBC are important tools to confirm the progress of the syndrome.

    2. Avoid stretching exercises and daily low-impact aerobics.

    3. Take ibuprofen (Motrin) 200 mg q4-6h prn for pain and amitriptyline (Elavil) 10 mg 1 to 2 hours before bedtime.

    4. Apply heat to or massage "trigger points" to reduce pain.

20. The nurse practitioner understands that chronic synovitis with pannus formation is the basic pathophysiologic finding in clients with:

    1. Systemic lupus erythematosus (SLE).

    2. Ankylosing spondylitis (AS).

    3. RA.

    4. Osteoarthritis.

21. The nurse practitioner is examining a client who is complaining of pain in her hips and knees. She has a history of osteoarthritis. On examination, the joints are painful to movement and are warm to touch. The best immediate therapy for this client is:

    1. Physical therapy for range of motion of affected areas.

    2. Decreased physical activity and immobilizing splints for affected joints.

    3. Moist heat and/or cold therapy on painful joints.

    4. ESR to determine level of activity.

22. The history of a client who may have contracted Lyme disease may include what characteristic?

    1. Erythematous rash on bridge of nose and cheeks with discoid patches on the trunk.

    2. Immediate development of arthritis symptoms, especially in the knees.

    3. Expanding rash with central clearing occurring within a month of being bitten.

    4. Early symptoms of meningitis and myocarditis.

23. The nurse practitioner understands that finding Heberden's nodes on physical examination of a client is a cardinal sign of:

    1. Septic arthritis.

    2. RA.

    3. Gouty arthritis.

    4. Osteoarthritis.

24. The nurse practitioner is teaching a client with a lower leg cast for a fractured tibia to begin crutch walking. Instructions for assisting the client to walk up the stairs with the crutches would include:

    1. Place both crutches on the upper step and step up with unaffected leg while balancing on crutches.

    2. Position the affected leg on the upper step and use the crutches to move up.

    3. Place the unaffected leg on the upper step and move affected leg and crutches up together.

    4. Position the affected leg and the crutch on the upper step and bring the unaffected leg up with the crutch.

25. Competing diagnoses for an adult male who presents with acute onset of unilateral inflammation, pain, and erythema of the first metatarsophalangeal joint could be:

    1. Gout, cellulitis, and osteoporosis.

    2. Cellulitis, RA, and gout.

    3. Osteoporosis, fibromyalgia, and cellulitis.

    4. Septic arthritis, RA, and osteoarthritis.

26. Diseases that often present as polyarthritic diseases include:

    1. Lyme arthritis, rheumatic heart disease, AS, and psoriatic arthritis.

    2. RA, gout, Reiter's syndrome, and osteoarthritis.

    3. Gonococcal arthritis, SLE, and septic arthritis.

    4. PMR, Lyme arthritis, pseudogout, and psoriatic arthritis.

27. The circumstances under which a common injury can most often cause a meniscus tear to occur are:

    1. The knee is almost completely extended and the tibia is externally rotated.

    2. An external force is applied and is strong enough to cause external rotation or hyperextension of the knee.

    3. Valgus or varus pressure on the knee occurs at full extension and at 30 degrees of flexion.

    4. The knee is simultaneously twisted and flexed.

28. Pain in lumbosacral strain typically begins:

    1. Immediately with the injury.

    2. 1 to 2 hours after injury.

    3. 6 to 8 hours after injury.

    4. 12 to 36 hours after injury.

29. Acute onset of pain that descends down to the lower leg and foot of a 25-year-old obese adult is likely to be a symptom of:

    1. Lumbosacral strain.

    2. Herniated intervertebral disk injury.

    3. Osteomyelitis.

    4. Osteoporosis.

30. When an injury or trauma causes a knee to "give out" and the client experiences severe pain and effusion, and later, "locking" of the knee with pivoting or turning, the diagnosis is probably:

    1. Patellofemoral stress syndrome.

    2. Growing pains.

    3. Shin splints.

    4. Patellar subluxation.

31. Quadriceps setting is one exercise recommended for clients with patellofemoral syndrome. Teach the client to:

    1. Lie supine on the floor with legs extended. Dorsiflex the foot. Push the thigh into the floor.

    2. Sit on the floor, leaning back on the elbows. Flex one knee to 90 degrees, and extend one leg completely and hold for 5 seconds.

    3. Lie on the floor and flex both knees to about 20 degrees with a rolled up towel underneath them. Extend one leg and hold for 5 seconds.

    4. Perform resistive exercises with an elastic band.

32. Which risk factor is associated with gout?

    1. Female.

    2. Age 20 years.

    3. Ingestion of salicylate medications.

    4. Overuse of the extremity.

33. In a third-degree ankle sprain, findings are:

    1. Minimal ecchymosis, moderate edema, and a stable joint.

    2. Moderate ecchymosis, moderate edema, and an unstable joint.

    3. Marked ecchymosis, marked edema, and a stable joint.

    4. Marked ecchymosis, marked edema, and an unstable joint.

34. A client with RA presents for follow-up. What is the best evaluative question the nurse practitioner can ask that will help determine the severity of disease?

    1. "Were you able to drive the car to your appointment today?"

    2. "Were you able to fix your dinner last night?"

    3. "How long does it take for your joints to loosen up after you get up in the morning?"

    4. "How many pounds can you carry?"

35. A 35-year-old female is seen with a complaint of diffuse musculoskeletal pain, stiffness, and fatigue for the past 3 months. The pain is worse in the morning and also with changes in weather. She states she wakes up in the morning feeling tired. Findings on physical exam are normal except for pain on digital palpation in 12 tender points. Laboratory results are unremarkable. The most likely diagnosis is:

    1. Fibromyalgia.

    2. Myofascial syndrome.

    3. RA.

    4. Depression.

36. When counseling a postmenopausal female client on prevention of osteoporosis, all of the following are therapeutic recommendations **except**:

    1. Quit smoking.

2. Take 200 mg of calcium and 40 IU of vitamin D daily.

3. Continue hormone therapy.

4. Monitor bone loss by dual-energy x-ray absorptiometry (DEXA) every 1 to 2 years.

37. A client tells the nurse practitioner that she has a "whiplash injury." The nurse practitioner understands that this is:

    1. Cervical facet joint dysfunction.

    2. Cervical flexion injury.

    3. Cervical-thoracic injury.

    4. Cervical strain.

38. A client presents with a complaint of sudden pain and swelling in the knee. He is also complaining of chills and fever. On exam, the knee is warm, tender, and swollen with evidence of effusion. The family nurse practitioner would:

    1. Splint the affected joint.

    2. Obtain sample of synovial fluid from the affected joint by aspiration.

    3. Initiate treatment with nonsteroidal antiinflammatory drugs (NSAIDs).

    4. Recommend rest, ice, compression, and elevation of affected joint.

39. In determining the specific cause of polyarticular complaints, the clinical clues most helpful for diagnosis are:

    1. Lab identification of antinuclear antibodies (ANAs) and sedimentation rate.

    2. X-ray film of affected joints.

    3. Affected joint pattern and presence or lack of inflammation.

    4. Sexual history of client.

40. A client with AS needs to be educated to manage disease by all **except**:

    1. Regular exercise program.

    2. Maintenance therapy with systemic corticosteroids.

    3. Using indomethacin (Indocin) for discomfort.

    4. Watching for signs and symptoms of iritis.

41. An adult client comes to the office complaining of foot pain. He can recall no specific injury but gives a history of being an occasional runner who drinks about 6 to 10 beers on weekends. What physical findings would the nurse practitioner expect?

    1. Redness, swelling, and warmth of the first metatarsophalangeal joint.

    2. Swelling, ecchymosis, and decreased range of motion.

    3. Swelling and decreased circulation.

    4. Decreased range of motion and obvious bone deformity.

42. Which of the diet selections indicate that the older client understands the health education regarding the prevention of osteoporosis?

    1. Chicken and baked potato.

    2. A glass of skim milk and a toasted cheese sandwich.

    3. Hamburger and salad.

    4. Ice cream sundae with whipped cream.

43. During the history, which of the following questions would best assist the nurse practitioner in diagnosing osteoarthritis versus RA?

    1. "Is your joint pain symmetrical and localized?"

    2. "Does your morning stiffness usually last several hours?"

    3. "Have you experienced fatigue, weakness, and weight loss?"

    4. "Is your joint pain asymmetrical and worse with movement and relieved by rest?"

44. The number one cause of disability in adults younger than 45 years is:

    1. Cancer.

    2. Fracture.

    3. Low back pain.

    4. Migraines.

45. The following is the most accurate statement about juvenile rheumatoid arthritis (JRA):

    1. Symptoms are much more severe than those of adult RA.

    2. Complete remission occurs in three fourths of clients.

    3. More than 90% of cases progress to severe joint destruction.

    4. Administration of cytotoxic drugs should be initiated as early as possible in the treatment regimen.

46. Primary treatment of joint injury involves:

    1. Rest, ice, compression, and elevation.

    2. Narcotic pain control and x-ray examination.

    3. Specialist referral and magnetic resonance imaging.

    4. NSAIDs and exercise.

47. The most common complaint in a client with back injury who has cauda equina syndrome, a surgical emergency, is:

    1. Urinary retention.

    2. Numbness below the level of injury.

    3. Weakness in the lower extremities.

    4. Pain.

48. Recognition of annular tears is important in the diagnosis of back pain because:

    1. They require immediate surgery.

    2. They are often misdiagnosed as strain or sprain, leading to herniation.

    3. They result in rapid paralysis.

    4. X-ray films would reveal them, but x-ray films are usually not ordered initially.

49. A chronic musculoskeletal problem that may occur after an injury and that is characterized by a 3-month history of pain on both sides of the body above and below the waist and tenderness in at least 11 of 18 specified points is:

    1. Chronic osteoarthritis.

    2. Reflex sympathetic dystrophy.

3. Tendinitis.

4. Fibromyalgia.

50. Which client is at greatest risk for osteoporosis?

    1. 55-year-old male smoker who is a retired athlete.

    2. 60-year-old white postmenopausal female switchboard operator weighing 105 lb.

    3. 42-year-old African American female intensive care nurse who is lactose intolerant.

    4. 50-year-old white obese female who lives on a farm and is mother of three.

51. A 38-year-old secretary complains of pain in her hands at night. On examination, the nurse practitioner notes wasting of the thenar eminence in both hands with dry skin on the thumb, index, and middle fingers. The nurse practitioner suspects:

    1. Carpal tunnel syndrome.

    2. Transient ischemic attack.

    3. Osteoarthritis.

    4. Raynaud's phenomenon.

52. A 53-year-old woman presents with complaints of morning stiffness in the neck and back. She also has pelvic and shoulder pain and fatigue. Her laboratory studies reveal an elevated ESR, a normal rheumatoid factor, a normal creatine phosphokinase level, and normochromic normocytic anemia. Physical examination reveals an elevated temperature, bilateral pain, and stiffness of the pectoral and pelvic muscles. According to this information, the best diagnosis is:

    1. Polyarteritis nodosa.

    2. Wegener's granulomatosis.

    3. PMR.

    4. RA.

53. A 55-year-old woman with a prior diagnosis of PMR presents with headache, low-grade fever, aching, stiffness, fatigue, malaise, and anorexia. On the basis of this information, the nurse practitioner would make a preliminary diagnosis of:

    1. Influenza.

    2. Pneumonia.

3. Temporal arteritis.

4. RA.

54. Children with JRA must be screened regularly for:

    1. Ulcerative colitis.

    2. Iridocyclitis.

    3. Diabetes mellitus.

    4. Adrenal insufficiency.

55. A client twisted his knee while playing sports. He complains of knee pain and also states that in the past few weeks his knee has "locked up" a couple of times. On examination, a positive McMurray's test response is elicited. This is consistent with a diagnosis of:

    1. Anterior cruciate ligament tear.

    2. Dislocated patella.

    3. Medial meniscus tear.

    4. Chondromalacia patella.

56. A man comes into the clinic complaining of low back pain that radiates down the lateral thigh. The pain began suddenly on the job after he lifted a heavy object. The nurse practitioner would further evaluate the client for:

    1. Compression fracture of lower lumbar vertebrae.

    2. A spinal cord injury.

    3. Compression of a lumbar disk.

    4. History of spinal cord injury.

57. An 80-year-old resident of a long-term care facility who has a history of multiinfarct dementia (MID) is alert but disoriented to person, place, and situation. His only health problems are MID and osteoarthritis. Over the past 2 weeks, he has become agitated, has demonstrated exit-seeking behavior, and has been noted to be continually rubbing his knees. The nurse practitioner suspects that this client is likely experiencing:

    1. Worsening dementia.

    2. Pain.

    3. Urinary tract infection (UTI).

    4. Acute infarct.

Pharmacology

58. The nurse practitioner is seeing a middle-aged woman with severe arthritis who has been receiving maintenance therapy of prednisone 10 mg/day for the past 6 weeks. She now presents as acutely ill with signs and symptoms of acute pneumonia. She complains of feeling fatigued and weak, she has a loss of appetite, and her blood pressure is lower than measurements on previous visits. Treatment should include:

    1. Immediate discontinuation of the prednisone.

    2. Increasing dosage to 60 mg/day and then tapering back to 10 mg/day.

    3. Gradual tapering of the prednisone from 10 mg/day to 1 mg/day.

    4. Maintaining dose of prednisone at 10 mg/day.

59. The primary drug of choice for a client with RA is:

    1. NSAIDs.

    2. Aspirin.

    3. Methotrexate.

    4. Hydrocortisone.

60. A client with RA begins taking prednisone 5 mg PO per day. In teaching the client about her medication, it would be important for the nurse practitioner to include what information?

    1. When the symptoms of arthritis subside, she will be able to quit taking her medication.

    2. It is important to take the medication as prescribed, even after the redness and swelling decrease.

    3. Increased fluid intake is important to prevent renal damage by the steroids.

    4. The medication should be taken about 30 minutes before eating.

61. A correct medication and dose for the treatment of an adult with an acute episode of gout is:

    1. Indomethacin (Indocin) 25 mg PO prn.

    2. Naproxen (Naprosyn) 100 mg PO bid.

    3. Colchicine 0.6 mg qid.

    4. Indomethacin (Indocin) 50 mg q8h for 6 to 8 doses, then decrease to 25 mg pm q8h until gout episode is resolved.

62. If a client's 24-hour urine collection indicates that the client is secreting too much uric acid (a result of >900 mg/day), the nurse practitioner would prescribe:

    1. Aspirin 325 mg PO per day.

    2. Tylenol 325 mg PO q4-6h prn.

    3. Indomethacin (Indocin) 25 mg PO q8h and then increase at weekly intervals by 25 mg daily.

    4. Allopurinol (Zyloprim) 100 mg PO × 1 week then increase the daily dose by 100 mg to a maximum of 300 mg/day.

63. Disease-modifying drugs for RA in adults include:

    1. Ibuprofen (Motrin, Advil), sulindac (Clinoril), and salicylates (aspirin, Disalcid).

    2. Corticosteroids (prednisone, methylprednisolone).

    3. Misoprostol (Cytotec).

    4. Hydroxychloroquine (Plaquenil), sulfasalazine (Azulfidine), methotrexate, and gold sodium thiomalate (Myochrysine).

64. Gold compounds are contraindicated in clients with all of the following **except**:

    1. Renal disease.

    2. Hepatic disease.

    3. RA.

    4. Blood dyscrasia.

65. The most appropriate medication used to control pain for a client with osteoarthritis would be:

    1. Acetaminophen.

    2. Systemic corticosteroids.

    3. Gold salts.

    4. Misoprostol.

66. What is a serious side effect of ibuprofen in the elderly client?

    1. Rebound headaches.

    2. Impairment of renal function.

    3. Neuropathy.

    4. Liver failure.

67. A client has been taking methotrexate (Rheumatrex) for 6 weeks. This was the medication of choice for her severe refractory RA. What tests should the nurse practitioner perform?

    1. Monthly platelet count, CBC, and differential.

    2. Urinalysis, blood sugar, and electrocardiogram (ECG) every 2 weeks.

    3. Monthly CBC, urinalysis, and electrolytes.

    4. Coagulation studies, electrolytes, and CBC every week.

68. A middle-aged male client presents with a complaint of waking up yesterday morning with his big toe swollen and painful. The client reports he has never had anything like this before and has not had any previous health problems. Physical exam reveals his big toe to be red, hot, and tender in the joint, with inflammation extending into the surrounding tissue. His temperature is 99.8° F (37.7° C) and the WBC count is mildly elevated. Needle aspiration of joint fluid reveals urate crystals. The best treatment the nurse practitioner could recommend for this client is:

    1. Bed rest, very-low-calorie diet, and increased fluid intake.

    2. Pharmacologic therapy with allopurinol (Zyloprim) 200 mg PO qd and education of the client about the need to continue to take this medication as maintenance therapy once symptoms resolve.

    3. Administration of naproxen (Naprosyn) 500 mg PO tid, instructing the client to continue full dose until symptoms resolve, and then tapering and discontinuation of naproxen over 72 hours.

    4. An injection of intraarticular corticosteroid therapy to the affected joint.

69. An elderly woman comes into the clinic complaining of "sores" in her mouth. The nurse practitioner observes several inflamed ulcers on her gums and lips. Which medication would the nurse identify as most likely to cause this problem?

    1. Propranolol (Inderal).

    2. Spironolactone (Aldactone).

    3. Fexofenadine (Allegro).

    4. Alendronate sodium (Fosamax).

10 Answers & Rationales

Physical Examination & Diagnostic Tests

1. **(2)** The goniometer is used to determine the degree of joint flexion and extension. It provides a means of measuring the degree of angle flexion and extension.

2. **(3)** Apley's sign, locking of the knee or the sound of clicks and pain, may indicate a loose body, such as torn cartilage. This test is performed to detect a torn meniscus. The drawer sign tests the cruciate ligaments with the client in sitting and lying positions, not prone. The McMurray's test is used to detect medial meniscus injury. In this test, the knee is fully flexed and the tibia is externally rotated. Varus pressure is applied to the knee while it is extended. For detection of a medial meniscus tear, the test is performed while valgus pressure is applied to the knee.

3. **(4)** Phalen's maneuver, when present, is suggestive of carpal tunnel syndrome. Tinel's sign is also a test for carpal tunnel syndrome but is performed by lightly percussing over the median nerve on the volar (palmar) side of the wrist; and an abnormal result would be tingling or shock-like sensations across the palm, thumb, and first two fingers. The drawer sign and McMurray's tests are used to assess the knee.

4. **(3)** The balloon sign occurs in instances when considerable fluid is in the suprapatellar pouch; ballottement of the patella is possible. The bulge sign is for testing fluid in the knee joint and is elicited with the knee extended by applying pressure to the medial aspect of the knee and watching for a bulge or fluid wave. A patellar tap suggests fluid in the knee as the

patella clicks against the femur. The drawer sign tests the cruciate ligaments with the client in a sitting and lying position. Kernig's sign, a sign of meningeal irritation, is the inability to extend the lower leg when that leg is flexed at the hip or the presence of resistance or pain during elicitation of the sign.

5. **(1)** Pain with gentle deviation of a fist in which the thumb is tucked under the four fingers to the ulnar side is a positive Finkelstein's sign and an indication of De Quervain's disease, which is swelling and tenderness over the volar portion of the "snuff box," resulting from chronic tenosynovitis. Treatment is usually a thumb splint, nonsteroidal antiinflammatory drugs (NSAIDs), and possible steroid injection into the area. A positive Tinel's sign (tapping gently over the carpal tunnel, causing tingling in the thumb, index finger, and middle and radial half of the ring finger) and a positive Phalen's maneuver (holding dorsum of the hands that are flexed to 90 degrees back to back with this same distribution of tingling) are indicative of carpel tunnel syndrome. A Lachman's sign is an indication of the stability of the cruciate ligament of the knee.

6. **(3)** The musculoskeletal system is examined by a visual inspection and palpation of bones, joints, and surrounding musculoskeletal soft tissue. Percussion is generally not done, and auscultation is not appropriate to the system being examined.

7. **(3)** Clients with polymyalgia rheumatica (PMR) have a rapid, dramatic clinical response to corticosteroid therapy. The serum protein

electrophoresis is used to rule out myeloma. The erythrocyte sedimentation rate (ESR) is elevated in a number of diseases and is not specific to PMR. The chest radiograph is used to diagnose diseases affecting the lungs and thorax.

8. **(3)** The wrist, metacarpophalangeal (MCP), and proximal interphalangeal (PIP) joints, along with other small joint of the hands and feet, are involved in rheumatoid arthritis (RA). The great toe is most often involved with gout. The large joints of the hip, knee, and shoulder along with the distal interphalangeal (DIP) joint and the base of the thumb are involved with degenerative joint disease (e.g., osteoarthritis).

9. **(2)** It would not be necessary to obtain a complete blood count (CBC). The hemoglobin A_{1c}(HgbA$_{1c}$) would be ordered to evaluate the relative control of diabetes. Electromyography (EMG) is most often performed to evaluate both nerve conduction and needle electrode examination. Many toxins and inflammatory processes are involved with polyneuropathy; hence, the sedimentation rate would be a helpful diagnostic tool.

10. **(4)** A thorough history is very important in assessing any client with injury, but in the event of a back injury, the mechanism of injury will provide the greatest clue as to the extent of injury and the proper path to take in diagnosis and treatment.

11. **(2)** Carpel tunnel syndrome, a compression neuropathy of the median nerve at the wrist, is commonly caused by repetitive finger and wrist motion and results in positive Tinel's sign and Phalen's maneuver. Tinel's sign is considered positive when tapping over the nerve with a reflex hammer causes tingling in the distribution of the nerve. Phalen's maneuver is performed by fully flexing the wrist passively and noting tingling in the thumb or fingers.

12. **(2)** The clinical findings point to a chronic inflammatory process such as RA. The dizziness, fatigue, lightheadedness, and weakness may be a problem with anemia. The anemia of chronic disease is either microcytic or normocytic. The value that differentiates the anemia of chronic disease from other anemias is the serum ferritin level (iron stores). The value will be either normal or high. The mean corpuscular volume (MCV) of 104 femtoliters indicates a macrocytic anemia, which would not include the anemia of chronic disease. The low serum ferritin level would not be considered a possibility with this disorder. The uric acid level would be elevated in gout. The white blood cell (WBC) count does not address the signs of anemia.

13. **(2)** Gentle inversion of the affected ankle in an ankle injury is compared with the unaffected ankle in the talar tilt test. Anterior ankle stability is tested in the anterior drawer test, in which the tibia is grasped by the examiner's one hand while the heel is firmly grasped and backward pressure is applied to the tibia with the examiner's other hand. In passive range of motion, the examiner inverts, everts, dorsiflexes, and plantar flexes the foot and ankle. The client puts the foot and ankle through complete range of motion in active range of motion.

14. **(2)** Varus pressure on a slightly flexed knee tests for lateral collateral ligament stability. Valgus pressure tests for medial collateral ligament stability. Cruciate ligaments are tested with the anterior drawer test. The McMurray's test is used to detect medial meniscus injury. In this test, the knee is fully flexed and the tibia is externally rotated. Varus pressure is applied to the knee while it is extended. The test is performed while valgus pressure is applied to the knee to detect a medial meniscus tear.

Disorders

15. **(3)** Impingement syndrome is usually caused by rotator cuff tendinitis, which occurs when internal/external rotation is impaired. Frozen shoulder can occur after a rotator cuff injury, especially if a sling is used for a prolonged period. With Adson's or Wright's maneuver, thoracic outlet syndrome would cause a decrease in or loss of the radial pulse when the client abducts the arm and holds a deep breath while simultaneously hyperextending the neck and turning the chin toward the raised arm.

16. **(3)** These are common symptoms of chondromalacia patella. With anterior cruciate tears, the client generally cannot bear weight on the extremity without it buckling or giving

way. With a dislocated patella, there would be severe pain associated with considerable effusion (loss of normal knee hollow on sides of patella), and possibly, a patellofemoral compartment.

17. **(1)** With a complete rotator cuff tear (rupture of the supraspinatus tendon), the client would have difficulty abducting the arm and impaired internal/external rotation. Touching the hand to the opposite shoulder is adduction.

18. **(4)** Anemia is common in PMR, along with an elevated ESR. There is a common complaint of morning stiffness; rheumatoid factor is negative. Option #1 is characteristic of systemic lupus erythematosus (SLE). Option #2 is characteristic of osteoarthritis. Option #3 is characteristic of ankylosing spondylitis (AS).

19. **(3)** Diagnostic studies are of little value and benefit, except to rule out other causes, such as PMR or hypothyroidism. Treatment is symptomatic; the usual drugs are amitriptyline (Elavil), NSAIDs, cyclobenzaprine (Flexeril), temazepam (Restoril), and triazolam (Halcion). Daily, slow, low-impact aerobics, preferably in the late afternoon or early evening, are encouraged. Heat and massage are helpful, but not on the "trigger points."

20. **(3)** The chronic inflammatory disorder of RA is associated with synovial hypertrophy from chronic synovitis and pannus formation that results in progressive destruction of the cartilage, ligament, tendons, and bone. AS usually involves the large peripheral joints (e.g., sacroiliac) and is characterized by extreme kyphosis. There is no inflammation with osteoarthritis (OA). SLE has a distribution of symptoms similar to that of RA, but no pannus formation.

21. **(3)** Moist heat or cold, whichever relieves the pain more effectively, is appropriate to use on acutely affected joints. Physical therapy is recommended after the acute involvement of the joint; care must be taken to decrease repetitive movements. Immobilization is avoided, because it tends to increase the stiffness of the joint. The ESR is not an appropriate indicator of activity of osteoarthritis.

22. **(3)** Expanding rash with central clearing may also be described as the "bull's eye" rash associated with Lyme disease. Option #1

describes the malar or "butterfly" rash of SLE. The arthritis symptoms and other complications (meningitis and myocarditis) occur later in the disease process, especially if the client is not treated with antibiotics (usually tetracycline, doxycycline, or amoxicillin).

23. **(4)** Deformities (bony protuberances) of the DIP are called Heberden's nodes and are cardinal signs of osteoarthritis. The DIP joints are seldom involved with RA. Gouty arthritis most often affects the great toe. Joints are warm, red, tender, and swollen with septic arthritis.

24. **(3)** The unaffected leg goes up the step first, then the crutches and affected leg follow. This allows for stability and weight bearing on the unaffected leg, with the crutches supporting the affected leg.

25. **(2)** Cellulitis usually presents with warm, erythematous, painful areas of the skin. Symptoms of erythema, edema, and pain in the first metatarsophalangeal joint are a common presentation of gout. Symptoms that can be present in RA are similar: red, swollen, painful joint(s). The inflammation of RA is usually symmetric but can present as erythematous, swollen joints. Systemic symptoms may also be present. Osteoporosis most often occurs in postmenopausal women as a result of bone loss that occurs with the decline of estrogen levels in the blood. Bone thinning leads to fractures, not inflammation of joints or skin. Osteoarthritis presents as pain and stiffness with decreased range of motion, stiffness in the morning for a few minutes, and occasionally joint effusions. Point tenderness in 11 of 18 sites with digital palpation is present in fibromyalgia. Joint swelling and erythema are not present. In septic arthritis, joint pain, inflammation, and erythema would be accompanied by systemic symptoms of fever and chills. It would be considered in the differential diagnosis for this client.

26. **(1)** Lyme arthritis, rheumatic heart disease, AS, psoriatic arthritis, RA, Reiter's syndrome, osteoarthritis, gonococcal arthritis, SLE, and PMR commonly occur as polyarthritic diseases. Most often gout, septic arthritis, and pseudogout occur as monoarthritis.

27. **(4)** A client who has sustained a meniscal tear can usually recall a twisting injury of the knee,

followed by pain and effusion over the joint line. A strong force or injury that causes external rotation or hyperextension of the knee is a common mechanism of collateral or cruciate ligament injury. A test for stability of the knee joint involves applying medial and lateral pressure to the knee during full extension and flexion of 30 degrees.

28. **(4)** As the soft tissue swells, pain onset usually occurs about 12 to 36 hours after injury.

29. **(2)** Herniated intervertebral disk pain typically descends to the lower leg and foot. Lumbosacral strain causes pain in the back, buttock, and sometimes the thigh. Osteomyelitis must be preceded by an event that permits an infectious agent to enter the bone. Osteoporosis occurs most commonly in postmenopausal women.

30. **(4)** At the time a patellar subluxation occurs, a traumatic event causes the knee to "give out," and the patella is usually laterally displaced. Severe pain and an effusion result. After the injury, the client will notice a locking sensation in the knee with pivoting or turning. Patellofemoral stress syndrome is a form of overuse syndrome. Pain of a dull, aching quality is present in the knee, sometimes with clicking. Long periods of sitting or activities that involve knee flexion as well as compression of the patella in the groove cause increased pain. Growing pains usually occur at night and resolve by morning. The pain is deep and does not involve the joints. In shin splints, inflammation of muscles along the medial shaft of the tibia from overuse causes aching pain. Rest relieves the pain. Improper warm-up exercises or a sudden increase in exercise by an unconditioned person, especially while wearing worn or improper athletic shoes, can lead to this pain.

31. **(1)** In quadriceps setting, with the foot dorsiflexed, the thigh is pressed down against the floor and held for 5 seconds. The straight leg raise involves lifting an extended leg while sitting on the floor and leaning back on the elbows with the opposite leg flexed to 90 degrees. A terminal arc extension requires that the client lie on the floor supine with extended legs flexed to 20 degrees over a rolled up towel. The client then extends one leg and holds for 5 seconds. The exercise is repeated with the opposite leg. All of the exercises can be used to stretch and strengthen the

quadriceps muscles in clients with patellofemoral stress syndrome. Resistive exercises with an elastic band are general exercises that can be done with the extremities.

32. **(3)** Gout generally affects men older than 30 years and is associated with obesity, lead intoxication, starvation, and use of some medications including salicylates, diuretics, pyrazinamide, and alcohol.

33. **(4)** A third-degree sprain is a complete tear of the ligament resulting in marked edema, ecchymosis, pain, and an unstable joint.

34. **(3)** Morning stiffness on activity and the length of time it takes for maximal improvement are two of the American Rheumatism Association Classification criteria for RA and can be used to measure effects of treatment. The other questions are good indicators of quality of activities of daily living but do not give a full, overall, measurable picture of the client's joint discomfort.

35. **(1)** This client meets the classification criteria for fibromyalgia based on history of widespread pain and pain in 11 of 18 tender points. Myofascial syndrome symptoms are more focal, and there is no associated fatigue or sleep disorder. Rheumatoid disease would have abnormal serologic test results. Depression may cause musculoskeletal pain and fatigue but would not have reproducible tender points.

36. **(2)** This is a subtherapeutic amount of calcium and vitamin D. The other choices are recommendations for prevention of osteoporosis.

37. **(4)** Most whiplash injuries are associated with a cervical neck strain caused by a motor vehicle accident. These injuries take a considerable time to heal, usually five times longer than a strain involving another part of the body.

38. **(2)** This client's symptoms are indicative of septic arthritis, which is a medical emergency; if not treated promptly, the joint may be severely damaged or destroyed. Examination of the joint fluid is the single most important diagnostic test. The other choices may provide some symptomatic relief, but the first goal of treatment is to determine whether the joint is septic.

39. **(3)** In developing a differential diagnosis, the history and physical exam will help narrow the differentiation. Other procedures are important in completing the evaluation, but the most important information is the pattern of joints affected and whether the disease is inflammatory or noninflammatory.

40. **(2)** Corticosteroids have limited value in treating AS, and long-term use is associated with many serious side effects. Important treatment includes regular exercise to strengthen supporting muscles and use of NSAIDs for pain. Approximately one third of clients have recurrent attacks of acute iritis.

41. **(1)** Trauma, increased alcohol intake on weekends, and physical stress have all been implicated in the occurrence of acute gout. Gout occurs primarily in adult men. Decreased circulation, ecchymosis, and bone deformity are not likely with acute gout.

42. **(2)** Calcium intake is important in minimizing the development of osteoporosis. Both of these foods contain calcium. The other options are not focused on calcium intake.

43. **(4)** Signs and symptoms of osteoarthritis include asymmetrical joint pain that is worse with movement and relieved by rest. Stiffness is of short duration (<15 minutes) after inactivity or in the morning. Pain may be described as aching and poorly localized. Options #1, #2, and #3 are indicative of RA.

44. **(3)** Low back pain is the number one cause of disability and accounts for 25% of disabling work-related injuries.

45. **(2)** Most do not have disease persistent into adulthood. Symptoms of juvenile rheumatoid arthritis (JRA) are very similar to those of adult arthritis. Most disease activity diminishes with age; although some clients with JRA do have some residual joint damage, the percentage is not this high. Aspirin is the treatment of choice, and cytotoxic drugs are reserved for clients for whom other therapy has failed.

46. **(1)** The RICE principle is used for initial treatment: **R**est, **I**ce, **C**ompression, and **E**levation. All other treatments mentioned may be appropriate, but not as the primary treatment.

47. **(1)** Although all of the symptoms may be associated with cauda equina syndrome, urinary retention is the most important clue to the immediate need for surgery.

48. **(2)** Annular tears are the first step toward herniation, and early recognition can help to prevent the need for surgical repair of a subsequent herniation.

49. **(4)** Fibromyalgia is a poorly understood condition that is very difficult to treat and can prolong the normal treatment course of an injury considerably. Osteoarthritis may follow an injury, as may reflex sympathetic dystrophy or tendinitis, but only fibromyalgia is associated with specified tender points.

50. **(2)** This example demonstrates five of the risk factors for osteoporosis, which include female, white or Asian, older than 45 years, low body weight, postmenopausal, sedentary lifestyle, low calcium intake, and smoker.

51. **(1)** Her occupation and symptoms are both suggestive of carpal tunnel syndrome. Initial treatment would involve night splinting, ice, and antiinflammatory medication.

52. **(3)** PMR is an inflammatory disorder of the proximal muscles presenting as described. Polyarteritis nodosa is an inflammatory disorder affecting the small arteries. It presents with muscle weakness, myalgias, headache, and subcutaneous nodules along the arteries in the extremities. Wegener's granulomatosis presents with mild anemia, dyspnea, cough, chest pain, hemoptysis, and abnormal findings on urinalysis.

53. **(3)** Up to 40% of clients with temporal arteritis have a history of PMR. Presenting complaints include headache, low-grade fever, aching and stiffness of joints, fatigue, malaise, and anorexia.

54. **(2)** Development of iridocyclitis may be insidious and asymptomatic, and if left untreated, it may cause blindness. Although children may have any of the other listed diseases, there is no correlation with JRA.

55. **(3)** A positive McMurray's test response (palpable click and pain when rotating the foot laterally and extending the leg) along with the symptoms are indicative of a medial meniscus tear. The drawer test evaluates for anterior cruciate ligament tears (i.e., knee flexed with foot on table; sit on foot and grasp both sides of

tibia at the knee; pull tibia forward; abnormal if movement of tibia away from the joint).

56. **(3)** The client is presenting with the classic symptoms of nerve root compression caused by pressure from a protruding lumbar disk. The sciatic stretch test (straight leg raise) maneuver will increase the radiation of pain down the hip.

57. **(2)** This client is likely experiencing an acute exacerbation of his osteoarthritis, since he is constantly rubbing his knees. Since 85% of the residents of long-term care facilities have uncontrolled pain, it is likely that this client has uncontrolled pain. Beginning routine administration of acetaminophen (Tylenol) would be an excellent start to pain management for this client. It is unlikely that the client's dementia is worsening, since this is an acute problem. While a urinary tract infection (UTI) is a good choice, the cues of rubbing the major joints would likely rule out a UTI as the problem. The client is not exhibiting any neurologic symptoms, which would rule out an acute infarct.

Pharmacology

58. **(2)** Clients receiving long-term steroid therapy should be evaluated for adrenal insufficiency during an acute illness, which increases stress. Signs and symptoms indicate subtle clinical manifestations of adrenal insufficiency. Empirical treatment is with stress-dose corticosteroid is recommended during acute illness. Stopping the medication or maintaining it at the same dose may precipitate acute adrenal insufficiency.

59. **(2)** Aspirin is the first choice. NSAIDs can be used, but the antiinflammatory and antipyretic effects of aspirin, plus low cost, make it the drug of choice. Methotrexate is used for severe cases that do not respond to either aspirin or NSAIDs. Steroids may be given but are not the drug of choice.

60. **(2)** The client needs to understand the importance of maintaining her dose of steroids. When symptoms decrease, the medication is effective. It is not influenced by fluids and it should be taken with food.

61. **(3)** This is the only effective dose listed for the treatment of an acute episode of gout. The other doses are incorrect and insufficient.

62. **(4)** Allopurinol works to keep the serum uric acid level lower. The goal of therapy is a serum uric acid level of <6.5 mg/dl. The other medications listed do not help to lower serum uric acid levels, and aspirin can precipitate a gout attack.

63. **(4)** These drugs modify the disease when NSAIDs (ibuprofen, sulindac, salicylates) have not worked. Corticosteroids can be used until the disease-modifying agents begin to work. Misoprostol (Cytotec) is used to prevent ulcer development related to long-term medication use.

64. **(3)** Gold is indicated for treatment of RA and is contraindicated in the presence of the other listed diseases.

65. **(1)** Acetaminophen or an NSAID is generally used for pain relief for clients with osteoarthritis. Systemic corticosteroids are not indicated in osteoarthritis. Gold salts may be one of several pharmacologic approaches to the treatment of RA. Misoprostol is used to minimize the development of NSAID-induced gastric ulcers.

66. **(2)** Renal function may already be reduced in the elderly, and ibuprofen can further impair renal function, which in turn can result in nephrosis, cirrhosis, and congestive heart failure.

67. **(1)** This client should be monitored for blood dyscrasias on a monthly basis. Women of child-bearing age should avoid pregnancy.

68. **(3)** NSAIDs are recommended treatment for an acute gout attack in clients able to take them. Allopurinol (Zyloprim) is contraindicated in an acute attack and can even precipitate an attack in the early stages of treatment. Low-calorie diets increase risks of gouty attacks. Joint injection would not be a first-line choice of treatment. However, in refractory cases in clients unable to take oral medication, it may be an option.

69. **(4)** Gastritis and oral ulcers are common adverse effects of Fosamax. The medication is used to increase calcium absorption in patients with osteoporosis. If these effects occur, the medication should be discontinued. The medications in the other options do not cause this problem.

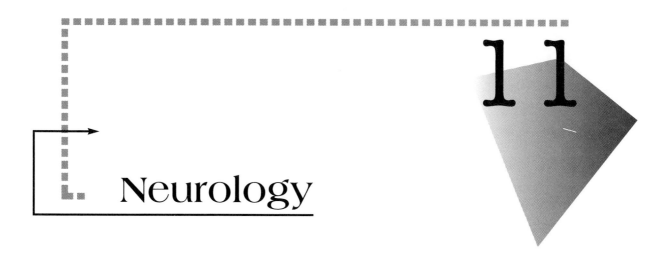

Neurology

Physical Examination & Diagnostic Tests

1. To evaluate the neurologic system for appropriate sensory system functioning in the geriatric client, it is appropriate to determine the presence of stereognosis. This is done by having the client:

   1. Rapidly touch the index finger and then the nose.

   2. Distinguish between a coin and a key by touch.

   3. Stand with heels together and eyes closed.

   4. Close eyes and identify familiar odors.

2. To determine cerebellar functioning in the geriatric client, the nurse practitioner evaluates:

   1. Ability of the client to balance on one foot, then on the other.

   2. Ability to discriminate between two familiar objects by sensation.

   3. Ability to recall names of three U.S. presidents.

   4. Range of motion and ability to move extremities.

3. What is considered a "soft" (or equivocal) neurologic sign?

   1. Positive Babinski's sign in an adult.

   2. Mirroring hand movements of the extremities.

   3. Brudzinski's sign.

   4. Kernig's sign.

4. A client is having problems controlling her seizures and is referred to have electroencephalography (EEG) performed. Before the test, the nurse practitioner explains to the client that:

   1. This test will cause some discomfort and she will be given a sedative before it begins.

   2. It will be important for her to take her regular dose of fluoxetine (Prozac) and phenytoin (Dilantin) before the test.

   3. The procedure is painless and she will not be in any discomfort or experience electrical shock during the procedure.

   4. After the test, bed rest will be required for 8 hours and she will be given full liquids for 12 hours.

5. Which cranial nerve is being tested when the nurse practitioner asks the client to raise his eyebrows, smile, frown, or puff out his cheeks?

　1. Hypoglossal nerve.

　2. Acoustic nerve.

　3. Glossopharyngeal nerve.

　4. Facial nerve.

6. The nurse practitioner notes an absent patellar reflex in a healthy individual. What might the nurse practitioner ask the client to do?

　1. Lift both arms above the head and count to 5 slowly as the reflex is tested.

　2. Raise both legs slowly and then lower them while the reflex is tested.

　3. Clench both hands together and pull while the reflex is tested.

　4. Close eyes and hold breath while examiner tests for the reflex.

7. With the client in the supine position, the nurse practitioner gently flexes the client's neck in the direction of the chin touching the chest. If there is pain and resistance to the flexion and the hips and knees flex at the same time, the nurse practitioner accurately describes this finding as:

　1. Phalen's sign.

　2. Romberg's sign.

　3. Kernig's sign.

　4. Brudzinski's sign.

8. The nurse practitioner understands that dysdiadochokinesia refers to:

　1. Trouble with speech.

　2. Memory impairment.

　3. Trouble with attempts at rapidly alternating movements.

　4. A neurologic triad of symptoms affecting gait, memory, and speech.

Disorders

9. The nurse practitioner understands that the most common form of facial paralysis in the adult client is:

　1. Facial nerve fasciitis.

　2. Trigeminal neuralgia.

　3. Bell's palsy.

　4. Herpes zoster.

10. A client has a history of injury at thoracic level 5 (T5) and his condition has stabilized. The nurse practitioner understands that with this level of injury, the client is most likely not going to be able to:

　1. Perform coordinated movements with his hands, such as writing.

　2. Achieve lower body strength and coordination for walking.

　3. Have upper body strength adequate to drive a car.

　4. Maintain upper body coordination required to feed himself.

11. An older client, who as a young child recovered very quickly after extensive initial impairment caused by poliomyelitis, is given a diagnosis of postpolio syndrome. The most common presentation is:

　1. Gastrointestinal upset, headache, and malaise.

　2. New onset of weakness, fatigue, and pain.

　3. Sudden onset of lower limb paralysis after an acute infection.

　4. Headache, fever, and elevated blood pressure and pulse.

12. A client has Parkinson's disease. The nurse practitioner is discussing safety measures for the home environment. It would be important for the nurse practitioner to include what information?

　1. Sleep on a firm mattress that is high off the floor to facilitate getting into and out of bed.

　2. Pour hot liquids with the cup or container placed on the table to avoid spilling.

　3. Place a sheepskin pad on the bed to decrease the development of decubiti.

　4. Perform passive and active range of motion twice daily to prevent contracture.

13. A client is admitted to a rural clinic after a diving accident. The nurse practitioner suspects a spinal cord injury at cervical level 5 (C5). While

awaiting emergency transport services, the nurse practitioner assesses for the development of complications by:

1. Checking for voluntary movement of extremities and sensation below the level of injury.

2. Assessing breath sounds and evaluating movement of the diaphragm with respirations.

3. Maintaining cervical flexion to facilitate airway until cervical traction is initiated.

4. Beginning neurologic checks with careful documentation of location of pain sensations.

14. Many clients who experience recurrent headaches have similar symptoms with each episode. Which is a sign that a headache may have a more serious cause?

1. It occurs on the right side.

2. Rhinorrhea occurs with the headache.

3. Headache becomes more and more painful.

4. The pain increases when the client bends over.

15. Epidemic meningococcal meningitis occurs rarely. This control is due to:

1. Use of active immunization.

2. Lower community carrier rates.

3. Improved socioeconomic conditions.

4. Earlier detection and recognition of outbreaks.

16. The nurse practitioner understands that benign paroxysmal positional vertigo:

1. Is described as vertigo and nystagmus with positional change and occurs most commonly in the elderly.

2. Is more common in the young and occurs suddenly and in episodes that include vertigo, tinnitus, hearing loss, and nausea and vomiting.

3. Follows a viral syndrome (upper respiratory tract or gastrointestinal); exacerbation of the vertigo occurs with position change but without hearing loss or tinnitus.

4. Involves gradual hearing loss and tinnitus along with vertigo; eventually facial numbness and weakness develop.

17. All of the following are included in the differential diagnosis of a client with facial paralysis **except**:

1. Herpes zoster.

2. Bell's palsy.

3. Trigeminal neuralgia.

4. Otitis media.

18. What instruction would be appropriate to include in the treatment plan for health promotion in a client with a diagnosis of multiple sclerosis?

1. Avoid aerobic exercise because of muscle weakness.

2. Keep warm (especially extremities) to improve neurologic function.

3. Avoid antioxidants (vitamins C and E, beta-carotene) because they contribute to loss of myelin sheath.

4. Consume a low-fat, high-fiber diet, with daily cranberry juice and a calcium supplement.

19. A client who has had a cerebrovascular accident is incontinent of urine. The family should be taught to:

1. Restrict fluid intake.

2. Insert a Foley catheter.

3. Establish a scheduled voiding pattern.

4. Reposition the client often to reduce the discomfort of urgency.

20. The best way to test the hearing of a client with Bell's palsy is to:

1. Stand out of sight of the client and ask the client to move or do something.

2. Use a tuning fork to test for lateralization of sound.

3. Stand in front of the client and whisper, "Raise your hand."

4. Snap your fingers next to the client's ear and ask whether the sound was heard.

21. The physical examination findings for a 50-year-old female client who wears a left lower leg brace are: weight 100 lb, height 65 inches, and vital signs within normal limits. Because this client has symptoms of postpolio syndrome, the nurse practitioner suggests that the client:

    1. Gain weight to prevent further disability.

    2. Exercise all muscle groups vigorously to prevent disuse syndrome.

    3. Avoid exposure to cold or chilling, because it may cause a loss of strength in the affected muscle.

    4. Reduce the amount of time using the brace for joint support to prevent further loss of strength.

22. Inflammation and swelling of the seventh cranial nerve with resultant unilateral facial muscle paralysis is called:

    1. Bell's palsy.

    2. Transient ischemic attack.

    3. Facial droop.

    4. Trigeminal neuralgia.

23. The nurse practitioner understands that the following is a trigger that helps to differentiate a migraine from a tension headache:

    1. Alcohol.

    2. Bright lighting and noxious stimuli.

    3. Stressful situations.

    4. Sleep pattern disturbances.

24. All of the following are true of migraine headache except:

    1. Migraine is likely related to the sensitization of trigeminal nerve fibers within the meninges.

    2. Migraine and related headaches are disorders of the inflammatory response.

    3. Genetic and environmental factors are influential in migraine.

    4. During migraine, serotonin levels decrease in the central nervous system (CNS).

25. A symptom that can occur in a client who has experienced a transient ischemic attack in the anterior cerebral circulation is:

    1. Bilateral vision disturbance and/or diplopia.

    2. Dysarthria (speech disturbance).

    3. Disorders of behavior and cognition.

    4. Motor and sensory problems on both sides of the body at once.

26. Many visits to emergency departments by adults are prompted by headaches. One symptom that may help the nurse practitioner differentiate a migraine headache from a headache that may be indicative of severe problems is:

    1. A migraine is preceded by an "aura."

    2. A migraine occurs mainly behind one eye and tends to be grouped.

    3. The onset of a migraine is sudden and accompanied by nuchal rigidity.

    4. A migraine occurs mainly on awakening.

27. An adult client presents with a complaint of facial paralysis that started suddenly. In making a diagnosis, the nurse practitioner considers the following symptoms of Bell's palsy.

    1. Concurrent paralysis of the opposite arm and leg.

    2. Pain in the (ipsilateral) ear that accompanied or preceded the paralysis.

    3. Loss of bowel control.

    4. Loss of hearing on the opposite side.

28. The nurse practitioner is evaluating an elderly client's tremor. Which finding would be most characteristic of an essential tremor rather than a parkinsonian tremor?

    1. The handwriting is not affected.

    2. The tremor occurs with purposeful movements.

    3. The tremor occurs at rest.

    4. The tremor gets worse with β-blockers or alcohol.

29. Which finding may be observed in a client with Parkinson's disease?

    1. Macrographia.

    2. Micrographia.

    3. Exaggeration of rapid successive movements.

    4. Increased swinging of arms while walking.

30. A client who was recently given a diagnosis of multiple sclerosis asks the nurse practitioner about the disease process. The nurse practitioner knows that:

    1. Ninety percent of clients have a quickly progressive form of the disease.

    2. Ninety percent of clients, after the first onset of symptoms, have relapses and remissions.

    3. Ten percent of clients will respond to corticosteroids.

    4. Ten percent of clients have problems with optic neuritis and sensory loss.

31. A 30-year-old female client has had several episodes of incontinence, weakness, loss of vision, and some ataxia. Physical exam reveals slight swelling of the optic disc on funduscopic exam, difficulty in walking heel-to-toe, lower extremity weakness, and 2+ deep tendon reflexes. The nurse practitioner suspects:

    1. Multiple sclerosis.

    2. Parkinson's disease.

    3. Amyotrophic lateral sclerosis.

    4. Postpolio syndrome.

32. Which is considered a likely cause of seizures in young adults?

    1. Congenital abnormalities and metabolic disturbances.

    2. Metabolic disorders, CNS infection, and fever.

    3. Idiopathic seizures, trauma, and substance abuse.

    4. Trauma, malignant tumor, and cerebral vascular accident.

33. A client has a history of recurrent headaches for the past 3 years, occurring one or two times per month and lasting 12 to 18 hours. When the client presents at the clinic, she has been using acetaminophen and has taken 6 g in the past 12-hour period and has had no relief. The nurse practitioner would:

    1. Refer the client to a neurologist for headache workup.

    2. Consider an analgesic rebound relative to the dose of acetaminophen taken.

    3. Order naproxen (Anaprox) for prophylactic treatment of the headaches.

    4. Order an electroencephalogram (EEG) and magnetic resonance imaging (MRI) to rule out pathologic conditions.

34. A client presents to the emergency department with the "worst headache of my life." The client reports that the headaches have not responded to the common over-the-counter headache remedies. What is most important for the nurse practitioner to rule out?

    1. Brain tumor.

    2. Migraine.

    3. Onset of newly diagnosed seizure disorder.

    4. Subarachnoid hemorrhage.

35. A client with a recent history of a left hemisphere stroke returns to the clinic for a checkup. What symptoms would the nurse practitioner anticipate the client to exhibit?

    1. Left-sided weakness.

    2. Bilateral weakness of lower extremities.

    3. Difficulty with speech.

    4. Left visual field deficit.

36. The nurse practitioner is evaluating a group of geriatric clients for risk factors for an embolic stroke. Which condition would be *least* likely to precipitate this type of stroke?

    1. Mitral valve disease.

    2. Atrial fibrillation.

    3. Endocarditis.

    4. Diabetes mellitus.

37. A client returns to the clinic for a follow-up visit. She has a history of simple, partial seizures. When questioning the client regarding the recurrence of seizures, the nurse practitioner would identify the recurrence of this seizure activity if the client reported:

    1. Short episodes during which she loses consciousness but does not fall.

    2. No loss of consciousness but jerking and tingling of her right leg, then right hand.

    3. Auditory hallucinations, unconsciousness, and urinary incontinence.

    4. Short period of unconsciousness, followed by period of confusion.

38. An elderly woman comes to the clinic complaining of having difficulty when she tries to do her needlework. She walks straight, although somewhat slowly, and no rigidity is noted on movement. She states that the shaking in her hands stops when she holds her hands in her lap. The nurse practitioner makes a tentative diagnosis of:

    1. Parkinson's disease.

    2. Transient ischemic attack.

    3. Benign essential tremor.

    4. Simple partial seizure activity.

39. A client with a history of myasthenia gravis presents with ptosis, facial weakness, dysphagia, and generalized weakness. What is important for the nurse practitioner to establish initially?

    1. When the symptoms first began and whether they have increased in severity.

    2. What medications the client is taking and when he last took them.

    3. What activity the client was participating in when the symptoms began.

    4. Whether the client has experienced any seizure activity with the increase in symptoms.

40. A client presents with miosis and ptosis with anhidrosis of the ipsilateral face and neck. The initial diagnosis would be:

    1. Horner's syndrome.

    2. Damage to cranial nerves III and IV.

    3. Menière's disease.

    4. Mycotic aneurysm.

41. The nurse practitioner is reviewing the records of a client who is recovering from a stroke (cerebrovascular accident). The records indicate the client is experiencing homonymous hemianopia. This is interpreted as:

    1. Partial loss of visual acuity in the peripheral area of the visual field.

    2. Diplopia in the eye contralateral to the cerebral lesion.

    3. Nystagmus in both eyes, but with dissimilar movements.

    4. Loss of vision in both eyes in either the right or left half of the visual field.

Pharmacology

42. An elderly patient is given a diagnosis of postherpetic neuralgia. All of the following are used initially to treat the associated pain except:

    1. Anticonvulsants.

    2. Tricyclic antidepressants.

    3. Nonsteroidal antiinflammatory drugs (NSAIDs).

    4. Opioids.

43. A client is taking antiepileptic medication. The nurse practitioner understands that antiepileptic medication:

    1. Must be taken indefinitely.

    2. Is usually discontinued after 4 years of no seizure activity and an EEG is used to confirm lack of seizure activity.

    3. Is usually given in combination with other antiepileptic agents or sedatives to reduce the seizure threshold.

    4. Must be given to all clients who experience a seizure.

44. The medication management of clients with peripheral vestibulopathy includes:

    1. Meclizine (Antivert) 100 mg PO qid.

2. Dimenhydrinate (Dramamine) 5 mg PO tid to qid.

3. Scopolamine transdermal disk (Transderm-Scop) 1 disk applied behind the ear and left in place for 3 days.

4. Prochlorperazine (Compazine) 25 to 50 mg PO q4h prn.

45. Which medication and dose can be used for abortive therapy for an adult client with symptoms of a migraine headache?

1. Sumatriptan (Imitrex) 6 mg IM.

2. Ergotamine (Ergostat) 2 mg SL.

3. Ketorolac (Toradol) 100 mg IM.

4. Amitriptyline (Elavil) 100 mg PO.

46. During a physical exam of a client given a diagnosis of chronic recurrent seizures who is currently receiving antiepileptic medication, the nurse practitioner notes hyperplasia of the gums. The nurse understands that hyperplasia of the gums is:

1. An unusual side effect of phenobarbital.

2. A common side effect of phenytoin.

3. A common occurrence with chronic recurrent seizures.

4. Caused by poor oral hygiene.

47. The family of a client with Parkinson's disease brings him to the clinic because he is experiencing increasing difficulty with ambulation. The nurse practitioner increases the frequency of carbidopa 25/levodopa 100 (Sinemet) administration from 3 to 4 times daily. What is important for the nurse practitioner to teach the family regarding the increase in the dose of this medication?

1. Sleep disorders and hallucinations are common side effects of Sinemet, and the last dose should not be given near bedtime.

2. Sinemet has shown efficacy in slowing disease progression.

3. Orthostatic hypotension can be problematic at higher dosing ranges.

4. The medication should be given on an empty stomach because of its altered absorption with meals, especially in conjunction with protein foods.

48. What is important teaching to provide to the client regarding the use of medications to treat trigeminal neuralgia?

1. Medication may cause seizure-like activity.

2. Therapeutic levels of the medication may take up to a month to be reached.

3. Relief of the symptoms should occur within 24 hours of starting the medication.

4. It is not necessary to monitor any blood levels.

11 Answers & Rationales

Physical Examination & Diagnostic Tests

1. **(2)** Stereognosis is the ability to determine familiar objects by shape rather than visual identification. Option #1 determines fine motor and coordination, Option #3 determines proprioception (balance, posture), and Option #4 determines the functioning of the first cranial nerve (i.e., olfactory).

2. **(1)** The cerebellar area controls gross motor movements and balance, as well as fine motor movements of the upper and lower extremities. Discriminatory sensation tests the sensory system, and a remote memory test is a mental status examination involving the cerebral cortex.

3. **(2)** Soft neurologic signs involve slight deviations of the central nervous system (CNS) that are present occasionally or inconsistently. Examples are short attention span, clumsiness, frequent falling (disturbances of gait), hyperkinesis, left-handed but right-footed, language disturbances, anisocoria, and mirroring movements of the extremities (when one hand performs a movement, the other is also in motion). The other three options indicate a CNS problem that occurs consistently (Brudzinski's and Kernig's signs indicate meningeal irritation; a positive Babinski's sign in an adult may indicate an upper motor lesion in the corticospinal tract).

4. **(3)** The procedure is painless and there is no danger of electrical shock. All anticonvulsants, antidepressants, stimulants (caffeine, tobacco), and alcohol should be stopped. There is no restriction on movement or diet after the procedure.

5. **(4)** The facial nerve is tested by facial movement, taste, sensation, and corneal reflex. The hypoglossal nerve is tested by the client sticking out his tongue. The acoustic nerve is tested by a hearing test. The glossopharyngeal nerve is tested by taste, gag reflex, and giving the client a drink and asking him or her to swallow.

6. **(3)** Augmentation of the patellar reflex can be obtained by having the client isometrically tense muscles not directly involved with the reflex arc being tested. This is called *Jendrassik's maneuver.*

7. **(4)** This describes Brudzinski's sign. Phalen's sign is elicited in carpal tunnel syndrome. Romberg's test is done to assess gross swaying by asking the client to stand with feet together and eyes closed for 5 seconds. Kernig's sign (inability to extend the lower leg when the leg is flexed at the hip or when there is resistance or pain during the process) along with Brudzinski's sign indicate meningeal irritation and should be further evaluated.

8. **(3)** Dysdiadochokinesia is trouble with attempts at rapidly alternating movements (e.g., finger to nose).

Disorders

9. **(3)** The most common form of facial paralysis is Bell's palsy, which is a disorder affecting the facial nerve and is characterized by muscle

flaccidity of the affected side of the face. Trigeminal neuralgia is a disorder of cranial nerve V characterized by an abrupt onset of pain in the lower and upper jaw, cheek, and lips. Herpes zoster affects the dermatomes and does not cause paralysis, but rather pain and possible postherpetic neuralgia.

10. **(2)** T5 injuries do not affect the coordination or capacity of the upper body, arms, and hands; the lower body is paralyzed. The client should be able to do all of the activities listed except walk.

11. **(2)** The cardinal signs of postpolio syndrome include onset of new weakness, fatigue, and pain along with hot or cold intolerance, and swallowing, speech, breathing, and/or sleep disturbances.

12. **(2)** Pouring liquids is frequently a complicated task for the client with Parkinson's disease because of tremors. If the cup or container into which the client is pouring the liquid is placed on a table, there is less chance of spilling the contents.

13. **(2)** At this level of injury (C5), the intercostal muscles and diaphragm can be affected and the client may have respiratory compromise. Airway maintenance and avoiding flexion of the neck are critical.

14. **(3)** If a headache becomes more and more severe, if there is new onset of severe headache in a client older than 35 years, if the headache's character or progression is different from that of other headaches, or if there is vomiting but no nausea, there could be a new and serious cause for the headache. The side on which the headache occurs and accompanying rhinorrhea may or may not be significant. Increasing pain when bending over is characteristic of sinus pressure or infection.

15. **(3)** Undoubtedly, improved sanitary and socioeconomic conditions have led to the marked reduction in the number of cases of epidemic meningitis. There is no research to support increased cases in communities with higher carrier numbers.

16. **(1)** Benign paroxysmal positional vertigo usually occurs in older clients. Younger persons who experience a sudden episode of vertigo, tinnitus, hearing loss, sensation of fullness, and nausea and vomiting typically have Menière's

disease. Peripheral vestibulopathy usually follows upper respiratory tract or gastrointestinal viral illness and involves nearly incapacitating vertigo that increases with positional changes, but not hearing loss or tinnitus. An acoustic neuroma should be suspected if gradual hearing loss, tinnitus, and vertigo occur before the development of facial numbness and weakness.

17. **(3)** The differential diagnosis for facial paralysis includes numerous problems: bacterial infections of the ears, Lyme disease, herpes zoster, mumps, temporal bone fracture, acoustic neuroma, other types of tumors, and demyelinating diseases. Trigeminal neuralgia is associated with intense facial pain, not paralysis.

18. **(4)** In addition to the factors listed, keeping cool, not warm, is associated with improvement of neurologic function. A regular exercise program is encouraged along with daily intake of a multivitamin, antioxidants, and low-dose aspirin (81 mg); maintaining ideal body weight, having rest periods or naps daily, and becoming informed about the disease process are important aspects of promoting health.

19. **(3)** Reestablishing regularity will assist in maintaining bladder control. A catheter exposes the client to infection. Fluids should not be restricted.

20. **(1)** Bell's palsy involves a sensorineural hearing loss. The client must be able to hear the direction of sound without any visual prompting. The tuning fork assists in differentiating between air and bone conduction of sound.

21. **(3)** In addition to encouraging the client to have regular health maintenance visits, the client should be advised to avoid gaining weight and exercising to the point of muscle pain. Cold temperatures can cause a loss of muscle strength in the affected muscle groups and should be avoided. Assistive or orthotic devices (canes, walkers, braces, etc.) should be used, and muscle strength and function should be periodically evaluated.

22. **(1)** The symptoms describe Bell's palsy, which is believed to be caused by a virus. This sudden onset of unilateral facial paralysis usually resolves within a couple of weeks but can endure for months. A few clients can have

residual problems. Transient ischemic attacks last <24 hours. Facial droop occurs with Bell's palsy as a result of paralysis of the muscles innervated by the facial nerve (seventh cranial nerve). Trigeminal neuralgia is sudden pain along the fifth cranial nerve.

23. **(4)** Sleep pattern disturbances, either too little or too much, may trigger a migraine headache. Lighting and noxious stimuli, as well as alcohol use and stress, may trigger both types of headaches.

24. **(2)** Headache disorders, including migraine, are disorders of neurovascular regulation. All other options are part of the current theory of migraine.

25. **(3)** A wide variety of changes in behavior and cognition can occur after a transient ischemic attack. Bilateral vision disturbance, diplopia, dysarthria (speech disturbance), and motor/sensory problems on both sides of the body are associated with a transient ischemic attack in the posterior cerebral circulation.

26. **(3)** Classic migraine headaches are accompanied by auras. Cluster headaches occur behind one eye and are grouped. Headaches associated with hypertension occur mainly on awakening. A sudden onset and nuchal rigidity may indicate a subarachnoid hemorrhage.

27. **(2)** Bell's palsy is typically preceded or accompanied by pain in the ear on the paralyzed side. The paralysis is confined to the face, and there is no effect on bowel control.

28. **(2)** The differentiating feature between the two tremors is that the essential tremor occurs with purposeful movements. Handwriting may be affected by both types of tremor. The tremor with Parkinson's disease occurs at rest. Essential tremors are reduced with the use of β-blockers or alcohol.

29. **(2)** Micrographia is a classic manifestation of Parkinson's disease. There is an impairment of rapid successive movements and a decrease in automatic movements such as swinging the arms while walking.

30. **(2)** Multiple sclerosis (MS) is characterized by exacerbations and remissions of the symptoms. Only 10% of patients with MS have a progressive form of the disease from onset.

Many clients (35%-40%) have problems of optic neuritis, sensory loss, and weakness and do respond to corticosteroids.

31. **(1)** Involvement of more than one area of the CNS, age 15 to 60 years, two or more separate episodes of symptoms involving different sites, and a gradual progression over at least 6 months are the criteria for multiple sclerosis.

32. **(3)** The most likely causes of seizures in adolescents and young adults are idiopathic disease, trauma, and substance abuse. Congenital abnormalities are the likely cause of seizures in newborns. In children <6 years old, metabolic causes, CNS infection, and fever can cause seizures. Trauma, malignant tumors, and cerebrovascular accidents (CVA) are likely causes of seizures in the elderly.

33. **(2)** The recommended dose of acetaminophen is no more than 4 g/day. This client may be experiencing an analgesic rebound headache. Appropriate prophylactic medications for migraine include β-blockers (propranolol), tricyclic antidepressants (amitriptyline), selective serotonin reuptake inhibitors (fluoxetine), anticonvulsants (topiramate), and calcium channel blockers (verapamil). It is not necessary to order expensive tests for clients with migraine or tension headaches. Usually, a careful, thorough history is sufficient.

34. **(4)** This is a common complaint of the client with subarachnoid hemorrhage headache. This client should be immediately referred to a neurologic surgeon.

35. **(3)** The speech center (Broca's area) is most often located in the left hemisphere. The client would experience weakness of the right side of the body and a right-sided visual deficit as well.

36. **(4)** Options #1, #2, and #3 all precipitate the development of an embolus that can result in an embolic stroke (cerebrovascular or brain accident). Diabetes will precipitate occlusive disease of the cerebral arteries and the possible development of a thrombotic stroke, not an embolic stroke.

37. **(2)** A simple partial seizure is characterized by unilateral paresthesia, numbness and tingling, and spastic movement of the extremities (old term is *jacksonian epilepsy*). There is no loss of consciousness or incontinence of bowel or bladder.

38. **(3)** The characteristics of a benign tremor are a fine to coarse rhythmic movement of the hands and feet that increases with activity and may be absent at rest. Frequently, the voice is also involved. An ingestion of a small amount of alcohol may decrease symptoms.

39. **(2)** It is important to determine whether the client has complied with his medication schedule. The symptoms may be the result of missed medication but may also occur because of too much medication. This is especially true with pyridostigmine bromide (Mestinon). This should be addressed first. The symptoms may also be exacerbated by exercise and heat.

40. **(1)** The clinical presentation is classic of Horner's syndrome, especially the lack of sweating, or anhidrosis, on the ipsilateral, or same, side of the face and neck as the eye symptoms. The client needs to be referred for further neurologic workup.

41. **(4)** Homonymous hemianopia is the loss of the vision in one half of the visual field. Either the right or left field of vision may be affected. It is most often caused by a lesion or disease in the optic tract or the occipital lobe.

Pharmacology

42. **(3)** Neuropathic pain is traditionally treated with a variety of medications including anticonvulsants, tricyclic antidepressants, and opioids. Sympathetic blockade may be used in recalcitrant cases. Nonsteroidal antiinflammatory drugs (NSAIDs) are not generally considered first-line treatment.

43. **(2)** Although most medication is discontinued after 4 years of no seizure activity, this should be confirmed by an electroencephalogram (EEG). Not all clients with seizures require medication; referral to and monitoring by a neurologist are appropriate.

44. **(3)** Scopolamine patches are placed behind the ear and provide medication for 3 days. Meclizine (Antivert) is given in doses of 12.5 to 25 mg PO tid to qid. The correct dose for dimenhydrinate (Dramamine) is 50 mg tid or qid. Compazine is given in doses of 5 to 10 mg q4h prn.

45. **(2)** The correct dose is ergotamine (Ergostat) 2 mg SL. Sumatriptan (Imitrex) is given SC or 100 mg PO. Ketorolac (Toradol) is given in doses of 30 to 60 mg IM. Amitriptyline (Elavil) is not used for abortive therapy.

46. **(2)** Hyperplasia of the gums is a common side effect of phenytoin (Dilantin). The client should practice regular dental prophylactic hygiene to deal with the problem.

47. **(3)** Sinemet induces a number of adverse reactions including hypotension, gastrointestinal (GI) upset, psychosis, and motor complications. It should be administered away from meals, despite GI side effects, for the best absorption. It exerts no known effect on slowing disease progression.

48. **(3)** The onset of the action of the medication and relief of the symptoms occur within 24 hours, usually within 4 to 6 hours. Monitoring of blood levels may be necessary, depending on the specific medication prescribed. Medications may be given to treat seizures.

12

Gastrointestinal & Liver

Physical Examination & Diagnostic Tests

1. The nurse practitioner is preparing to examine the abdomen of a client. What is the correct sequence in which to conduct the examination?

   1. Inspection, palpation, percussion, auscultation.
   2. Palpation, percussion, auscultation, inspection.
   3. Percussion, palpation, auscultation, inspection.
   4. Inspection, auscultation, percussion, palpation.

2. When obtaining a history from a young female adult client with abdominal pain, the following priority areas must be assessed:

   1. Food preferences and dislikes.
   2. The location of the pain and associated symptoms.
   3. The client's medical history and medication history.
   4. The first day of the client's last menstrual period.

3. To test for a positive obturator sign in a client with abdominal pain, the nurse practitioner:

   1. Passively internally rotates the right hip from the 90-degree hip/knee flexion position.
   2. Asks the client to take a deep breath while applying pressure in the area of the gallbladder.
   3. Percusses over the costovertebral angles.
   4. Percusses at the right midclavicular line, right below the umbilicus and continues upward.

4. Diagnosis of acute hepatitis B includes the following results:

   1. Positive HBsAg, anti-HBc, HBeAg, IgM anti-HBc.
   2. HBeAg-positive and HBsAg-positive.
   3. HBeAg-negative and HBsAg-negative.
   4. IgM anti–HBc-negative (high titer) and HBsAg-negative.

5. The nurse practitioner is performing a new patient physical examination on a 51-year-old man. The history reveals that the client's father died of colon cancer. What priority diagnostic tests are used to screen this client?

   1. Barium enema and upper gastrointestinal (GI) series.

   2. Carcinoembryonic antigen (CEA) titer and sigmoidoscopy.

   3. Proctoscopy, biopsy, and colonoscopy.

   4. Fecal occult blood testing and flexible sigmoidoscopy.

6. The anti-HCV test is used to diagnose which condition?

   1. Acute hepatitis C.

   2. Chronic hepatitis C.

   3. Resolved hepatitis C.

   4. Acute, chronic, or resolved hepatitis C.

7. The diagnosis of early acute pancreatitis will be considered by the nurse practitioner on the basis of physical findings and the following laboratory test result:

   1. A white blood cell (WBC) count of 10,300/ mm^3.

   2. A serum amylase level of 75 U/L.

   3. A serum amylase level of 300 U/L.

   4. A serum lipase level of 75 U/L.

8. A middle-aged woman who is overweight has right upper quadrant pain that radiates to her right subscapular area and is severe and persistent. She is also experiencing anorexia, nausea, and a fever. Her most recent meal consisted of a double quarter-pound hamburger with cheese, French fries, and a vanilla shake. On the basis of this information, the nurse practitioner examines the abdomen and percusses for costovertebral angle tenderness. The abdomen is tender in the right upper quadrant and, if there is a positive:

   1. Obturator sign, the client has appendicitis.

   2. Costovertebral angle tenderness, the client has a urinary tract infection.

   3. Murphy's sign, the client has cholecystitis.

   4. McBurney's sign, the client has a strangulated hernia.

9. The nurse practitioner notes that a patient has a positive *Helicobacter pylori* test result. The nurse practitioner interprets this finding as an infection associated with:

   1. Gastroesophageal reflux disease (GERD).

   2. Irritable bowel syndrome (IBS).

   3. Duodenal ulcer.

   4. Infectious esophagitis.

10. When assessing a client with a complaint of severe abdominal pain, the nurse practitioner notes that the abdomen is flat and firm with no bowel sounds and the client has positive guarding. What diagnostic study should be ordered immediately?

    1. Complete blood count (CBC) and differential.

    2. Serum electrolytes.

    3. Hemoglobin S.

    4. Coombs' antiglobulin test.

Disorders

11. Diarrhea is often associated with:

    1. Infectious gastroenteritis, inflammatory bowel disease, diverticulitis.

    2. Diseases of the colon or rectum.

    3. Fever and abdominal pain in sexually transmitted diseases.

    4. Dysuria and flank pain in urinary tract infections.

12. Esophageal pain may radiate to the:

    1. Infrascapular area.

    2. Right shoulder.

    3. Neck and left arm.

    4. Periumbilical area.

13. In adults, viral gastroenteritis that has a short incubation period (18-72 hours) and short duration (24-48 hours); is characterized by abrupt onset of nausea and abdominal cramps, followed by vomiting and or diarrhea; and is often accompanied by headache and myalgia is caused by:

    1. Enteric adenovirus.

    2. Enteric calicivirus (Norwalk).

3. Rotavirus.

4. Cytomegalovirus.

14. The nurse practitioner suspects peritonitis in a client. The best action is to:

    1. Percuss over the costovertebral angle and watch for signs of pain.

    2. Perform a rectal exam and test the stool for blood.

    3. Auscultate the abdomen for decreased bowel sounds.

    4. Palpate for a tense, hard abdomen and check for a positive obturator sign.

15. Which of the following suggests an emergent condition?

    1. Pain in a young adult that is rated as 5 on a scale of 1 to 10 and is relieved by having a bowel movement.

    2. Localized pain that steadily increases for more than 6 hours with rebound tenderness and guarding.

    3. Pain in a young adult female that is sudden in onset and localized in the right lower quadrant and lasts 14 to 36 hours.

    4. Pain that follows the onset of vomiting and diarrhea.

16. Under what circumstances should peptic ulcer disease (PUD) be treated empirically before diagnostic studies are done? When the client's ulcer pain:

    1. Occurs with blood in the stool.

    2. Can be relieved by food, antacids, or vomiting.

    3. Is accompanied by weight loss.

    4. Is atypical or occurs with anemia.

17. A careful history of a client with a chief complaint of diarrhea reveals that this adult has recurrent abdominal pain and diarrhea that alternates with constipation. The most likely diagnosis is:

    1. Drug-induced diarrhea.

    2. Inflammatory bowel disease.

    3. Giardiasis.

    4. IBS.

18. What are the assessment characteristics of clients with dysphagia?

    1. Usually have more difficulty swallowing solids than liquids.

    2. Can have a stricture caused by esophagitis following a long history of reflux disorder.

    3. Have dysphagia for both solids and liquids.

    4. Can have marked weight loss.

19. The pathogenesis of GERD is:

    1. Frequent and excessive retrograde movement of stomach contents into the esophagus caused by abnormal lower esophageal sphincter (LES) function.

    2. A hiatal hernia that leads to esophageal irritation and inflammation.

    3. Reflux of the gastric contents after meals when a client is in the upright position, often after a period of vigorous exercise.

    4. Initiated by erosion of the GI mucosa into the LES, causing weakening of LES pressure and a burning sensation in the stomach.

20. A client comes to the urgent care center concerned about pain and swelling in his groin. He tells the nurse practitioner that his doctor told him that he has an incarcerated hernia. The examination of the client reveals a hernia that:

    1. Easily moves back and forth across the abdominal wall.

    2. Protrudes from the groin area and cannot be reduced into the abdomen.

    3. Is very painful to palpation with significant abdominal swelling.

    4. Decreases in size when the client increases intraabdominal pressure.

21. Which of the following findings would indicate a need for endoscopy in clients with PUD?

    1. All new cases of dyspepsia.

    2. Symptoms persisting after 8 to 12 weeks of therapy.

    3. Dyspepsia in all clients who smoke and use alcohol.

    4. Good response to empiric treatment after 7 to 10 days.

22. The nurse practitioner's understanding of which principle will be helpful in educating clients with GERD?

    1. A hiatal hernia is always a coexisting and major contributing factor.

    2. The LES has become a poor antireflux barrier.

    3. The amount of acid reflux is dependent on a familial tendency for GERD.

    4. Overeating and use of caffeine and alcohol cause GERD.

23. Inflammatory toxigenic GI illness is characterized by:

    1. No fecal leukocytes, secretory diarrhea, site: colon.

    2. No fecal leukocytes, watery diarrhea, site: distal small bowel.

    3. Fecal leukocytes, secretory diarrhea, site: colon.

    4. Fecal leukocytes, watery diarrhea, site: colon.

24. Which of the following statements accurately describes irritable bowel syndrome (IBS)?

    1. Affects men more then women.

    2. Affects children more than young adults.

    3. Affects women more than men.

    4. Predominantly affects elderly clients.

25. The nurse practitioner understands that hepatitis B can be transmitted by blood and blood products. Another common mode of transmission of hepatitis B is:

    1. Respiratory contact.

    2. Contaminated fluid.

    3. Fecal-oral route.

    4. Perinatal exposure.

26. A young adult client presents to the nurse practitioner's office with the chief complaint of intermittent heartburn, which becomes worse after eating and at night and is relieved temporarily by taking antacids. The client also states that several times in the last 14 days he has regurgitated very bitter tasting material into his mouth. Findings on physical examination by the nurse practitioner are unremarkable. The nurse practitioner's most likely diagnosis is:

    1. Viral esophagitis.

    2. IBS.

    3. GERD.

    4. Carcinoma of the esophagus.

27. What two forms of viral hepatitis are transmitted primarily by the fecal-oral route?

    1. Hepatitis A and B.

    2. Hepatitis B and C.

    3. Hepatitis A and D.

    4. Hepatitis A and E.

28. What are the characteristics of an indirect inguinal hernia?

    1. A portion of the bowel or omentum protrudes directly through the floor of the inguinal canal and exits through the external inguinal ring.

    2. Occurs mainly in middle and later years.

    3. Is due to a weakness in abdominal structure.

    4. Passes through the internal abdominal ring, traverses the spermatic cord through the inguinal canal, and exits at the external inguinal ring.

29. Which is true of enterobiasis?

    1. The parasite is in the soil and enters the body through the feet. It can cause anemia.

    2. The parasite causes pruritus around the anus because the gravid females exit through the anus at night and lay eggs on the skin. Humans are the only hosts of this parasite.

    3. The eggs of this parasite enter the body by direct ingestion of dirt (pica) or ingestion of dirt on unwashed vegetables or by consumption of water that contains eggs.

    4. This parasite is a protozoan. The source is usually contaminated water but infection is spread from person to person by oral-fecal contamination.

30. Which diet represents therapeutic modification for GERD?

1. Low-energy and low-calorie diet.

2. Energy-controlled and calorie diet.

3. High-energy and hemodynamically stabilized diet.

4. Avoidance of acidic and fatty foods, chocolate, and peppermint.

31. Nonpharmacologic management of GERD includes which of the following?

1. Weight reduction and sleeping with head of bed elevated 4 to 6 inches with blocks.

2. Lying down and resting after meals and weight reduction.

3. Drinking large amounts of fluids with meals and avoiding alcohol.

4. Avoiding mint, orange juice, and milk and following an increased protein diet.

32. An organism associated with the etiology of PUD is:

1. *Streptococcus pneumoniae.*

2. *Helicobacter pylori.*

3. *Moraxella catarrhalis.*

4. *Staphylococcus aureus.*

33. The most common causes of cirrhosis are:

1. Hepatitis A and hepatitis B.

2. Hepatitis B and Wilson's disease.

3. Hepatitis D and congestive heart failure.

4. Chronic hepatitis B and C and alcohol.

34. Prolapse of a vascular anal cushion through the anal canal with resultant entrapment by the internal anal sphincter describes:

1. Prolapse of the rectal mucosa.

2. Hemorrhoid.

3. Tumor.

4. Inguinal hernia.

35. An acute febrile illness with jaundice, anorexia, malaise, and an incubation period of 45 to 160 days; having a chronic and an acute form; and transmitted by parenteral, sexual, and perinatal routes best describes which condition?

1. Hepatitis A.

2. Hepatitis B.

3. Hepatitis C.

4. Hepatitis D.

36. Several clients present to the nurse practitioner's office with a history of cholelithiasis. Which client complaining of increased pain would require immediate admission to the hospital for possible prompt intervention?

1. A client who is human immunodeficiency virus–positive (HIV+).

2. A 75-year-old client with diabetes.

3. A client who is 5 weeks pregnant.

4. A client who is vomiting and has a slight fever.

37. An older adult male presents to the nurse practitioner for evaluation of "heartburn" and recent significant weight loss. The client states that he has been taking antacids and an oral histamine (H_2) blocker for 4 weeks, with no relief of symptoms. The client states that after eating, he feels like there is a problem with solid food digestion in his stomach. He also gives a history of cigarette smoking and he drinks alcohol daily. What differential diagnosis must the nurse practitioner consider first?

1. Gastric ulcer.

2. Acid reflux.

3. Esophageal tumor.

4. Lung tumor.

38. An older adult male presents to the nurse practitioner complaining of weakness and vomiting. The client gives a history of "several" drinks per day for the past 12 years and cirrhosis. The nurse practitioner observes that the client's lips appear to have dark blood on them. What emergent condition does the nurse practitioner suspect?

1. Seizure disorder.

2. Cerebral hemorrhage.

3. Pancreatitis.

4. Esophageal varices.

39. A usually benign diagnosis that can result in small bowel obstruction and infarction and that requires immediate referral to a surgeon is:

    1. Gastric ulcer.

    2. Endometriosis.

    3. Hernia.

    4. Ectopic pregnancy.

40. A young adult female presents to the nurse practitioner for evaluation of 2 days of increasing crampy, abdominal pain. She states that she also has some mild nausea and anorexia and a low-grade fever. The client states that the pain is periumbilical. Her CBC reveals a slightly elevated WBC count but is otherwise normal. The nurse practitioner's next step for the care of this client is:

    1. Referral to a gynecologist for evaluation of a possible ectopic pregnancy.

    2. Referral to surgeon for evaluation of possible appendicitis.

    3. Observation of the client overnight and reassessment the next day.

    4. Instructing the client to follow a clear liquid diet and watch for increasing symptoms.

41. The nurse practitioner's adult client has early alcoholic cirrhosis as determined by liver biopsy. In teaching the client about her disease, it is important that the nurse practitioner inform her that the disease is most likely irreversible at this point but that which of the following will generally halt the progression of the disease?

    1. Vitamin B supplements.

    2. Long-term, low-dose corticosteroid therapy.

    3. Abstinence from alcohol.

    4. Maintenance of a nutritious diet.

42. An elderly client presents with fever, leukocytosis, lower left quadrant pain, and diarrhea alternating with constipation. The nurse practitioner would make the diagnosis of:

    1. Appendicitis.

    2. Diverticulitis.

    3. IBS.

    4. Pancreatitis.

43. Which clients would be at lowest risk for developing diverticular disease?

    1. Vegetarians with high-fiber diets.

    2. Obese clients with high-cholesterol diets.

    3. The elderly on small-meal diets.

    4. Fad dieters on low-sugar diets.

44. The nurse practitioner knows that the following symptom is characteristic of left-sided colon cancer:

    1. Anemia.

    2. Tenesmus.

    3. Bright red rectal bleeding.

    4. Change in bowel habits.

45. The nurse practitioner knows that in clients with ulcerative colitis in whom the disease is proximal to the sigmoid colon, careful surveillance is required because of an increased risk of:

    1. Colon cancer.

    2. PUD.

    3. Depression.

    4. Perforation.

46. Which is true of PUD in the elderly?

    1. Smoking does not increase the risk of PUD.

    2. Duodenal ulcers are more common in the elderly.

    3. Perforation is a rare complication.

    4. Weight loss and anorexia are often the only symptoms.

47. Which is true of early cancer of the esophagus in the elderly client?

    1. Alcoholism and smoking increase the risk for cancer of the esophagus.

    2. It is usually an adenocarcinoma.

    3. Dysphagia for liquids, cough, and hoarseness are early symptoms.

    4. A boring-type midchest pain indicates mediastinal involvement and requires immediate surgery.

48. A client has a history of colon polyps. The nurse practitioner knows that:

    1. Polyps of the cecum are most likely to be malignant.

    2. Polyps <1 cm are more suggestive of malignancy.

    3. Villous polyps are rarely malignant.

    4. Sessile polyps are more likely to be malignant than pedunculated polyps.

49. The nurse practitioner identifies which of these conditions as most conducive to the development of metabolic alkalosis?

    1. Severe anxiety resulting in hyperventilation.

    2. Excessive vomiting related to gastroenteritis.

    3. Depressed respirations from excessive narcotic ingestion.

    4. Decreased renal function with glomeruli damage.

50. An adolescent client is brought to the nurse practitioner by his mother for evaluation after a dirt-bike accident. The client states that the bike flipped over and struck him on the abdomen. There is a hematoma noted just below the left anterior rib area. In this case, the nurse practitioner must be particularly aware of the possibility of:

    1. Ruptured bowel caused by blunt trauma.

    2. Bladder trauma.

    3. Hypovolemia caused by a ruptured spleen.

    4. Arrhythmias.

Pharmacology

51. A 28-year-old male has been given a diagnosis of hepatitis C and begins receiving ribavirin therapy. The nurse would:

    1. Instruct the client to take Tylenol 30 minutes before each treatment.

    2. Caution the client about the necessity of not fathering children during therapy or 6 months afterward.

    3. Encourage the client to use herbal therapy with gingko to decrease feelings of depression.

    4. Instruct the client to eat three well-balanced high-calorie meals daily.

52. An adult client has been treated on and off for PUD for the past 12 years. He has always responded quickly to ranitidine (Zantac) and antacids. He continues to smoke. He presents to the nurse practitioner's office with severe epigastric pain, weakness, and feelings of lightheadedness. The stool guaiac test result is positive and his hemoglobin level is 11.2 g/dl. His weight has decreased slowly over the past 6 months for unknown reasons. On the basis of this information, what should the nurse practitioner do next?

    1. Refill his medications.

    2. Give medications and refer to smoking cessation clinic.

    3. Discontinue cimetidine and start omeprazole (Prilosec).

    4. Consult with physician.

53. The nurse practitioner is examining a 30-year-old obese man who is complaining of indigestion and heartburn with a strong acid taste in his mouth about an hour after meals. The history is negative for chronic illnesses. A diagnosis of GERD is made. What is the best initial treatment for this client?

    1. Lie down after meals; eat five smaller meals per day.

    2. Take Pro-Banthine 15 mg tid, 30 minutes before eating.

    3. Decrease weight, and take ranitidine (Zantac) 150 mg bid.

    4. Take omeprazole (Prilosec) 40 mg once a day, and use antacids as needed.

54. Which of the following would be prescribed as initial treatment for uncomplicated PUD?

    1. Clarithromycin 500 mg bid.

    2. Doxepin (Sinequan) 25 mg qhs.

    3. Omeprazole (Prilosec) 20 mg qd.

    4. Pirenzepine 50 mg tid.

55. Which drug would be most useful for the nurse practitioner to prescribe for an adult client to prevent ulcers caused by nonsteroidal antiinflammatory drugs (NSAIDs)?

    1. Celecoxib (Celebrex).

    2. Cimetidine (Tagamet).

    3. Doxepin (Sinequan).

    4. Pirenzepine.

56. After percutaneous or permucosal exposure to an HBsAg-positive source:

    1. In an unvaccinated person, begin the hepatitis B vaccine series.

    2. In a known hepatitis B responder with an adequate response, no treatment is necessary.

    3. In a known hepatitis B responder with inadequate antihepatitis B surface antigen, give hepatitis B immune globulin (HBIG) and initiate a new hepatitis B vaccine series.

    4. In an unknown hepatitis B responder who completed the entire hepatitis B vaccine series, give a hepatitis B booster.

57. *Helicobacter pylori* has been found to be a causative factor in many cases of PUD. Which regimen is most likely to be successful treatment for an adult client?

    1. Combination of clarithromycin (Biaxin), amoxicillin (Amoxil), and omeprazole (Prilosec).

    2. Combination of Pepto-Bismol, cephalexin (Keflex), and metronidazole (Flagyl).

    3. Combination of lifestyle changes, Pepto-Bismol, and cimetidine (Tagamet).

    4. Combination of H_2 blocker, amoxicillin (Amoxil), and antacid.

58. A primary therapy for clients with mild ulcerative colitis is:

    1. Metronidazole (Flagyl).

    2. Sulfasalazine (Azulfidine).

    3. Amoxicillin (Amoxil).

    4. Cephalexin (Keflex).

59. The stepwise approach to management of GERD for an adult client includes lifestyle changes and which medication?

    1. Antacids as needed and cimetidine (Tagamet) 800 mg qhs.

    2. Antacids as needed plus ranitidine (Zantac) 150 mg bid.

    3. Antacids as needed plus omeprazole (Prilosec) 20 mg qd.

    4. Cisapride (Propulsid) 10 mg taken 15 minutes before meals and at bedtime.

60. After exposure to household or sexual contacts with hepatitis A, the nurse practitioner would:

    1. Give immunoglobulin 0.02 mg/kg as soon as possible but no later than 2 weeks after exposure.

    2. Give one dose of HBIG and immunoglobulin 0.02 mg/kg as soon as possible.

    3. Give immunoglobulin 0.02 mg/kg and two doses of HBIG.

    4. Understand that no injections are needed.

61. Shigellosis is treated by:

    1. No medication intervention, careful toileting and bathroom sanitation, and keeping the perineal area clean.

    2. Symptomatic treatment and antidiarrheal agents such as Loperamide as needed.

    3. Symptomatic treatment and trimethoprim-sulfamethoxazole (Septra) in doses appropriate for age and weight bid × 7 to 10 days.

    4. Boiling water and quinacrine (Atabrine) 100 mg PO tid × 5 days.

62. Pharmacologic management of nausea and vomiting includes:

    1. Emetrol 15 to 30 ml PO.

    2. Promethazine (Phenergan) 25 mg.

    3. Hydroxyzine hydrochloride (Vistaril) 1 mg IM.

    4. Trimethobenzamide (Tigan) 10 mg PO prn.

63. The two major factors that lead to disruption of the GI mucosa with subsequent development of an ulceration are:

    1. Alcohol consumption and use of NSAIDs.

    2. Use of NSAIDs.

    3. Use of NSAIDs and *Helicobacter pylori* infection.

    4. *Helicobacter pylori* infection and smoking.

64. A young woman presents with a history of recent unprotected sexual activity with a partner who now has a diagnosis of hepatitis B. She is currently asymptomatic and she does not recall having a vaccine in the past. The best action for the nurse practitioner is:

    1. Draw blood for a hepatitis B e antibody test (anti-HBe).

    2. Administer one dose of HBIG.

    3. Administer two doses of HBIG and initiate vaccination.

    4. Administer one dose of HBIG and initiate vaccination.

65. What condition is a contraindication for the administration of the hepatitis B vaccine?

    1. Pregnancy.

    2. Breastfeeding.

    3. Severe hypersensitivity.

    4. Age >60 years.

66. A 78-year-old client is given a diagnosis of enterocolitis and the physician prescribes vancomycin (Vancocin) 125 mg PO qid. The nurse practitioner will follow the progress of the client. What areas will be monitored with regard to medication tolerance?

    1. CBC, platelet count, clotting studies.

    2. Serum creatinine, blood urea nitrogen (BUN), hearing changes.

    3. Serum electrolytes, urinalysis, ataxia.

    4. Changes in bowel habits, diarrhea, electrocardiographic changes.

67. A client with PUD is treated with a regimen that includes bismuth subsalicylate (Pepto-Bismol), tetracycline, and metronidazole (Flagyl). The client calls the nurse practitioner to report that his stools are unusually dark. He is not experiencing any gastric discomfort, orthostatic hypotension, or increased lethargy. The nurse practitioner's interpretation of this information is:

    1. He is probably bleeding and should come in immediately.

    2. He ate something that affects the color of his stool.

    3. His stools are dark because of the Pepto-Bismol.

    4. The stool discoloration is due to the metronidazole (Flagyl).

68. A patient with a history of arthritis and gastric ulcers comes to the clinic complaining of severe GI distress. The client has been taking Zantac 150 mg bid. The nurse practitioner would ask all of the following questions. Which would be considered the most important?

    1. Are you taking the Zantac with food?

    2. Are you taking the Zantac with water?

    3. Have you changed your eating habits recently?

    4. What medication are you using for the arthritis?

69. When teaching a client with hepatitis C who is receiving interferon and ribavirin therapy, the nurse would encourage the client to eat:

    1. Small frequent meals, high in carbohydrates.

    2. Small frequent meals, high in protein.

    3. Three well-balanced meals daily, high in calories.

    4. Three well-balanced meals daily, but with minimal fluid intake.

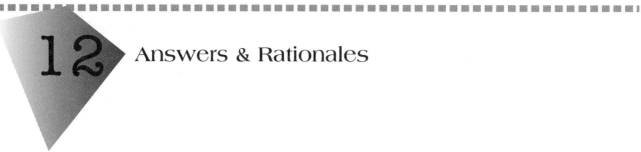

Answers & Rationales

Physical Examination & Diagnostic Tests

1. **(4)** Inspection and auscultation should be conducted first to prevent undue guarding. The nurse practitioner should auscultate and listen to the abdomen before percussing and palpating it, because palpation may alter the frequency of bowel sounds. If the examination is painful initially, the client is going to be very uncomfortable with allowing the examiner to continue.

2. **(4)** Although all of the information is important in sorting out the cause of abdominal pain, for a young female client of child-bearing age, ascertaining whether the client is pregnant is a priority. The nurse practitioner should obtain a gynecologic history including dates of last two normal menstrual periods, condom use, whether client is sexually active, and timing of last sexual intercourse. The location and character of the pain may help identify its origin. Abrupt onset of pain usually has a different cause than pain that develops over hours. Whether the pain has changed since onset can help in determining whether a larger area of the abdomen is becoming involved or whether the pain is subsiding. Both visceral and parietal pain can be referred to remote sites along shared nerve pathways. Aggravating and alleviating factors can provide clues to the origin of the pain. Medical history and medication history can give clues to known conditions and to medications that may be causing the symptoms or are being used for conditions that can cause abdominal pain. For example, a client taking ranitidine (Zantac) may fail to mention a history of gastroesophageal reflux disease (GERD).

3. **(1)** If abdominal pain results from passive internal rotation of the right hip from the 90-degree hip/knee flexion position, the client has a positive obturator sign, which is suggestive of appendicitis. In a positive Murphy's sign (Option #2), pain and a brief inspiratory arrest result when a client takes a deep breath while the examiner applies pressure over the gallbladder. This is suggestive of cholecystitis. Percussion over the costovertebral angles that elicits pain is positive costovertebral angle tenderness, which is suggestive of pyelonephritis. Percussion over the right midclavicular line below the umbilicus and continuing upward is a technique for locating the liver.

4. **(1)** Hepatitis B surface antigen (HBsAg) is found in active or chronic hepatitis B disease. In acute illness, the two factors in serum are HBsAg and antibody to the hepatitis B core antigen (anti-HBc). When the client has made a recovery, HBsAg is usually negative and evidence of surface antibody (anti-HBs) is found. Hepatitis B e antigen (HBeAg) indicates active replication of the virus. IgM anti-HBc–negative results indicate chronic disease. Positive HBsAg indicates chronic disease. Negative HBsAg indicates prior exposure.

5. **(4)** These are standard diagnostic tests used for screening a client with a high risk of colon cancer. The carcinoembryonic antigen (CEA) titer is used more to determine recurrence of cancer; barium enema, upper gastrointestinal (GI) series, and proctoscopy do not provide sufficiently reliable information for detecting a malignancy. The earliest marker of colon

carcinoma is a guaiac-positive stool detected with a Hemoccult test. Fecal occult blood testing is a protocol for collecting and testing six samples from three consecutive stools at the patient's home. Flexible sigmoidoscopy is a procedure that allows direct visual examination of the distal portions of the colon and rectum by a trained examiner using a flexible endoscope after cleansing of the descending and sigmoid colon and rectum. This procedure identifies 80% of neoplasms in the colorectal area. The American Cancer Society's guidelines (2001) recommend fecal occult blood testing annually and sigmoidoscopy every 5 years for adults older than 50 years. All positive test results should be followed up with a colonoscopy. A colonoscopy is a procedure that allows direct visual examination of the entire colon and rectum with a colonoscope.

6. **(4)** This is the surface marker for hepatitis C. At present, there is no way to differentiate the diffuse forms of hepatitis C, because the viremia level is well below the threshold of most assays.

7. **(3)** Options #2 and #3 are almost identical. (*Note*: *use the testing strategy; both are wrong or one is the correct answer*.) In acute pancreatitis the serum amylase level increases within 3 to 6 hours of onset. The serum lipase level is elevated after the increase in the amylase level. (Normal levels of serum amylase in adults are 50 to 180 U/L; normal levels of serum lipase are 55 to 417 U/L.)

8. **(3)** The history, right upper quadrant pain that radiates to the right subscapular area, and a positive Murphy's sign are all commonly associated with cholecystitis. A positive obturator sign at McBurney's point is associated with appendicitis. Clients with strangulated hernias have colicky abdominal pain, nausea, vomiting, abdominal distention, and hyperperistalsis. Those with reducible hernias are asymptomatic or have only mild pain.

9. **(3)** *Helicobacter pylori* appears to be associated with the majority of duodenal and gastric ulcers not attributed to long-term nonsteroidal antiinflammatory drug (NSAID) use. Prevalence of infection in clients with duodenal ulcers is about 70% to 75%. Factors that contribute to GERD include incompetent lower esophageal sphincter (LES) and abnormal esophageal clearance. The most common pathogens in clients with infectious esophagitis are *Candida albicans,* herpes simplex, and

cytomegalovirus. Infectious esophagitis is usually seen in immunosuppressed clients. Irritable bowel syndrome (IBS) is a chronic functional disorder without structural or biochemical abnormalities.

10. **(1)** The client is demonstrating classic symptoms of appendicitis. The nurse practitioner would want to obtain a CBC with differential. Hemoglobin S is specific for sickle cell anemia. Coombs' antiglobulin test shows the presence of antigen-antibody complexes.

Disorders

11. **(1)** Diarrhea is a common symptom in infectious gastroenteritis, inflammatory bowel disease, diverticulitis, and early intestinal obstruction. Diseases of the colon or rectum are often associated with constipation that clearly precedes the onset of abdominal pain. With sexually transmitted diseases, abdominal pain can often occur with vaginal discharge or bleeding and sometimes irregular menses. Dysuria, flank pain, hematuria, and urinary frequency are common signs and symptoms of upper or lower urinary tract infections or ureteral calculi.

12. **(3)** Esophageal pain may radiate to the neck and left arm. Gallbladder pain can radiate to the infrascapular area; diaphragm pain, to the right shoulder; and the pain of appendicitis, to the periumbilical area.

13. **(2)** Gastroenteritis is a common cause of abdominal pain in children. Symptoms vary depending on the type of viral infection. Rotavirus affects mainly infants between 3 and 15 months of age in the winter months. Rotavirus causes voluminous watery diarrhea without leukocytes. Enteric adenoviruses are the second most common cause of viral infection in infants. The symptoms are similar to those of rotavirus, but the duration of illness may be longer. Enteric calicivirus, or Norwalk virus, causes chiefly vomiting, but some diarrhea, in older children and adults. Duration of symptoms is short, usually 24 to 48 hours. Cytomegalovirus, which rarely causes diarrhea, is common after bone marrow transplantation and in the late stages of human immunodeficiency virus (HIV) infection.

14. **(4)** A tense, hard abdomen; verbal refusal or severe pain when asked to jump; and a positive obturator sign are positive signs of peritonitis. Costovertebral angle tenderness is a sign of a renal disorder. Examination of stool for occult blood is not a test for peritonitis. Decreased bowel sounds could be present in appendicitis or bowel obstruction but are not a sign of peritonitis.

15. **(2)** Localized pain that steadily increases for 6 or more hours with rebound tenderness and guarding could be caused by an emergent condition, such as appendicitis or ruptured ectopic pregnancy. Pain in an adolescent girl that is relieved by having a bowel movement could be constipation; pain that is sudden in onset and is in the right lower quadrant, lasting 14 to 36 hours, could be mittelschmerz, if the girl is midway through her menstrual cycle. Pain that follows the onset of vomiting and diarrhea usually occurs in gastroenteritis.

16. **(2)** Pain that awakens a client early in the morning from sleep or is relieved or worsened by food ingestion is typical of peptic ulcer pain. Atypical pain or pain that occurs with anemia or weight loss could be caused by a disorder other than peptic ulcer, such as gastric cancer. Anemia may also indicate acute blood loss from a bleeding ulcer or chronic blood loss (less commonly). The client's ulcer could be bleeding, which would be indicated by blood in the stool.

17. **(4)** IBS presents with abdominal pain and/or altered bowel habits. These symptoms can be exacerbated by psychological stresses. Symptoms disappear during sleep. Bacterial or viral gastroenteritis presents as abdominal pain with diarrhea and vomiting of abrupt onset. Drug-induced diarrhea follows initiation of drug therapy, and in this situation, there is no mention of previous drug therapy. In inflammatory bowel disease, nocturnal diarrhea, and abdominal pain are often accompanied by rectal fistula, fever, and/or skin lesions. Diarrhea occurring with giardiasis is malodorous. Weight loss occurs over a period of weeks.

18. **(3)** Dysphagia for both liquids and solids and repeated swallowing or performance of a rapid Valsalva maneuver that helps food or liquid pass into the stomach are reported by clients with dysphagia caused by a motility disorder. It is episodic, nonprogressive, and unpredictable. Those with dysphagia caused by obstruction have more difficulty swallowing solids than liquids, may have a stricture from esophagitis, have progressive dysphasia, may have chronic heartburn, and may report marked weight loss if an esophageal cancer is present.

19. **(1)** Esophageal inflammation caused by excessive reflux that overpowers the normal mucosal defense mechanism leads to symptoms of reflux. People with and without a hiatal hernia can experience gastroesophageal reflux. Physiologic or normal reflux occurs in most people after eating when they are in an upright position, especially during vigorous exercise, but its low frequency and small volume do not lead to symptoms. Symptoms of PUD are initiated by erosion of the gastrointestinal (GI) mucosa.

20. **(2)** The most common hernia is an inguinal hernia, protruding at the inguinal canal. *Incarcerated* means the hernia cannot be reduced or returned to the abdominal cavity. A reducible hernia easily moves across the abdominal wall. There should be no abdominal swelling, and if the hernia is particularly painful and associated with nausea and vomiting, strangulation should be considered.

21. **(2)** All cases of recurrent, not new, dyspepsia indicate a need for endoscopy. Endoscopy is reserved for those clients with no response to empiric therapy after 7 to 10 days and symptoms persisting after 8 to 12 weeks of therapy. Dyspepsia can be characterized by fullness, belching, and regurgitation and can be associated with PUD and GERD. Smoking should be discontinued and alcohol intake should be decreased to a moderate level in clients with PUD and GERD, but endoscopy is not indicated for these clients.

22. **(2)** The factor contributing most to reflux is an incompetent LES, the antireflux barrier. Hiatal hernia is not believed to play an important role in the etiology of reflux. Hiatal hernias usually cause no symptoms; however, in clients with reflux, they can be associated with higher amounts of reflux and delayed esophageal acid clearance. Reflux occurs after meals in the upright position and may be exacerbated by meals, but overeating is not a direct cause. Alcohol and excessive use of caffeine may affect the LES pressure.

23. **(3)** The etiologic agents that produce inflammation and cause diarrhea are

characterized by positive fecal leukocytes. Viral diarrhea is free of pus; thus no fecal leukocytes would be found on the smear. Noninflammatory diarrhea is usually caused by rotavirus. Toxigenic bacteria cause diarrhea by elaborating toxins that have been released after bacterial growth in the intestine. The term is indicative of colonic involvement by invasive bacteria or parasites or toxin production that affects the large bowel. These poisonous substances result in secretory diarrhea.

24. **(3)** The female-to-male ratio for IBS is 4:1. It is a disease of young or middle-aged adults, frequently appearing at age 20 to 25 years.

25. **(4)** A common means of hepatitis B transmission is from mother to baby during the perinatal period. Other mechanisms of transmission are exposure to infected body fluids, sexual contact, and transfusion of blood or blood products. Hepatitis E virus is spread in contaminated water. Hepatitis A's mode of transmission is fecal-oral and person-person.

26. **(3)** The client is presenting with the most reliable symptoms of GERD. GERD is most often related to inappropriate relaxation of the LES, which allows reflux of gastric acid and pepsin into the distal esophagus. Common presentations of IBS are differentiated by cramping, abdominal pain, or altered bowel habits predominating. Clients with esophagitis complain of the acute onset of chest pain, dysphagia, and odynophagia. Bleeding is associated with carcinoma.

27. **(1)** Hepatitis A and E are transmitted by the fecal-oral route. Hepatitis A spreads rapidly in households and day care centers for children. Risk is higher in day care centers with young children who wear diapers. Outbreaks can also be caused by ingestion of food and water contaminated with human sewage. Hepatitis B is transmitted by blood transfusion, needle-sharing, sexual contact, and vertical (perinatal) transmission. Hepatitis B is not primarily transmitted by the fecal-oral route. Hepatitis C is primarily transmitted through parenteral exposure to blood or blood products. Hepatitis D occurs as a coinfection with hepatitis B; mode of transmission is parenteral exposure to blood or blood products, sexual contact (with hepatitis B also present), or injection of drugs. Hepatitis E is transmitted through the fecal-oral route.

28. **(4)** Because indirect hernias are due to a congenital defect in which the processus vaginalis remains patent, they occur more often in younger persons. A portion of the bowel and/or the omentum comes through the internal abdominal ring, traverses the spermatic cord through the inguinal canal, and exits at the external inguinal ring. In a direct hernia, the omentum or bowel protrudes directly through the floor of the inguinal canal and exits through the external inguinal ring. Because this type of hernia is due to a weakness in the abdominal structures, it occurs more often in middle and later years of life.

29. **(2)** Enterobiasis parasites reside in the intestine. Females lay eggs on the skin outside the anus, which results in extreme pruritus. Humans are the only hosts. Hookworm larvae reside in the soil, enter the body through the feet, and can cause anemia. When dirt containing roundworm eggs is ingested as a result of pica or its presence on unwashed vegetables or when contaminated water is consumed, an intestinal infestation occurs. Giardiasis results from ingestion of the protozoan *Giardia lamblia* through contaminated water or via oral-fecal transmission.

30. **(4)** Certain acidic and fatty foods such as chocolate, peppermint, and orange juice should be avoided. Low-energy diets are used for weight loss in obesity. Energy-controlled diets are used for clients with diabetes mellitus for increased glucose tolerance. High-energy and hemodynamically stabilized diets are used for clients with anorexia for increased weight and fat. Severe cases may require parenteral feeding.

31. **(1)** The major nonpharmacologic intervention for GERD is to advise the client not to lie down within 3 hours after meals, the period of greatest reflux. Management of GERD also includes weight reduction, avoidance of lying down after meals, avoidance of large meals, avoidance of exercise after meals, and elevation of the head of the bed. Certain foods and drink such as alcohol, mint, and orange juice should be avoided because they delay gastric emptying. Acidic foods such as tomato products and spicy foods should be avoided, since they may cause symptoms of heartburn. The client should be taught to avoid bending after meals. Drinking large amounts of fluids with meals does not influence GERD.

32. **(2)** *Helicobacter pylori* has been implicated in the etiology of ulcer disease. The three main causes of peptic ulcer disease (PUD) are use of NSAIDs, chronic *H. pylori* infection, and acid secretory states such as Zollinger-Ellison syndrome. The other organisms listed are implicated in other types of infections, such as acute otitis media and skin infections. *Streptococcus pneumoniae and Moraxella catarrhalis* have been implicated as causative agents in pneumonia.

33. **(4)** Chronic hepatitis B and C and alcohol are the most important causes of cirrhosis in the United States. Especially in men, consumption of one six-pack of beer or 4 to 6 glasses of wine daily significantly increases the risk for long-term hepatic injury leading to cirrhosis. The corresponding amount for women is about half that. Hepatitis A is a self-limited infection without a known chronic state. Hepatitis D acute infections do not directly result in a high incidence of cirrhosis. Wilson's disease is a rare autosomal metabolic disease that may lead to cirrhosis, but the incidence of cirrhosis associated with Wilson's disease is lower than that associated with alcoholism and hepatitis B and C. Wilson's disease usually occurs between the ages of 10 and 30 years and is characterized by excessive deposition of copper in the liver. In advanced cases of cirrhosis, hemochromatosis may be associated with congestive heart failure.

34. **(2)** A hemorrhoid results when a vascular anal cushion prolapses through the anal canal and is entrapped by the internal anal sphincter. In a rectal mucosa prolapse, the wall of the rectum prolapses. A tumor is not a vascular anal cushion. An inguinal hernia is a result of trapped peritoneal fluid in the tunica vaginalis of the testis. When the vaginalis is open, an abdominal structure may be forced into it, resulting in an inguinal hernia. Hemorrhoids become symptomatic as a result of activities or conditions that increase venous pressure, such as prolonged sitting, straining on stool, and pregnancy.

35. **(2)** These characteristics describe hepatitis B, which is prevalent among intravenous drug users and homosexuals. Hepatitis A has similar symptoms but can usually be transmitted by the fecal-oral route and has an incubation period of 15 to 50 days (averages 30 days) and no chronic form. Hepatitis C infection rarely causes jaundice. It is transmitted parenterally and has an incubation period of 14 to 140 days (averages 42-49 days) and a chronic form. Hepatitis D coexists with hepatitis B, is transmitted parenterally, and can also become chronic. Hepatitis E is characterized by oral-fecal transmission associated with contaminated food and water and has an incubation period of 14 to 60 days and no chronic disease state.

36. **(2)** Although most clients with cholelithiasis need eventual intervention, those who are elderly and have diabetes are at increased risk for complications and should be hospitalized for prompt diagnosis, administration of intravenous fluids, pain control, and surgical consultation. Clients with diabetes mellitus and cirrhosis have an increased risk of cholelithiasis.

37. **(3)** A typical description of a solid food dysphagia is given by clients who have esophageal tumors. The symptom of heartburn caused by either gastric ulcer or acid reflux should be controlled with an H_2 blocker or proton pump inhibitor. Weight loss and progressive solid food dysphagia are clinical findings of esophageal cancer. Esophageal cancer usually develops in men (ratio of men to women is 3:1) between the ages of 50 and 70 years. Long-term tobacco and alcohol use increase the risk. Solid food dysphagia is present in more than 90% of clients. Clients with PUD have a history of NSAID use, smoking, and nonspecific epigastric pain. Alcohol does not appear to cause ulcers. Clinical manifestations of lung cancer include cough, hemoptysis, dyspnea, chest pain, and weight loss.

38. **(4)** Esophageal varices are dilated submucosal veins that may result in upper GI bleeding. One third of clients have upper GI bleeding. Clients with a history of heavy alcohol intake are at increased risk for cirrhosis and portal hypertension, which may result in variceal bleeding. These clients often present clinically with bleeding, spontaneous "coffee ground" or bright red blood, hypotension, and eventual shock. Esophageal varices are found in half of clients with cirrhosis. Clients with seizure disorders have seizures for 30 to 90 seconds; they may have a history of head trauma and eye deviation during the seizures. Pancreatitis usually presents with pain in the epigastrium. Clients with cerebral hemorrhage have neurologic deficits that gradually progress in a stepwise fashion.

39. **(3)** A strangulated hernia is irreducible, and the blood supply to the trapped bowel is compromised, resulting in bowel infarction. Ulcers, endometriosis, and ectopic pregnancy can cause abdominal pain and can be surgical emergencies, but they do not cause bowel obstruction.

40. **(2)** Increasing crampy abdominal pain that starts as periumbilical pain, anorexia, and fever are classic symptoms of appendicitis. The client should be evaluated by a surgeon to decrease the risk of rupture of the appendix. Although ectopic pregnancy should always be a consideration in young females with abdominal pain, the characteristics of the pain and other symptoms are not typical of an ectopic pregnancy.

41. **(3)** Abstinence from alcohol will stop the progression of cirrhosis and is the most important treatment in cirrhosis. The diet for the patient should be nutritious, with adequate protein and calories. Salt should be restricted if the client has fluid retention. Vitamin supplementation is needed, but an adequate amount is obtained through diet and multivitamins without extra vitamin B supplements. Ferrous sulfate is given for iron deficiency anemia. Dietary protein should be restricted during acute episodes of cirrhosis. Long-term corticosteroid therapy is not used in long-term disease management. For selected clients, liver transplantation is indicated.

42. **(2)** Diverticular disease presents with change in bowel habits (diarrhea alternating with constipation) and blood in the stool; if diverticulitis develops, flatus, low-grade fever, and leukocytosis may be present. Clients with diverticulitis have a range of mild to severe disease. Abdominal pain in the left lower quadrant ranges from mild to moderate with frequent nausea and vomiting. Appendicitis may present with pain in the right lower quadrant and may not be severe until perforation occurs. Other signs—including nausea and vomiting, leukocytosis, and fever—may or may not be present. IBS may present with aching or cramping periumbilical or lower abdominal pain, often precipitated by meals and relieved by defecation. Pain may radiate to the left side of the chest or left arm. There may be alternating episodes of diarrhea and constipation. Pancreatitis may present with epigastric pain or tenderness that lasts for hours and may radiate to the back, fever,

nausea and vomiting, mental confusion, and jaundice.

43. **(1)** A high-fiber diet is the treatment for this disease, and vegetarians who eat increased amounts of fruits, vegetables, grains, and cereals are in the lowest risk category. Clients mentioned in Options #2, #3, and #4 are at higher risk. Low-sugar diets and high-cholesterol diets do not influence the incidence of diverticular disease.

44. **(4)** Colorectal cancer occurs most commonly in individuals older than 50 years. A change in bowel habits with reduced caliber of stool and blood mixed with the stool are characteristic of cancer in the left side of the colon, which is the most common site. Anemia is found with right-sided lesions. Bright red rectal bleeding and tenesmus are characteristic of rectal cancer.

45. **(1)** Colon cancer risk in clients with ulcerative colitis increases by 0.5% to 1% per year after the tenth year following diagnosis. Folic acid 1 mg/day assists in decreasing the risk. Colonoscopies are recommended every 1 to 2 years for 8 to 10 years after diagnosis. PUD is associated with NSAID use, *H. pylori* infection, and acid hypersecretory states. Perforation is associated with diverticulitis, an intraabdominal infection, which is the result of perforation of a colonic diverticulum. Risk factors for depression include genetic factors, developmental problems, and social stresses.

46. **(4)** PUD in the elderly often does not cause the usual pain and indigestion associated with the disease in younger individuals. Smoking does increase the risk and, without the pain as a warning sign, perforation is common. Gastric ulcers are more commonly seen in the elderly.

47. **(1)** Cancer of the esophagus is found mostly in elderly men. Alcoholism and smoking are the primary risk factors for cancer of the esophagus. The cell type is usually squamous cell. Dysphagia for liquids, cough, and hoarseness, as well as midchest pain, indicate late disease, which does not usually respond to any treatment, including surgery.

48. **(4)** Flexible sigmoidoscopy and colonoscopy are screening tools for colorectal cancer, recommended after age 50. They are useful for identifying adenomatous polyps, which are considered premalignant. Sessile or flat polyps are more suggestive of malignancy. Polyps of

the cecum and polyps <1 cm are less likely to be malignant, and villous polyps are often malignant.

49. **(2)** Excessive vomiting with loss of acid and gastric juice is the most common cause of metabolic alkalosis. Respiratory problems do not precipitate primary metabolic acid-base imbalance, and renal disease most often causes metabolic acidosis. Severe anxiety resulting in hyperventilation results in respiratory alkalosis. Hyperventilation results in an increase in pH.

50. **(3)** The location of the injury indicates the possibility of a ruptured spleen. While bowel and bladder problems are possible with blunt trauma to the abdomen, the upper abdominal location makes a spleen injury more likely. Older children may complain of dizziness, fatigue, chest pain, and palpitations caused by arrhythmias; but hematomas are not usually present.

Pharmacology

51. **(2)** Ribavirin has been associated with birth defects. Tylenol is not recommended because it can be hepatotoxic. Ginkgo is not recommended because it decreases platelet aggregation. It is recommended for the client to eat frequent small meals because of the nausea associated with hepatitis C.

52. **(4)** For clients with recurring symptoms after a course of treatment for PUD, the nurse practitioner should consult the physician. The client is having symptoms of active bleeding, and endoscopy may be indicated at this point. The physician should be consulted regarding the next step. Omeprazole (Prilosec), a proton pump inhibitor that inhibits acid secretion, is useful for hypergastrinemia and may be useful in clients with PUD not controlled by H_2 antagonists in the absence of active bleeding.

53. **(3)** H_2 blockers, changes in diet, and weight reduction are the first-line treatment for GERD. The client should be advised to sit up after meals and sleep with his head elevated. Anticholinergics (Pro-Banthine) may increase the problem by lowering the LES pressure. Omeprazole is not recommended for the first phase of treatment and is indicated for clients whose symptoms persist after 6 weeks of standard doses of H_2-receptor antagonist therapy.

54. **(3)** Goals of PUD treatment include relief of pain, healing of ulcer, and cost-effectiveness. The proton pump inhibitors heal 90% of duodenal ulcers after 4 weeks and 90% of gastric ulcers after 8 weeks. Proton pump inhibitors such as omeprazole are recommended for ulcers because these drugs provide faster pain relief and more rapid healing than H_2-receptor antagonists. The anticholinergic drugs, doxepin (Sinequan) and pirenzepine, are useful when used with the H_2-receptor antagonists but are limited by side effects and used only in Canada and Europe at this time. Clarithromycin is used in the active treatment of *Helicobacter pylori*–associated ulcers as part of the eradication therapy. The eradication therapy is prescribed for 10 to 14 days.

55. **(1)** Therapy with a COX-2 selective agent (celecoxib, rofecoxib) is recommended for the majority of clients at high risk of NSAID-induced complications. The prostaglandins, such as misoprostol (Cytotec), are also used to decrease recurrent ulcerations in clients who require NSAIDs. They have not, however, been shown to increase ulcer healing. Cimetidine (Tagamet) has been shown to increase healing. Doxepin (Sinequan) and pirenzepine are not prescribed in the United States as of this date.

56. **(2)** If a person exposed to a client known to be positive for hepatitis B has sufficient immunity to hepatitis B, no treatment is necessary. If this same person had not been vaccinated, in addition to initiation of the hepatitis B vaccine series, hepatitis B immune globulin (HBIG) 0.06 ml/kg IM is also administered. If an exposed person has had an inadequate immune response to the hepatitis B vaccine series, a hepatitis B booster is to be given. There is no need to repeat the series. If the response to the hepatitis B vaccine series is unknown, test the exposed person's HBsAg level and decide what intervention, if any, is needed.

57. **(1)** Clients with refractory ulcers caused by *H. pylori* are successfully treated with the triple-drug therapy of omeprazole (Prilosec), amoxicillin (or metronidazole if allergic to penicillin), and clarithromycin. An H_2-receptor antagonist may be substituted for the proton pump inhibitor (omeprazole) for less expensive

therapy. Treatment should be given for 10 to 14 days. After completion of *H. pylori* eradication therapy, treatment should continue with a proton pump inhibitor or H_2-receptor antagonist for 4 to 8 weeks to promote healing of the ulcer.

58. **(2)** Sulfasalazine (Azulfidine) therapy for clients with mild ulcerative colitis results in symptomatic improvement in 50% to 75% of cases. If no response is seen after 2 to 4 weeks, the addition of prednisone is recommended. This drug prevents relapse of ulcerative colitis once remission is induced. The other drugs listed are not recommended as first-line treatment.

59. **(2)** Since 25% of clients are effectively treated with lifestyle changes, therapy should begin with use of these measures. If these are not completely effective, an H_2-receptor antagonist can be added. Twice-daily dosing is recommended. Omeprazole (Prilosec) is recommended only for refractory cases after 6 weeks of standard doses of H_2-receptor antagonists. Cisapride (Propulsid) is not recommended because of the possible cardiac side effects. Lifestyle changes and antacid tablets as needed are the recommended starting points for therapy.

60. **(1)** Immunoglobulin 0.02 ml/kg should be given as soon as possible after exposure to minimize the risk of a contact developing hepatitis A. It has not been shown to be effective if administered more than 2 weeks after exposure.

61. **(3)** Treatment with sulfamethoxazole and trimethoprim shortens the course and prevents further spread of the organism. Prevention of dehydration that can result from the diarrhea is accomplished through symptomatic treatment (clear liquids for 24-48 hours, no dairy products, electrolyte-rich sports drinks, advance diet as tolerated). Antidiarrheal medications are not recommended because intestinal motility is important in recovery. Option #4 would be appropriate treatment for nonpregnant adults who have giardiasis.

62. **(1)** The Emetrol dose for adults is 15 to 30 ml. Phenergan 25 mg can be given to children older than 12 years (not 6 years old) and adults. The older child and adult dose for hydroxyzine hydrochloride (Vistaril) is 25 to 100 mg. Trimethobenzamide (Tigan) is dosed at 200 mg, not 10 mg.

63. **(3)** NSAIDs are more often associated with mucosal disruptions causing gastric ulcers. *H. pylori* is associated with mucosal disruption that leads to PUD. Alcohol and smoking are not causes of GI mucosal disruption.

64. **(4)** For unvaccinated clients with exposure to hepatitis B, administer one dose of hepatitis B immune globulin (HBIG) and initiate the hepatitis B vaccine series. HBIG may be protective or may attenuate the severity of the illness, if given within 7 days of exposure (adult dose of 0.06 ml/kg body weight). If the client thinks the individual may have been vaccinated but does not know whether there was a response, the nurse practitioner may have prevaccination antibody testing done. The hepatitis B e (HBe) antibody test is done to determine the potential for transmission; the HBe antibody generally appears about 3 months after the onset of the infection.

65. **(3)** The only contraindication to the hepatitis B vaccine is a prior anaphylaxis or severe hypersensitivity to the vaccine or components of the vaccine.

66. **(2)** This medication causes problems with nephrotoxicity and ototoxicity (eighth cranial nerve). Laboratory tests to monitor renal function should be done on a regular basis. The client should be frequently evaluated for any hearing loss. The geriatric client is particularly susceptible to complications and toxic effects.

67. **(3)** This is a common observation for a client taking Pepto-Bismol. He or she may also experience a problem.

68. **(4)** H_2 blockers are not effective in preventing ulcerations caused by NSAIDS. If the client is using NSAIDS to control the pain from arthritis, the nurse practitioners should consider changing to a prostaglandin (misoprostol and/or a proton pump inhibitor, omeprazole), which prevent NSAID-induced ulcers.

69. **(1)** Small frequent meals are recommended because of the drug's side effects of nausea, vomiting, and fatigue.

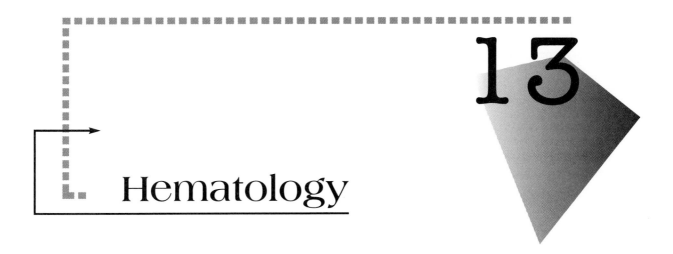

Hematology

Physical Examination & Diagnostic Tests

1. On physical examination, a palpable, firm, non-tender supraclavicular lymph node is noted on the left side of the body. This finding is consistent with a diagnosis of:

   1. Bacterial infection draining from the internal jugular chain.

   2. Thoracic or abdominal malignancy.

   3. Inflammation of the tonsils and adenoids.

   4. Non-Hodgkin's lymphoma.

2. Which test is most important for diagnosing iron deficiency anemia?

   1. Direct Coombs' test.

   2. Serum folate level.

   3. Serum ferritin level.

   4. Red blood cell (RBC) count.

3. The term *shotty* is commonly used to describe lymph nodes that are:

   1. Tender, mobile, and >5 mm.

   2. Small and pellet-like.

   3. Discrete and cystic.

   4. Irregular, soft, and fixed to surrounding tissue.

4. A macrocytic, normochromic anemia is diagnosed in an elderly man. The next test(s) that should be ordered is (are):

   1. Serum iron level and total iron-binding capacity (TIBC).

   2. Bone marrow biopsy.

   3. Colonoscopy.

   4. Vitamin B_{12} and RBC-folate levels.

5. The nurse practitioner would suspect disseminated intravascular coagulation (DIC) if the client's laboratory results indicated:

   1. Increased prothrombin time (PT), decreased platelet count, decreased fibrinogen level.

   2. Decreased PT, increased hematocrit, increased fibrinogen level.

   3. Increased platelet count, decreased hematocrit, increased PT.

   4. Increased platelet count, increased hematocrit, decreased PT.

6. After confirming the diagnosis of iron deficiency anemia in an adult client on the basis of complete blood count (CBC), peripheral smear, serum iron, TIBC, serum ferritin level), what would be the next essential test for the nurse practitioner to order?

   1. Stool guaiac test ×3.

   2. Prothrombin time (PT)/partial thromboplastin time (PTT).

   3. Liver function tests.

   4. Endoscopy.

7. Evaluation of an elderly male client reveals a macrocytic, normochromic anemia. Subsequent testing shows a folate level that is normal and a decreased vitamin B_{12} level. Further evaluation could include:

   1. Referral to a hematologist for a bone marrow biopsy.

   2. Schilling test.

   3. Upper gastrointestinal (GI) series.

   4. No tests are indicated at this time.

8. The most sensitive test for the diagnosis of sickle cell anemia is:

   1. CBC with a peripheral smear.

   2. Bone marrow biopsy and aspiration.

   3. Hemoglobin electrophoresis.

   4. Hemoglobin and hematocrit.

9. An elderly man presents to the nurse practitioner's office with complaints of fatigue, dizziness, decreased activity tolerance, and occasional bounding heart rate. Physical examination reveals pallor (including mucous membranes), tachycardia, and general appearance of lethargy. The following tests are ordered: CBC with differential, peripheral smear, serum iron, TIBC, and serum ferritin level. These tests are ordered because there is a high index of suspicion of:

   1. Sideroblastic anemia.

   2. Pernicious anemia.

   3. Folic acid deficiency anemia.

   4. Iron deficiency anemia.

10. Anemia of chronic disease would reveal which of the following lab findings?

    1. Decreased iron, decreased TIBC, and decreased serum ferritin.

    2. Decreased iron, decreased TIBC, and increased serum ferritin.

    3. Decreased iron, increased TIBC, and decreased serum ferritin.

    4. Decreased iron, increased TIBC, and increased serum ferritin.

Disorders

11. Sickle cell anemia is caused by:

    1. Exposure to ionizing radiation.

    2. A genetically induced production of abnormal hemoglobin S.

    3. A deficiency of dietary folic acid.

    4. Long-term use of thiazide diuretics.

12. An adult client presents to the nurse practitioner with a history of erythrocytosis. One common complaint that could cause a serious complication for this client is:

    1. A laceration.

    2. Vomiting and diarrhea.

    3. Coughing.

    4. Dizziness.

13. A client has a folic acid deficiency anemia. The nurse practitioner teaches the client to eat foods rich in folic acid, such as:

    1. Green leafy vegetables, nuts, and liver.

    2. Carrots, salmon, and avocados.

    3. Cottage cheese, yogurt, and skim milk.

    4. Lima beans, brussels sprouts, and potatoes.

14. Which of the changes occur in the RBC indices for pernicious anemia?

    1. Microcytic, normochromic.

    2. Microcytic, hypochromic.

    3. Normocytic, normochromic.

    4. Macrocytic, normochromic.

15. Which statement is true concerning thalassemia?

    1. It is characterized by defective lymphocyte synthesis.

    2. Thalassemia minor does not require pharmacologic treatment.

    3. Thalassemia major is associated with high RBC counts and elevated serum iron levels.

    4. It is characterized by an acute onset of symptoms leading to leukocytosis.

16. Iron deficiency anemia is an example of:

    1. Macrocytic, normochromic anemia.

    2. Macrocytic, hypochromic anemia.

    3. Microcytic, hypochromic anemia.

    4. Normocytic, normochromic anemia.

17. An adult client with pernicious anemia may present with which signs and symptoms?

    1. Paresthesias, unsteady gait, lethargy, and fatigue.

    2. Hepatomegaly, jaundice, and right upper quadrant pain.

    3. Hypertension, angina, and peripheral edema.

    4. Blurred vision, diplopia, and decreased visual acuity.

18. Anemia of chronic disease is a:

    1. Normochromic, normocytic anemia.

    2. Normochromic, microcytic anemia.

    3. Hypochromic, microcytic anemia.

    4. Hypochromic, macrocytic anemia.

19. A young adult presents to the clinic for a routine checkup. History is unremarkable, and on physical exam, an enlarged (2-cm) mobile, nontender, and rubbery lymph node is palpated on the left posterior cervical chain. The nurse practitioner's next step is to:

    1. Order a throat culture and Monospot test.

    2. Refer the client to a surgeon for a lymph node biopsy.

    3. Order a STAT chest x-ray study.

    4. No intervention is necessary at this time.

20. The nurse practitioner understands that "B" symptoms associated with non-Hodgkin's lymphoma include:

    1. Bruising and bleeding.

    2. Peripheral edema, shortness of breath, and ascites.

    3. Fever, night sweats, and unexplained weight loss (>10% of body weight).

    4. Headache, fatigue, and weakness.

21. In teaching a client with anemia to include foods rich in iron in the diet, the nurse practitioner encourages the client to eat:

    1. Cheese, milk, and yogurt.

    2. Red beans, whole-grain bread, and bran cereal.

    3. Tomatoes, cabbage, and citrus fruits.

    4. Beef, spinach, and peanut butter.

22. Anemia of chronic disease is associated with:

    1. Malnutrition and vitamin B_{12} deficiency.

    2. Infections, inflammation, and neoplasms.

    3. Traumatic injuries and folate deficiency.

    4. Excessive menstrual flow, trauma, and heredity.

23. The nurse practitioner understands that most adult clients with Hodgkin's disease present with:

    1. Nausea, vomiting, and diarrhea.

    2. Night sweats, weight loss, and fever.

    3. Painless, movable mass in the neck, axilla, or groin.

    4. Hepatosplenomegaly with a painful mass in the mediastinum.

24. What is the most common leukemia found in the older adult, typically asymptomatic and characterized by a median survival rate of approximately 10 years?

    1. Acute myelogenous.

    2. Chronic myelogenous.

    3. Acute lymphocytic.

    4. Chronic lymphocytic.

25. Folic acid deficiency most commonly results from:

    1. Lead exposure.

    2. Poor dietary habits.

    3. GI bleeding.

    4. Genetic defect.

Pharmacology

26. The nurse practitioner determines that an adult male client has an iron deficiency anemia and has ruled out GI bleeding as the cause. The nurse practitioner:

    1. Refers the client to a hematologist.

    2. Administers iron dextran 50 mg IM weekly ×4 weeks.

    3. Prescribes ferrous sulfate 300 mg PO tid and has the client return in 1 month for repeat CBC, serum iron level, and TIBC.

    4. Has the client return in 6 months for additional stool guaiac testing.

27. Teaching clients regarding the treatment of vitamin B_{12} deficiency includes:

    1. The client will take vitamin B_{12} tablets twice a day for 1 year.

    2. Oral folic acid supplements will be taken daily for the client's lifetime.

    3. Monthly cyanocobalamin (vitamin B_{12}) injections will be given for the client's lifetime (after being given weekly for the first month).

    4. Iron supplementation and monthly blood transfusions will be required until the deficiency is corrected.

28. Treatment of anemia of chronic disease should include:

    1. A folic acid supplement, 1 mg PO qd.

    2. Iron sulfate ($FeSO_4$) supplement, 300 mg PO tid.

    3. Treatment of the underlying condition.

    4. Weekly epoetin alfa (Epogen) injections.

29. After initiating vitamin B_{12} therapy, the nurse practitioner would expect which of the following during a 2-week follow-up visit to the clinic?

    1. Ferritin level of 40 ng/ml.

    2. Reduced RBCs, white blood cells (WBCs), and platelets.

    3. Increased macrocytosis and anisocytosis.

    4. Increased hemoglobin, hematocrit, and reticulocyte count.

30. It is recommended to administer a 0.5-ml (25-mg) test dose of which medication?

    1. Nascobal (intranasal vitamin B_{12} gel).

    2. Folic acid.

    3. Iron dextran.

    4. Ferrous sulfate (Feosol).

31. What is the prophylactic treatment regimen for adult clients without infection or fever who have neutropenia?

    1. Trimethoprim-sulfamethoxazole, acyclovir (Zovirax), and fluconazole (Diflucan).

    2. Zithromax pack and fluconazole (Diflucan).

    3. Trimethoprim-sulfamethoxazole and dexamethasone (Decadron).

    4. No medication is needed for clients who do not have a fever or infection.

13 ▷ Answers & Rationales

Physical Examination & Diagnostic Tests

1. **(2)** A Virchow's node in the left supraclavicular region is of concern because of the high correlation with abdominal or thoracic malignancy. Infections and inflammatory conditions produce tender, inflamed lymph nodes.

2. **(3)** The serum ferritin level correlates with total body iron stores, since it is the major iron storage protein. Its value is reduced in iron deficiency anemia. The direct Coombs' test measures in vivo red blood cell (RBC) coating by immunoglobulins, and the result is positive in autoimmune hemolytic anemia, blood transfusion reactions, and drug-induced hemolysis. The serum folate level indicates the amount of folic acid in the serum.

3. **(2)** Shotty, or small and pellet-like, lymph nodes that are movable, cool, nontender, discrete, and up to 3 mm in diameter are usually considered normal.

4. **(4)** It is important to determine which type of macrocytic anemia a client has, so that the appropriate therapy can be ordered. Therefore the vitamin B_{12} and RBC-folate levels would be ordered. These tests would determine whether the client has a pernicious anemia (the most common type) or a folate deficiency (also common in the elderly). A serum iron level and total iron-binding capacity (TIBC) would be ordered if an iron deficiency anemia were suspected (it is not in this case because this is a microcytic anemia). There is no indication for a colonoscopy. It would be premature to order a bone marrow biopsy at this point, without performing initial testing and thereby potentially overlooking an easily treated condition (e.g., pernicious anemia, folate deficiency anemia).

5. **(1)** Disseminated intravascular coagulation (DIC) is a complication of infection, malignancy, and sometimes trauma. DIC is the inappropriate accelerated systemic activation of the coagulation cascade, resulting in simultaneous hemorrhage and thrombosis. The lab results would show increased prothrombin time (PT) and a decrease in platelets and fibrinogen in response to the hemorrhage and clotting.

6. **(1)** A stool guaiac test would identify blood loss from the gastrointestinal (GI) tract, the most common cause of iron deficiency anemia. The other tests should be done if the stool guaiac test result is positive. Finding the cause of the iron deficiency is paramount, and the stool guaiac test is an easy, noninvasive method of ruling out bleeding as the cause.

7. **(2)** The Schilling test will determine the cause of the vitamin B_{12} deficiency. It will distinguish among inadequate intake, an intrinsic factor deficiency, and a malabsorption problem. This will allow the practitioner to prescribe the most appropriate therapy for the client. A bone marrow biopsy and an upper GI series are not indicated at this time.

8. **(3)** Normal and abnormal hemoglobins can be detected by electrophoresis, which matches hemolyzed RBC material against standard bands for the various known hemoglobins, including hemoglobin S (the abnormal

hemoglobin that is associated with sickle cell anemia). A complete blood count (CBC) with peripheral smear and hemoglobin/ hematocrit would not yield enough information to diagnose sickle cell anemia. Bone marrow biopsy would not be necessary and would not indicate the presence of hemoglobin S.

9. **(4)** This client's clinical picture is a classic presentation of anemia. Further testing would be needed to determine the type of anemia involved. The most common cause in elderly men is GI bleeding, which would cause an iron deficiency anemia. The tests that were ordered would confirm or rule out this diagnosis; the peripheral smear is especially important in determining the specific type of anemia. If the smear ruled out the diagnosis of iron deficiency anemia, it would lead the practitioner to other diagnoses (including the remaining choices) and appropriate laboratory tests required for confirmation.

10. **(2)** Normal to increased iron stores (serum ferritin) with concurrent low serum iron levels are the hallmarks of anemia of chronic disease. The serum iron level is decreased along with the TIBC. Options #1 and #4 contain incorrect information for the anemias. Option #3 contains the findings for iron deficiency anemia.

Disorders

11. **(2)** Sickle cell anemia is a genetic disorder characterized by the production of hemoglobin S, an anemia associated with shortened erythrocyte survival, microvascular occlusion by sickle-shaped erythrocytes, and an increased susceptibility to certain infections. Exposure to ionizing radiation has been associated with the development of certain malignancies, especially leukemia. A deficiency of dietary folic acid does not cause sickle cell anemia, although folic acid is used in the treatment of these clients to help increase hematopoiesis and aid in recovery from aplastic events. Long-term use of thiazide diuretics has been implicated in the development of hemolytic or aplastic anemias in very rare cases.

12. **(2)** Erythrocytosis (or polycythemia) can be worsened by dehydration from any cause.

Coughing and dizziness will have no effect on the condition, and a laceration may actually improve the symptoms because of the blood loss.

13. **(1)** Green leafy vegetables, nuts, and liver are excellent sources of folic acid. Also, cereals and breads are now fortified with folic acid. The other foods are not significant sources of folic acid.

14. **(4)** A macrocytic (mean cell volume [MCV] >100), normochromic anemia resulting from atrophic gastric mucosa not secreting intrinsic factor is the definition of pernicious anemia. These indices could also include folic acid deficiency anemia. Options #1 and #2 could include iron deficiency anemia or anemia of chronic disease. Option #3 could also include anemia of chronic disease.

15. **(2)** Thalassemias are chronic, inherited anemias characterized by defective hemoglobin synthesis leading to a decreased RBC count, profound microcytosis, a normal serum iron level, and normal RBC distribution width index (RDW) in thalassemia minor, which does not require pharmacologic treatment. Clients with thalassemia minor should not be given iron supplements to resolve anemia. Clients with thalassemia major are usually treated by a hematologist.

16. **(3)** Iron deficiency anemia is a microcytic, hypochromic anemia. The RBCs are smaller (microcytic) because of the decrease in hemoglobin production caused by inadequate amounts of iron. This also makes the cells appear pale (hypochromic). The other selections describe other types of anemia, which would be determined by the peripheral smear.

17. **(1)** A deficiency in vitamin B_{12} can cause neurologic signs and symptoms including paresthesias, an unsteady gait, lethargy, and fatigue. These findings are specific to pernicious anemia and so must always be assessed for in any client who presents with an anemia. The other signs and symptoms are not characteristic of pernicious anemia.

18. **(1)** Anemia of chronic disease is a chronic normochromic, normocytic anemia. Production of hemoglobin and maturation of RBCs are normal.

19. **(2)** A client with lymphadenopathy as described, without evidence of infection, should always be referred to a surgeon for biopsy, because biopsy is the only definitive test with which to rule out a malignancy (a frequent cause of lymphadenopathy not caused by infectious processes). There are no signs or symptoms to suggest the need for a throat culture, Monospot test, or chest x-ray study. Not intervening is not appropriate because the cause of lymphadenopathy needs to be determined.

20. **(3)** This constellation of symptoms (fever, night sweats, weight loss) is used in the staging of non-Hodgkin's lymphoma (NHL); the presence of these symptoms is considered to be an indicator of poor prognosis. The other symptoms may occur, depending on the amount of disease involvement, but they are not considered "B" symptoms (also known as *constitutional symptoms*).

21. **(4)** Beef, spinach, and peanut butter are iron-rich foods. Options #1, #2, and #3 are examples of foods rich in calcium, fiber, and vitamin C, respectively.

22. **(2)** Anemia of chronic disease is associated with infections (e.g., tuberculosis), chronic inflammatory conditions (e.g., systemic lupus erythematosus, rheumatoid arthritis), and malignancies. Excessive blood loss from menstrual flow or traumatic injuries would more likely cause an iron deficiency anemia. Malnutrition can contribute to iron, vitamin B_{12}, and folate deficiencies.

23. **(3)** Most clients present with a painless, movable mass in the neck, axilla, or groin. Older clients may present with fatigue, weight loss, or persistent fever and night sweats. Often, there is pain in diseased areas after consumption of alcohol (an unexplained finding). Hepatosplenomegaly presents with advanced disease.

24. **(4)** Chronic lymphocytic leukemia (CLL) is found primarily in middle-aged and older adults; fewer than 10% of all clients are younger than 50 years. Acute myelogenous leukemia (AML) incidence increases with age, and approximately 50% of clients are younger than 50 years. Chronic myelogenous leukemia (CML) occurs most often at a median age of 45 years. Acute lymphocytic leukemia (ALL) is most common in children and gradually increases in frequency in later life.

25. **(2)** Folic acid deficiency most commonly results from dietary deficits and frequently affects the elderly, the chronically ill, food faddists, and alcoholics. Pregnancy requires an increase in folic acid, as do disease states such as cancer, chronic inflammation, Crohn's disease, rheumatoid arthritis, and malabsorption syndromes.

Pharmacology

26. **(3)** Treatment with iron, administered orally for at least 6 months, is necessary to correct both the anemia and the depleted body iron stores. The client should have the hemoglobin value, hematocrit, iron level, and TIBC rechecked after 1 month of iron supplementation. If improvement is not observed in all measurements, most notably a rise in the hemoglobin level by 1 g/dl, the client should be referred to a hematologist. There is no need to refer the client to a GI specialist or repeat the stool guaiac test, because there is no indication that this client's condition is caused by bleeding. Iron dextran may be used if the client is unable to take PO medications.

27. **(3)** If the deficiency is not due to inadequate intake, the client will require lifetime supplementation with vitamin B_{12}. It must be given in the form of an intramuscular or subcutaneous injection to ensure absorption. Oral folic acid supplements, iron supplementation, and blood transfusions would not treat the cause of the deficiency, and therefore the resulting anemia would not be corrected.

28. **(3)** Treatment of the underlying condition leads to resolution of the anemia of chronic disease. Folic acid and iron supplements are indicated for folate and iron deficiency anemias, respectively. Epoetin alfa (Epogen) injections are indicated for those conditions that affect erythropoiesis, namely, chronic renal failure, chemotherapy-induced anemia, and acquired immunodeficiency syndrome. Clients with underlying iron deficiency anemia **and** anemia of chronic disease may benefit from a trial of iron therapy.

29. **(4)** In addition to a sense of well-being, improved appetite, and reduction of neurologic symptoms (gait disturbances, paresthesias,

numbness and tingling in the fingers, extreme weakness, etc.), the hemoglobin value, hematocrit, and reticulocyte count should increase with vitamin B$_{12}$ therapy.

30. **(3)** The use of IM or IV iron dextran is for clients who cannot tolerate oral supplementation or who have GI disease that limits the oral absorption of oral preparations and treatment should be initiated with a test dose of 0.5 ml (25 mg) so that clients can be observed for anaphylaxis.

31. **(1)** Adult clients with neutropenia should be treated with prophylactic antibiotics, antivirals, and an antifungal when they have no infection or fever. Broad-spectrum antibiotic treatment is ordered for neutropenic fever when the organism responsible for the infection is not known. After blood cultures are obtained, a regimen including cephalosporin, an aminoglycoside, and extended-spectrum penicillin is started.

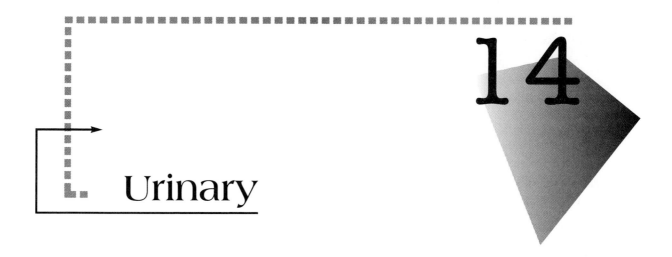

Urinary

Physical Examination & Diagnostic Tests

1. Which urinalysis findings suggest a urinary tract infection (UTI)?

   1. Protein only.

   2. Alkaline pH and positive nitrite and leukocyte esterase.

   3. Hematuria and pyuria only.

   4. Red color without the presence of red blood cells (RBCs).

2. What do an intravenous urography and voiding cystourethrography assist in diagnosing?

   1. Congenital anomalies, stone formation, or foreign bodies.

   2. Renal size and the presence of stones.

   3. A problem in the urethra, prostate, or bladder.

   4. Inflammation of the ureter and renal pelvis.

3. According to the Agency for Health Care Policy and Research (AHCPR) Guideline Panel, the basic continence evaluation for the primary care provider includes:

   1. History, physical examination, measurement of postvoid residual volume, and urinalysis.

   2. Measurement of postvoid residual volume and blood urea nitrogen (BUN) and serum creatinine levels and urinalysis.

   3. History; physical examination; measurement of serum glucose, BUN, and serum creatinine levels; and urinalysis.

   4. Urodynamic, endoscopic, and imaging tests; urinalysis; and measurement of serum creatinine level.

4. Which of the following clients would be a good candidate for urodynamic studies?

   1. Client with a history of stress incontinence and urge incontinence.

   2. Client who had recent surgery for bladder suspension.

   3. Client with initial incontinence episode after total knee replacement.

   4. Elderly male client with residual volume of 45 ml after a 250-ml voiding.

5. The nurse practitioner is evaluating results of serum blood studies for a client who is experiencing a slight increase in blood pressure (BP). The client has no history of high BP and no other chronic diseases. Which serum lab value would the practitioner be most concerned about?

   1. Serum creatinine level of 5.2 mg/dl.

   2. BUN level of 30 mg/dl.

   3. Serum potassium level of 4.5 mEq/L.

   4. Serum osmolarity of 290 mOsm/kg.

6. When taking a history on voiding patterns in adults, the nurse practitioner knows:

   1. Adults normally void q2-3h in a 24-hour period (8-12 times a day).

   2. The first sensation to void occurs when the bladder fills to 200 to 300 ml.

   3. Normally, 15 to 20 minutes passes between the first urge to void and the time that functional capacity is reached.

   4. Adults typically reach functional (comfortable) capacity at 200 to 300 ml and may experience some leakage if voiding is delayed.

7. The nurse practitioner expects which findings on examination of an older client with dehydration?

   1. Tongue furrows and skin tenting on the forehead.

   2. Specific gravity of urine 1.004.

   3. Pulse rate 58 bpm strong and regular; BP 100/62 mm Hg.

   4. Geographic tongue and reduced saliva pool.

8. Which diagnostic test is considered **essential** in the preliminary workup of a client with incontinence?

   1. Urinalysis (UA) with culture and sensitivity (C & S).

   2. Bedside urodynamic studies.

   3. Intravenous pyelogram (IVP) and retrograde pyelogram.

   4. Renal sonogram.

Disorders

9. A young adult female client explains to the nurse practitioner that she has been having frequent and painful urination. The nurse practitioner orders a clean-catch urine for routine urinalysis and culture and sensitivity. The laboratory culture and sensitivity report is as follows: 10^5 *Escherichia coli* and 10^4 *Staphylococcus epidermidis* per milliliter. The nurse practitioner would:

   1. Treat the *E. coli*.

   2. Order penicillin (Amoxicillin)

   3. Treat the *S. epidermidis*.

   4. Encourage client to drink citric fruit juices.

10. An elderly female client is incontinent of urine. Her perineal area is red and excoriated. What would the nurse practitioner advise the family caregiver to avoid using on the skin in the perineal area?

    1. Petrolatum.

    2. Moisture-barrier films.

    3. Mild soap and water.

    4. Zinc oxide ointment.

11. A young adult comes to the student health clinic complaining of severe abdominal discomfort and bloody urine. A priority in the diagnostic workup would include:

    1. Intravenous pyelography to rule out a kidney stone.

    2. Straining all urine.

    3. Microscopic urine exam.

    4. A 24-hour urine culture.

12. Which plan would be most appropriate for an older client with functional incontinence?

    1. Evaluate need for pads.

    2. Limit fluid intake in the evenings.

    3. Perform Credé's maneuver.

    4. Provide a bedside commode.

13. A 60-year-old male client presents with recurrent UTIs. What is the most likely cause?

    1. Balanitis.

    2. Epididymitis.

    3. Chronic bacterial prostatitis.

    4. Benign prostatic hypertrophy.

14. A possible cause of transient urinary incontinence, which can be reversed, is:

    1. Poor pelvic support causing hypermobility of the base of the bladder in females.

    2. Lower urinary tract problems, such as carcinoma.

    3. Cystocele or uterine prolapse in women.

    4. Ingestion of certain medications, such as sedatives, diuretics, anticholinergic agents, and α-adrenergic agents.

15. Which is the best definition of functional incontinence?

    1. Leakage of urine during activities that increase abdominal pressure, such as coughing, sneezing, laughing, or other physical activities.

    2. Mainly caused by factors outside the urinary tract, primarily immobility, that prohibit proper toileting habits.

    3. Inability to delay urination, with an abrupt and strong desire to void.

    4. Occurrence of incontinence with overdistention of the bladder.

16. What are the two most common pathogens in community-acquired UTIs?

    1. *Klebsiella pneumoniae* and *Proteus mirabilis*.

    2. *Staphylococcus saprophyticus* and *Escherichia coli*.

    3. *Proteus mirabilis* and *Staphylococcus saprophyticus*.

    4. *Escherichia coli* and *Proteus mirabilis*.

17. What is the usual clinical presentation of an adult client with cystitis?

    1. No symptoms noted.

    2. Acute onset of chills, fever, flank pain, headache, malaise, and costovertebral angle tenderness.

    3. Complaints of dysuria, urgency, frequency, nocturia, and suprapubic heaviness.

    4. Signs and symptoms of fever, irritability, decreased appetite, vomiting, diarrhea, constipation, dehydration, and jaundice.

18. Recurrent UTIs in females are due to relapse or reinfection. The nurse practitioner understands that relapse:

    1. Is less common than reinfection and occurs within 2 weeks of the completion of drug therapy for the infection.

    2. Is responsible for most recurrent UTIs in females.

    3. May be caused by residual urine after voiding as a result of a prolapsed uterus or bladder or a lack of estrogen.

    4. Can be treated with the same medication regimen as the original infection.

19. The nurse practitioner understands that the treatment of pyelonephritis:

    1. In females is suggestive of a structural problem.

    2. Requires hospitalization, parenteral antibiotic therapy, and an intravenous voiding pyelogram in males.

    3. In females requires hospitalization, parenteral antibiotic therapy, and an intravenous voiding pyelogram.

    4. Requires no follow-up.

20. What is the term given to the type of urinary incontinence associated with conditions such as Parkinson's disease, Alzheimer's disease, and stroke?

    1. Stress incontinence.

    2. Urge incontinence.

    3. Functional incontinence.

    4. Overflow incontinence.

21. A 40-year-old white male presents to the clinic with a history of uric acid renal calculi. The nurse practitioner knows that the alkaline-ash, low-purine diet is very difficult for a patient to adhere to. What other options can be considered?

    1. Monitor the client for another episode.

    2. Discuss the alkaline-ash, low-purine diet with the client.

    3. Start administration of allopurinol (Zyloprim) and monitor the serum uric acid level.

    4. Refer the client to a urologist.

22. A male client presents with complaints of blood in his urine; he has no pain and no difficulty with urination. The nurse practitioner obtains a urinalysis to confirm the presence of blood, and there are no bacteria present. What is the priority diagnosis that must be ruled out for this client?

    1. Cancer of the prostate.

    2. Prerenal failure.

    3. Renal calculi.

    4. Cancer of the bladder.

23. The nurse practitioner is taking the history of a client who has been given a diagnosis of renal calculi. What information in the history would the nurse practitioner identify as a precipitating factor in the development of renal calculi?

    1. Increased incidence of UTIs over the past 3 years.

    2. Drinking 6 to 8 oz of milk daily.

    3. History of fractured femur and prolonged bed rest.

    4. High intake of citrus fruits and high-fiber carbohydrates.

24. A client has a diagnosis of renal failure, and the origin of the problem is thought to be postrenal. What would the nurse practitioner identify as a possible precipitating cause of this client's renal failure?

    1. History of myocardial infarction with severe hypotensive episode.

    2. Advanced prostatic hypertrophy with hematuria.

    3. Renal vascular changes associated with a long history of diabetes.

    4. Exposure to carbon tetrachloride at his job site.

25. A nurse practitioner recognizes what factors as contributing to the development of prerenal failure?

    1. History of an anaphylactic reaction that rendered the client unconscious.

    2. Extended treatment of an infection with gentamicin (Garamycin).

    3. Acute pyelonephritis, and consequently, glomerulonephritis.

    4. Renal vascular changes that occur as a result of atherosclerotic disease.

26. The nurse practitioner is teaching a female client guidelines regarding bladder health, which include all **except**:

    1. Drink at least 6 to 8 glasses of water per day.

    2. Avoid doing Kegel exercises.

    3. Avoid constipation.

    4. Consider estrogen replacement after menopause.

27. A 75-year-old white female client presents to the clinic with her husband, who is her primary caregiver. She has a history of multiinfarct dementia, likely from a long history of untreated hypertension. Her husband reports that for the past 2 days she has had increasing confusion, he has not been able to redirect her, and she has been agitated. He denies any addition of new medications or use of any new over-the-counter or herbal supplements. The nurse practitioner suspects:

    1. New infarct.

    2. Worsening of dementia.

3. UTI.

4. Underlying caregiver stress, seeking help.

Pharmacology

28. A client is diagnosed with benign prostatic hypertrophy. Which medication should be recognized by the nurse practitioner as likely to exacerbate this condition?

    1. Glyburide (DiaBeta).

    2. Oral buspirone (BuSpar).

    3. Inhaled ipratropium (Atrovent).

    4. Ophthalmic timolol (Timoptic).

29. Which of the following agents can be useful for treating stress incontinence?

    1. Propantheline (Pro-Banthine) 7.5 to 30 mg, three to five times a day.

    2. Oxybutynin (Ditropan) 2.5 to 5 mg tid to qid.

    3. Doxepin (Sinequan) 10 to 25 mg qd/bid/tid initially, to a maximum total daily dose of 25 to 100 mg.

    4. Conjugated estrogen (Premarin) 0.3 to 1.25 mg/day, orally or vaginally, and medroxyprogesterone (progestin) 2.5 to 10 mg/day, either continuously or intermittently.

30. To decrease the production of uric acid stones, the nurse practitioner orders what medication?

    1. Allopurinol (Zyloprim).

    2. Potassium citrate (Urocit-K).

    3. Bethanechol (Urecholine).

    4. Phenazopyridine (Pyridium).

31. A 70-year-old woman is treated with oxybutynin (Ditropan) for her urinary frequency and urgency. The nurse practitioner would explain to the client she will probably experience:

    1. Increased sensitivity to sunlight.

    2. Dizziness when she stands up.

    3. A dry mouth and increased thirst.

    4. Increased bruising.

32. All of the following medications can cause urinary incontinence in the older adult **except**:

    1. Hypnotics.

    2. Antibiotics.

    3. Sedatives.

    4. Antidepressants.

33. The nurse practitioner has selected nitrofurantoin (Macrodantin) for treatment of a chronic UTI in a female geriatric client. What should be evaluated before the administration of this medication?

    1. Creatinine clearance (should be >50 ml/min).

    2. Levels of serum alanine aminotransferase.

    3. Any current medications that include anticoagulant agents.

    4. History of allergic reactions to sulfa-based medications.

34. A 46-year-old man with a history of renal calculi presents with complaints of severe flank pain radiating to his groin area; he is also experiencing nausea and vomiting. His temperature is 99° F (37.2° C). What is the best initial order for the nurse practitioner to give at this time?

    1. Morphine sulfate 10 mg SC now.

    2. Ibuprofen (Advil) 600 mg PO now and q6h.

    3. Increase fluid intake and strain all urine.

    4. Trimethobenzamide (Tigan) 250 mg PO now.

35. The nurse practitioner is prescribing nitrofurantoin (Macrodantin) for a woman who is experiencing problems with UTIs. What specific directions are given to this client regarding the administration of this medication?

    1. Medication should be taken with food; anticipate the urine to have brown discoloration.

    2. Do not take medication with milk products; take on empty stomach for better absorption.

    3. Take the medication four times a day until the symptoms have subsided for at least 24 hours.

    4. Acetaminophen (Tylenol) and/or ibuprofen (Advil) should not be taken with this medication.

36. A young woman presents with complaints of burning on urination, frequency, and urgency. Phenazopyridine (Pyridium) is prescribed by the nurse practitioner. What specific directions are given to the client regarding this medication?

    1. May discolor contact lenses; if sclera begin to turn yellow, return to the office.

    2. Always take the medication on an empty stomach to increase absorption.

    3. Do not take any medication containing aspirin or salicylate.

    4. May interfere with effectiveness of the mini pill for birth control.

37. Before prescribing oxybutynin (Ditropan) for the client with overactive bladder symptoms, which disorder in the client's medical history must the nurse practitioner consider?

    1. Diabetes.

    2. Cough.

    3. Narrow-angle glaucoma.

    4. Gallstones.

38. Angiotensin-converting enzyme (ACE) inhibitors are recommended for slowing the progression of chronic renal disease but are contraindicated in the following disorder:

    1. Cardiovascular disease.

    2. Hypertension.

    3. Diabetes.

    4. Renal artery stenosis.

Answers & Rationales

Physical Examination & Diagnostic Tests

1. **(2)** Alkaline pH and positive nitrite and leukocyte esterase are the test results that indicate the presence of a urinary tract infection (UTI). Proteinuria alone suggests glomerulonephritis. Hematuria and pyuria without bacteria may indicate chlamydia, gonorrhea, viral infection, or less commonly, tuberculosis. If the result of a dipstick test is negative for red blood cells (RBCs) but the urine is red, a substance that can change the color of the urine is likely the cause.

2. **(1)** In intravenous urography and voiding cystourethrography, congenital anomalies, stone formation, and foreign bodies can be identified. Renal size and the presence of stones can be seen in flat plate and upright films of the abdomen. In a cystoscopy, the urethra, prostate, and bladder can be visualized. Urethroscopy can be used to visualize the ureter and renal pelvis.

3. **(1)** The 1996 Agency for Health Care Policy and Research (AHCPR) Guideline Panel encourages primary health care providers to initiate the basic evaluation of urinary incontinence by performing a history and physical examination, measurement of postvoid residual volume, and urinalysis. The other tests may be performed on the basis of findings from the initial evaluation.

4. **(1)** The optimal clients for urodynamic studies include those who have not had prior incontinence surgery or who have clear symptoms of stress or urge incontinence. It is not unexpected to find postvoid residual urine in an elderly male client.

5. **(1)** The primary concern for this client is the markedly elevated serum creatinine level of 5.2 mg/dl. All of the other serum lab values are within normal limits. This client should be referred to a nephrologist immediately, because her serum creatinine level is nearing the value (6.0 mg/dl) at which dialysis should be considered. While waiting for the referral, the nurse practitioner should order the following lab tests for her appointment with the nephrologist: whole parathyroid hormone (PTH) level, liver function tests, lipid panel, renal panel, magnesium level, and calcium level. Having these laboratory tests completed will assist the nephrologist in determining the cause of the client's renal failure. A complete review of the client's medications should be initiated to determine whether she is taking any medication that may cause renal failure (e.g., an angiotensin-converting enzyme [ACE] inhibitor [Captopril]). Additionally, a review of the client's family history would be appropriate to rule out a familial kidney disorder (e.g., Alport's syndrome).

6. **(2)** Adults normally void four to six times in a 24-hour period (q4-6h). Most adults usually do not get up in the middle of the night, unless they have a medical problem (e.g., benign prostatic hypertrophy or urge incontinence) or are taking diuretics. The feeling of the bladder filling occurs around 90 to 150 ml, with first urge occurring at 200 to 300 ml. Normally, 1 to 2 hours pass between the first urge to void and the time that functional capacity is reached. Adults typically reach functional (comfortable) capacity at 300 to 600 ml and should *never* experience leakage if voiding is delayed.

7. **(1)** The signs of dehydration in the older adult are skin tenting on the forehead, concentrated urine (specific gravity >1.025), oliguria, sunken eyes, lack of axillary moisture, orthostatic blood pressure changes, tachycardia, dry mucous membranes of the mouth and nose, and absent or small saliva pool. In the obese elder client who has lost weight, tenting of the forehead is not always a reliable clinical sign because of excessive loss of subcutaneous fat from weight loss. As the elder client becomes dehydrated, there will also be a decrease in the aqueous humor of the eye. Gentle palpation of the eyeball will reveal a boggy eyeball versus a firm eyeball. This can be a useful assessment tool for this type of client. It is important to examine the mouth, because it provides reliable assessment data in the older adult suspected of having dehydration. A geographic tongue (patchy papillary loss giving rise to a map-like appearance) should not be confused with tongue furrows and tongue coating.

8. **(1)** Urinalysis with culture and sensitivity is an essential part of an incontinence workup and can be done in the primary care office before more discriminating tests are performed to evaluate bladder storage and emptying. A symptomatic or asymptomatic UTI can cause symptoms of urgency and frequency, which are associated with incontinence.

Disorders

9. **(1)** *Escherichia coli* is the most common organism causing UTIs in the young adult female, and counts of 10^5 are diagnostic of a UTI. *E. coli* will likely respond to trimethoprim-sulfamethoxazole (Bactrim DS) or any suitable, sensitive antiinfective agent; and the client should be treated for the UTI. *Staphylococcus epidermidis* is normal skin flora and is likely a contaminant caused by inappropriate clean-catch specimen collection technique.

10. **(2)** Although moisture-barrier films are very effective in protecting healthy skin from urine, they contain alcohol an can burn and irritate denuded skin; therefore they should be used sparingly. If the perineal area is already red and excoriated, use of a moisture-barrier film is contraindicated. Each time the client is changed, the caregiver should cleanse the perineal area with mild soap and water and then apply a thin layer of either petrolatum or zinc oxide to treat the irritant dermatitis. The addition of vitamin C, 250 mg, daily, and zinc, 220 mg, daily, will aid the healing process. Once the perineal area is healed, the vitamin C and zinc should be discontinued.

11. **(3)** The nurse practitioner suspects a UTI and needs to confirm the diagnosis with a microscopic examination of urine for the presence of white blood cells and bacteria. Also considered in the differential diagnosis would be a kidney stone. If no white blood cells or bacteria are found on microscopic examination, an abdominal x-ray should be ordered to rule out the presence of a kidney stone.

12. **(4)** Functional incontinence is the inability to toilet appropriately because of impaired mobility. Ensuring that the client has the appropriate equipment available at home (i.e., bedside commode, walkers, wheelchairs, accessible bathrooms, and clothing that is easily removed) will assist him or her in maintaining independence. Discussing the option of using products such as Depends while on outings may also provide a sense of independence for the client. This client may also benefit from scheduled toileting every 2 hours, to eliminate the frequency of accidents. Often, clients with functional incontinence become socially isolated and depressed because of their fear of having an "accident" while in public. The nurse practitioner should explore all options available. Evaluating the need for pads is effective with stress incontinence. Limiting fluid intake in the evenings to reduce nocturnal incontinence is appropriate for urge incontinence. Performing the Credé's maneuver is appropriate for overflow incontinence.

13. **(3)** This client likely has chronic bacterial prostatitis, and it is difficult to treat because the bacteria is harbored in the prostatic calculi and the corpora amylacea. Chronic bacterial prostatitis requires 3 to 4 months of treatment with trimethoprim-sulfamethoxazole (Septra or Bactrim DS); a quinolone (Cipro) may be necessary to prevent urinary symptoms.

14. **(4)** Sedative-hypnotics, diuretics, anticholinergic agents, α-adrenergic agents, and calcium channel blockers can cause transient reversible urinary incontinence. Poor pelvic support is a possible cause of stress incontinence. Urge incontinence, or the inability

to delay urination with a sudden and powerful urge to void, is a possible result of lower urinary tract problems. A prolapsed uterus or bladder can cause overflow incontinence with overdistention of the bladder.

15. **(2)** Functional incontinence is the inability to toilet appropriately because of impaired mobility. Stress incontinence is leakage from the bladder during activities that increase intraabdominal pressure and therefore increase the pressure on the bladder, forcing urine leakage. An inability to delay urination, with a strong, abrupt urge to void, is urge incontinence and is due to bladder hyperactivity or a hypersensitive bladder. The client often has little warning before urine passes out of the bladder. Incontinence with overdistention of the bladder is called *overflow incontinence* and is due to an underactive detrusor or one that will not contract or to bladder outlet or urethral obstruction. It is characterized by frequent urination in small amounts.

16. **(2)** *Escherichia coli* is the pathogen in 80% to 90% of community-acquired infections. Gram-positive *Staphylococcus saprophyticus* is the second most common pathogen. *Klebsiella pneumoniae* and *Proteus mirabilis* are also possible common pathogens. In hospital settings, *E. coli* is less prevalent.

17. **(3)** Cystitis in adults usually presents with dysuria, urgency, frequency, nocturia, and suprapubic heaviness. Acute onset of chills, fever, flank pain, headache, malaise, and costovertebral angle tenderness are common in pyelonephritis in adults.

18. **(1)** Relapse is an uncommon cause of recurrent UTIs in women and occurs within 2 weeks of completion of antibiotic therapy. It may need to be treated for 2 to 12 weeks. Reinfection is the cause of most UTIs in women and may be due to residual urine resulting from a prolapsed uterus or bladder or to lack of estrogen in perimenopausal women. If the client has two or fewer UTIs in a year, the single-dose or 3-day regimen of antibiotic therapy may be used.

19. **(2)** Pyelonephritis in men is suggestive of a structural abnormality and is usually an indication for hospitalization, parenteral antibiotics, and an intravenous voiding pyelogram. Pyelonephritis in women is usually

a result of invasion of the urinary tract by bacteria that have ascended the urethra from the introitus of the urethra. If bacteremia is suspected, women need to be hospitalized also. Suggested follow-up is by telephone contact within 12 to 24 hours of initiation of antibiotic therapy and at 2 weeks and 3 months for posttreatment urine cultures.

20. **(2)** Urge incontinence is associated with conditions such as Parkinson's disease, Alzheimer's disease, and stroke that involve the central nervous system, causing detrusor motor and/or sensory instability.

21. **(3)** While discussing the alkaline-ash, low-purine diet with the client is appropriate, most clients, when they learn how difficult it is to follow, will be noncompliant with the diet, even though they realize they run the risk of developing another uric acid renal calculus. Starting administration of allopurinol (Zyloprim) 100 mg qd PO and monitoring the serum uric acid level and ensuring that the level remains at normal levels will control the incidences of uric acid stones, while allowing the client freedom without such strict dietary restrictions. Monitoring the client for another episode is inappropriate, since the serum uric acid is likely elevated and a repeat incident is likely imminent. Referral to an urologist is inappropriate at this time because there is no acute episode.

22. **(4)** Painless hematuria is the most common presenting symptom in the client with bladder cancer. Painless hematuria often occurs early in the course of bladder cancer and is often the only symptom the client will exhibit. There is no evidence of renal failure (oliguria, edema). Renal calculi would be characterized by both hematuria and flank pain, and cancer of the prostate will often present with the other symptoms of benign prostatic hypertrophy.

23. **(3)** A sedentary lifestyle or episodes of immobilization can predispose a client to the development of renal calculi. UTIs usually do not precipitate problems with renal calculi; however, the presence of renal calculi will predispose the client to UTIs. Six to eight ounces of milk daily is not excessive and will not predispose a client to renal calculi, and the increased intake of citrus and high-fiber carbohydrates is good for the client's dietary needs.

24. **(2)** Postrenal failure results because of the development of a complication that presents an obstructive problem distal to the kidney, as seen in advanced prostatic hypertrophy with hematuria. A severe hypotensive episode, commonly seen after an acute myocardial infarction, is considered prerenal. The vascular changes caused by diabetes and the exposure to nephrotoxic chemicals are considered intrarenal.

25. **(1)** The precipitating factor in prerenal failure is most often an incident that precipitated renal ischemia, that is, a shock situation. Treatment with nephrotoxic medications such as gentamicin (Garamycin), pyelonephritis, and renal vascular changes are all causes of intrarenal failure.

26. **(2)** Performing Kegel (pelvic floor) exercises routinely assists in maintaining strong pelvic floor musculature. Weak pelvic floor musculature may contribute to urinary incontinence, especially with activity. Additionally, the nurse practitioner should include teaching about avoiding dietary substances that can irritate the bladder such as caffeine, alcohol, and spicy foods.

27. **(3)** The acute onset of increased confusion, inability to redirect, and increased agitation indicates the presence of an infection in the elder client with dementia. The culprit is likely a UTI. The nurse practitioner should obtain a urinalysis and empirically treat for a UTI until the results of the urinalysis are received. Since there are no neurologic symptoms (weakness, flaccidness, etc.), it is unlikely that there is a new infarct. Acute confusion is not a sign of worsening dementia, because dementia is a gradual process. Underlying caregiver stress would not present with the caregiver bringing the client in with an acute problem. Caregiver stress usually presents with the person presenting to his or her own primary care provider complaining of stress.

Pharmacology

28. **(3)** Benign prostatic hypertrophy is a common cause of urinary retention in older men. Inhaled ipratropium (Atrovent) is an atropine-like bronchodilator that is used to treat chronic bronchitis, and its anticholinergic agent may exacerbate urinary retention. Neither glyburide (DiaBeta), an oral antihyperglycemic agent, nor buspirone (BuSpar), an oral antianxiety agent, has an effect on the urinary system. Timolol (Timoptic) is a topical agent used for the treatment of glaucoma and does not have a systemic effect.

29. **(4)** Combination hormone replacement therapy with conjugated estrogen (Premarin) 0.3 to 1.25 mg/day, administered orally or vaginally, and medroxyprogesterone (progestin) 2.5 to 10 mg/day, given either continuously or intermittently, can be useful for management of stress incontinence. Propantheline (Pro-Banthine) and oxybutynin (Ditropan) may be useful in treating urge incontinence; research on the use of these drugs for urge incontinence is limited. Doxepin (Sinequan) is a tricyclic antidepressant and is used infrequently for stress incontinence today.

30. **(1)** A urinary alkylating agent such as allopurinol (Zyloprim) is frequently used to decrease the formation of uric acid stones. As a standard of practice, the nurse practitioner should check the client's serum uric acid level monthly for 3 months to ensure that levels are decreasing to normal ranges. Once the serum uric acid levels are normalized, serum uric acid levels can be checked annually.

31. **(3)** Oxybutynin (Ditropan) produces anticholinergic effects, and dry mouth is a common side effect. Since this is an elderly client, she may be taking other medications that may exacerbate this side effect. The nurse practitioner should review the client's list of medications to verify that the client is taking no other medications present that will exacerbate this side effect. If she is taking medications that will increase this side effect (e.g., diuretics), the nurse practitioner should advise the client of methods to relieve the dry mouth, such as sucking on hard candy or chewing gum. It is also possible that the client may be taking other medications with anticholinergic side effects and the addition of Oxybutynin (Ditropan) could increase anticholinergic effects to the point that the client could be at risk for falls. Careful review of the client's medication list is essential before a new medication is added. The other reactions listed are not consistent with Oxybutynin (Ditropan).

32. **(2)** Sedatives and hypnotics lead to sedation and muscle relaxation in all populations, but particularly in the elderly population because of the effects of aging on the central nervous system (CNS) that lead to increased muscle relaxation. The combined effects of sedatives and hypnotics and age-related changes often lead to urinary incontinence. Antidepressants have anticholinergic effects and lead to sedation. When the effects of aging on the CNS are combined with the anticholinergic side effects of antidepressants, the elder client experiences increased muscle relaxation, which contributes to urinary incontinence. Antibiotics have not been implicated in the development of urinary incontinence in the elder client.

33. **(1)** Nitrofurantoin (Macrodantin) is contraindicated if there is any impairment of renal function, if the antibacterial concentration in the urine is inadequate, or if there is an increased risk of toxic effects. For a chronic UTI, the nurse practitioner would consider treatment with nitrofurantoin (Macrodantin), 100 mg, PO, qhs, as prophylaxis. When this dose is used for the elder client, there should be no serum or tissue accumulation of the medication. Liver function studies may be indicated if the elder client experiences adverse reactions to the medication. Anticoagulants and sulfa-based medications have not been reported to produce any significant drug interactions.

34. **(1)** The severe pain of renal calculi should be addressed before other treatments or diagnostics. The severe pain needs to be treated as soon as possible with morphine sulfate 10 mg SC or meperidine (Demerol). The ibuprofen (Advil) may be used for beginning pain. Trimethobenzamide (Tigan) can be used, but only after pain relief has been initiated.

35. **(1)** In teaching the client about nitrofurantoin (Macrodantin), the most important side effects are gastrointestinal upset, which can be decreased if the medication is taken with food or milk and discoloration of the urine, which is a very common occurrence. The client should also be told to continue taking this medication for at least 3 days after a sterile urine specimen is obtained and that the medication may interfere with the efficacy of her birth control pills if she is using them.

36. **(1)** The nurse practitioner should advise the client that if she experiences yellow discoloration of the sclera while taking phenazopyridine (Pyridium), she is to return to the office immediately. This may indicate poor renal excretion and requires a renal workup (renal panel; parathyroid hormone [PTH], magnesium, thyroid-stimulating hormone, and serum calcium levels; 24-hour urine collection for determination of creatinine clearance) and possible referral to a nephrologist. Phenazopyridine (Pyridium) should be administered with food, and there is no drug interaction with aspirin or with birth control pills.

37. **(3)** Oxybutynin (Ditropan) is contraindicated in clients with narrow-angle glaucoma. Clients with open-angle glaucoma may take this medication.

38. **(4)** ACE inhibitors increase the pressure within the kidneys in renal artery stenosis, causing an increase in serum creatinine and potassium levels. ACE inhibitors have protective properties for clients with cardiovascular disease, hypertension, and diabetes.

Male Reproductive 15

Physical Examination & Diagnostic Tests

1. Which organ is **not** palpable on physical examination of a male client?

   1. Vas deferens.

   2. Testes.

   3. Epididymis.

   4. Cowper's glands.

2. A review of a lab report with an elevated serum gonadotropin level would raise suspicion of which disorder?

   1. Seminal vesiculitis.

   2. Vas deferens disease.

   3. Testicular disease.

   4. Benign prostatic hypertrophy (BPH).

3. Which of the following structures can be palpated during an external examination of a male client?

   1. Epididymis.

   2. Cowper's ducts.

   3. Seminal vesicles.

   4. Ejaculatory ducts.

4. What would be most helpful in diagnosing gynecomastia?

   1. History and physical examination.

   2. Liver function test.

   3. Thyroid function test.

   4. Mammogram.

5. The correct position in which to place a healthy, adult male client for examination of the rectum and prostate is:

   1. Left lateral Sims' position with right knee flexed and left leg extended.

   2. Supine position with hips and legs flexed and feet positioned on the examining table.

   3. Modified knee-chest position with client prone and knees flexed under hips.

   4. Leaning over the examination table with chest and shoulders resting on the table.

6. Which test is a tumor marker used to diagnose advanced prostate cancer?

  1. α-Fetoprotein (AFP) test.

  2. Prostate-specific antigen (PSA) test.

  3. Prostatic acid phosphatase (PAP) test.

  4. Human chorionic gonadotropin (hCG) test.

7. Which statement is correct about the PSA test?

  1. The PSA level can be elevated in clients with BPH.

  2. The PSA level is not elevated in clients with prostatitis.

  3. Prostatic massage will not elevate PSA levels.

  4. PSA does not increase in reoccurrence of prostate cancer.

8. Which procedure is used in screening males (age 40) for prostate cancer but is not diagnostic?

  1. PSA test.

  2. Digital-rectal exam (DRE).

  3. Urinalysis and complete blood count (CBC).

  4. PSA and DRE.

9. When examining the scrotum of an adult Hispanic male, a normal finding is:

  1. Symmetric scrotal sac with two movable testes.

  2. Smooth, rubbery, sac-like surface that is sensitive to gentle compression.

  3. Asymmetric sac with the left side lower than the right side.

  4. A reddened color that is darker than body skin with sebaceous cysts.

Disorders

10. A 49-year-old male smoker presents to the clinic with complaints of painless gross hematuria. What is the most serious problem that needs to be considered by the nurse practitioner?

  1. Bladder cancer.

  2. BPH.

  3. Erectile dysfunction.

  4. Urinary tract infection.

11. What finding is indicative of testicular torsion?

  1. Scrotal swelling with tenderness that occurs only after age 40.

  2. Sudden onset of pain with a firm, tender mass in the scrotum.

  3. Positive Prehn's sign.

  4. Cremasteric reflex.

12. During a routine physical examination, the client expresses concern over the observation that one side of his scrotum is larger than the other. He states that it has been getting larger for the past few months; the scrotum is smaller in the morning and gets larger throughout the day. He has felt a heaviness in the scrotum, denies any acute pain but does confirm some discomfort in his lower back. He denies any history of trauma to the scrotal area. On examination, the nurse practitioner confirms the enlargement, and on further examination, determines that the scrotum will transilluminate and that manual manipulation of the scrotum does not cause pain. The initial diagnosis for this client is:

  1. Hydrocele.

  2. Orchitis.

  3. Epididymitis.

  4. Traumatic injury.

13. Which statement is correct concerning circumcision?

  1. Circumcision is helpful in preventing phimosis.

  2. Circumcision is a cause of paraphimosis.

  3. Balanoposthitis is the direct result of circumcision in older men.

  4. Circumcision increases the incidence of cancer of the penis.

14. Acute epididymitis is characterized by:

  1. Absence of dysuria.

  2. Nonenlarged scrotum.

  3. Tenderness over the epididymis.

  4. Lack of abdominal pain.

15. Which one of the following is correct about hypogonadism?

    1. Usually presents with impotence.

    2. May cause increased libido.

    3. Is not associated with gynecomastia.

    4. Does not contribute to infertility.

16. Which of the following is a true statement about impotence?

    1. Impotence can be caused by antihypertensives.

    2. Impotence is caused by infections only.

    3. Impotence is not the result of multicausal factors.

    4. Impotence is not the result of vascular problems.

17. Circumcision can prevent which of the following?

    1. Paraphimosis.

    2. Epididymitis.

    3. Sexually transmitted diseases.

    4. Prostatitis.

18. Which statement is true about the prostate?

    1. Secretes fluid that is acid.

    2. Secretes fluid that is alkaline.

    3. Secretes androgens.

    4. Produces sperm.

19. An elderly man presents to the clinic with complaints of difficulty voiding and hematuria. The rectal examination reveals a very firm prostate about 5 cm in diameter, asymmetric, with firm nodules. The PSA level is 14 ng/ml. The next action is to:

    1. Medicate with finasteride (Proscar), 5 mg PO daily and reevaluate in 3 months.

    2. Advise client to avoid caffeine, alcohol, and over-the-counter decongestants.

    3. Obtain a urinalysis to determine presence of infection and amount of hematuria.

    4. Refer to urologist for biopsy and diagnostic evaluation for prostatic cancer.

20. A 20-year-old male presents with complaints of severe scrotal pain for the past 2 hours. The scrotum is swollen and extremely tender; palpation of the epididymis is not possible. The nurse practitioner knows that the immediate treatment is:

    1. Narcotic analgesics and bed rest.

    2. Warm packs and scrotal support.

    3. Antibiotics, ice packs, and analgesics.

    4. Referral to a surgeon for exploration.

21. A 20-year-old male client presents with scrotal pain. A suspected diagnosis that requires immediate referral is:

    1. Testicular torsion.

    2. Hydrocele.

    3. Epididymitis.

    4. Inguinal hernia.

22. An adult male client is being evaluated for dysuria, fever, and perineal pain. The physical exam by the nurse practitioner reveals a distended bladder. Further physical exam should **not** include:

    1. A urine culture.

    2. Prostate massage.

    3. Cultures for gonorrhea and chlamydia.

    4. Measurement of blood urea nitrogen (BUN) and creatinine levels.

23. An older adult male presents with a history of burning on urination and difficulty urinating that has been increasing over the past few days. A STAT urinalysis reveals the presence of leukocytes and bacteria. The primary diagnosis considered by the nurse practitioner is:

    1. Bladder cancer.

    2. Testicular torsion.

    3. Benign prostatic hyperplasia.

    4. Renal failure.

24. The client with localized prostate cancer will exhibit which symptoms?

    1. Hesitancy, frequency, and dysuria.

    2. Fatigue, severe constipation, and dysuria.

    3. Hematuria, nocturia, and weight loss.

    4. Myalgia, confusion, and lethargy.

25. A young male client presents with a complaint of a feeling of fullness in the scrotum. Physical examination reveals a round, soft, nontender, nonadherent bluish discolored testicular mass resembling a "bag of worms"; there is no variation in size with respiration or the Valsalva maneuver. The mass transilluminates and is located anterior to the testes. The most likely diagnosis is:

    1. Varicocele.

    2. Hernia.

    3. Tumor.

    4. Spermatocele.

26. An uncircumcised male client presents with a complaint of not being able to retract the foreskin over the glans penis. What is the most likely diagnosis?

    1. Lateral phimosis.

    2. Phimosis.

    3. Peyronie's disease.

    4. Paraphimosis.

27. A middle-aged male client complains of a tight band causing a lateral curvature of the penis during erection and painful intercourse. What is the most likely diagnosis?

    1. Phimosis.

    2. Lateral phimosis.

    3. Lateral paraphimosis.

    4. Peyronie's disease.

28. A middle-aged uncircumcised client presents with red pinpoint pustules and papules on the prepuce and glans. The most likely diagnosis is:

    1. Peyronie's disease.

    2. Balanitis.

    3. Phimosis.

    4. Paraphimosis.

29. A male client is diagnosed with balanitis; the most likely cause is:

    1. Candidiasis.

    2. Herpes genitalis.

    3. Lichen planus.

    4. Psoriasis.

30. A male client presents with a complaint of sexual dysfunction. The nurse practitioner understands that sexual dysfunction is impairment of:

    1. Erection only.

    2. Emission only.

    3. Ejaculation only.

    4. Erection or emission or ejaculation.

31. A client presents with a complaint of dysuria, enlarged scrotal tenderness over the epididymis, and abdominal pain. The most likely diagnosis is:

    1. Testicular torsion.

    2. Vas deferens inflammation.

    3. Epididymitis.

    4. Balanitis.

32. The nurse practitioner knows that erectile dysfunction is:

    1. Primarily psychological in origin.

    2. Primarily associated with the 70+ older male.

    3. The persistent inability to achieve and maintain an erection adequate for sexual intercourse.

    4. The physiologic dysfunction when smooth muscle contracts, causing a lack of adequate amount of blood in the penis to render a rigid, larger penis.

33. Priapism is classified as which type of sexual dysfunction?

    1. Erection.

    2. Emission.

    3. Ejaculation.

    4. None of the above.

34. In response to a male client's question concerning a possible cause of prostate cancer, which is correct?

    1. Syphilis.

    2. Gonorrhea.

    3. Cryptorchidism.

    4. Balanitis.

35. A male client complains of impotence. Which one may be a contributing factor?

    1. Antihypertensives.
    2. Intercourse.
    3. Smoking.
    4. Masturbation.

36. A young male presents for a sports physical examination. In addition to examining the client for hernias, it would be appropriate for the nurse practitioner to do which of the following?

    1. Teach testicular self-exam.
    2. Perform a PSA test.
    3. Examine for prostate cancer.
    4. Perform a PSA test and a DRE.

37. An older male presents with gynecomastia. The most likely cause is:

    1. Cirrhosis.
    2. Diabetes mellitus.
    3. Hypergonadism.
    4. Peptic ulcer disease.

38. Concerning the male breast, which is a correct statement?

    1. Gynecomastia is the result of low levels of estrogen and normal levels of testosterone.
    2. Most breast cancers in men are estrogen-receptor–positive.
    3. Breast cancer in males is very common.
    4. Gynecomastia is a nonhormonal or tissue alteration.

39. Which is true of prostate cancer?

    1. Rarely diagnosed in men >50 years of age.
    2. Soft, indiscrete, symmetric nodules of the prostate.
    3. Rarely has obstructive symptoms.
    4. Asymmetric, discrete, hard nodules of the prostate.

40. Which symptoms would suggest a possible diagnosis of prostate cancer in a male older than 50 years?

    1. Hesitancy, dribbling, and urgency.
    2. Decreased force of urinary stream.
    3. Pain and feeling of a full bladder.
    4. Rapid onset of obstructive symptoms of urinary output.

41. Which statement is correct concerning testicular cancer?

    1. It is a very common problem in men older than 50 years.
    2. This problem is directly related to testicular trauma.
    3. Testicular cancer presents suddenly with pain.
    4. Testicular cancer is primarily found in young men.

42. Which statement is correct about acute bacterial prostatitis?

    1. Characterized by recurrent urinary tract infections.
    2. Ascending infection of urinary tract.
    3. Always occurs in men younger than 30 years.
    4. Usual treatment is a 12-week course of antibiotics.

43. Which finding is indicative of orchitis?

    1. Extremely painful scrotum.
    2. No history of parotitis.
    3. No evidence of systemic viral infection.
    4. Decreased serum amylase level.

44. A client has nongonococcal urethritis (NGU). The nurse practitioner understands that:

    1. No related problems occur if it is untreated.
    2. It is often asymptomatic.
    3. It is easily differentiated from gonococcal urethritis on physical examination.
    4. There is a very purulent discharge with a foul odor.

45. What organism is the most common cause of NGU in men?

    1. *Chlamydia trachomatis.*

    2. *Neisseria gonorrhoeae.*

    3. *Escherichia coli.*

    4. *Streptococcus faecalis.*

46. Cryptorchidism is defined as:

    1. Testicular underdevelopment.

    2. Imbalance of estrogen/androgen ratio.

    3. Undescended testicles.

    4. Absence of spermatogenesis.

47. Which test is a useful tumor marker for testicular cancer?

    1. α-Fetoprotein (AFP) test.

    2. PSA test.

    3. Prostatic acid phosphatase test.

    4. Alkaline phosphatase (ALP) test.

48. The most common causative agent of orchitis is:

    1. Arbovirus.

    2. Echovirus.

    3. Mumps.

    4. Rubeola.

49. What are common symptoms of BPH?

    1. Dribbling, hesitancy, loss of stream volume and force, and recurrent urinary tract infections.

    2. Dysuria, urgency, frequency, nocturia, and suprapubic heaviness or discomfort.

    3. Obstructive symptoms, such as a weak urinary stream, abdominal straining to void, hesitancy, incomplete bladder emptying, and terminal dribbling.

    4. Acute onset of fever, chills, flank pain, headache, malaise, costovertebral angle tenderness, and possibly hematuria.

50. A 25-year-old client with a history of sickle cell disease complains of a sudden problem with erections that are not sexually oriented. He is currently experiencing a painful erection and he is unable to void. The nurse practitioner knows that the treatment of choice is:

    1. Meperidine (Demerol) and bed rest.

    2. Immediate referral to a urologist.

    3. Increased hydration for sickle cell crisis.

    4. Determination of PSA level.

51. A 65-year-old, uncircumcised man presents to the clinic with complaints of penile tenderness, inability to retract the foreskin, and serosanguineous drainage from beneath the foreskin. The nurse practitioner must first consider the possible diagnosis of:

    1. Balanitis.

    2. Penile cancer.

    3. Herpes.

    4. Penile trauma.

52. What is considered a major contributing factor in erectile dysfunction?

    1. Diet high in vitamin C.

    2. Diabetes mellitus.

    3. Allergies.

    4. Low-sodium diet.

Pharmacology

53. A client has been taking doxazosin (Cardura) 2 mg PO daily for 3 weeks for treatment of his BPH. He returns to the clinic and is complaining of feeling dizzy when he stands up. The nurse practitioner:

    1. Determines the client's blood pressure with client lying down, standing, and sitting.

    2. Orders a urinalysis to determine the presence of hematuria and bacteremia.

    3. Reviews with the client his symptoms over the past 3 weeks.

    4. Performs a rectal exam to determine whether the prostate is smaller than previously noted.

54. In planning the treatment for a client with balanitis, the nurse practitioner orders:

    1. Rest, ice, and elevation.
    2. Massage.
    3. Antifungals.
    4. Emergency circumcision.

55. A 28-year-old male presents with complaints of fever, low back pain, perineal pain, and intense pain on voiding. Rectal exam reveals a tender, swollen, firm, warm prostate. On the basis of the client's symptoms, the treatment of choice is:

    1. Trimethoprim-sulfamethoxazole (TMP-SMX; Septra DS) 1 tablet bid, × 30 days.
    2. Tetracycline (Achromycin) 250 mg qid × 10 days.
    3. Amoxicillin (Amoxil) 500 mg tid × 14 days.
    4. Erythromycin (Ilosone) 250 mg q6h × 24 days.

56. A 70-year-old man complains of scrotal pain with dysuria and frequency that has been increasing over the past 2 weeks. Physical examination reveals extreme tenderness and swelling of the scrotum, there is a urethral discharge, and the testes are normal in size and position. A urinalysis reveals pyuria. On the basis of the client's symptoms, the treatment of choice for this client is:

    1. Nitrofurantoin (Macrodantin) 100 mg PO qid × 14 days.
    2. Trimethoprim-sulfamethoxazole (Septra DS) 1 tablet PO bid × 10 days.
    3. Doxazosin (Cardura) 1 mg PO qd × 10 days.
    4. Oxybutynin (Ditropan) 5 mg PO tid × 10 days.

57. Finasteride (Proscar) is prescribed for a 50-year-old man who is experiencing a problem with urination caused by an enlarged prostate. The nurse practitioner would teach this client that while taking this medication, it is important for him to:

    1. Increase his fluid intake.
    2. Refrain from sexual activity.
    3. Use contraceptives.
    4. Increase intake of folic acid.

58. A 75-year-old client is diagnosed with chronic bacterial prostatitis and the nurse practitioner selects TMP-SMX (Septra DS) as the treatment. How should the TMP-SMX be prescribed for this client?

    1. 2 tablets bid × 10 weeks.
    2. 1 tablet tid × 3 days then 2 tablets × 10 days.
    3. 2 tablets qid × 2 days, then 1 tablet bid × 14 days.
    4. 1 tablet bid for 30 days.

59. What might be considered as the initial treatment for Peyronie's disease?

    1. Surgery
    2. A trial of vitamin E, 400 IU, bid.
    3. Circumcision.
    4. Oxybutynin

Answers & Rationales

Physical Examination & Diagnostic Tests

1. **(4)** Cowper's glands (bulbourethral glands) are located near the prostate and beside the urethra near the base of the penis. These glands are part of the internal and nonpalpable genitalia, which consist of glands and ducts. The testes, vas deferens, and epididymis are part of the external genitalia.

2. **(3)** The gonadotropin level is elevated in testicular disease, whereas the prostate-specific antigen (PSA) level is elevated in diseases of the prostate, such as benign prostatic hypertrophy (BPH).

3. **(1)** The epididymis is part of the external genitalia, whereas the ducts and glands are part of the internal genitalia. The epididymis is palpated on the posterolateral surface of each testis and is a comma-shaped structure. The seminal vesicles (pair of glands) lie behind the urinary bladder in front of the rectum. These vesicles join the ampulla of the vas deferens to form the ejaculatory duct.

4. **(1)** A complete history and physical exam will usually reveal the cause of gynecomastia without further testing, since gynecomastia can be caused by medication; starving and refeeding; or lack of androgen production (atrophying testes), which changes the estrogen/androgen ratio.

5. **(4)** For client comfort and ease of examination, the healthy, ambulatory adult client is asked to lean over the examination table with his chest and upper body resting on the table. Although Option #1 is correct, it is the position used for examining a client who is confined to bed.

6. **(3)** Prostatic acid phosphatase (PAP) is an enzyme marker. An increased value is the result of increased metabolism and catabolism of cancer cells of the prostate; in three fourths of clients, the cancer arises in the posterior lobe of the prostate. This marker is also used to monitor therapy with antineoplastic drugs and cancer metastatic to bone (osteoblastic lesions). α-Fetoprotein (AFP) (oncofetal antigen) is produced by fetal liver, yolk sac, and intestinal epithelium and disappears from the blood soon after birth; it is not present in healthy individuals. The AFP level is increased in patients with primary hepatocellular cancer, embryonal cell (nonseminomatous germ cell) cancer, testicular tumors, and other types of cancer. PSA (protein marker), which is more sensitive than PAP, increases in prostate cancer and in BPH. Human chorionic gonadotropin (hCG) (hormone marker), produced by placental syncytiotrophoblasts, is not usually found in sera of healthy, nonpregnant women but increases in seminomatous and nonseminomatous testicular cancer.

7. **(1)** The PSA level can be elevated in clients with BPH and those with prostatitis, as well as after prostate gland massage, and it does increase with the increasing burden of the tumor, as in the reoccurrence of prostate cancer.

8. **(2)** Recommended screening for prostate cancer should begin at the age of 40 years with digital-rectal exam (DRE), and PSA testing should begin at age 50 if there are no risk factors or symptoms. Urinalysis and complete blood count (CBC) are used in an annual physical exam as screening procedures but are not indicated in

screening for prostate cancer. *The PSA test and DRE are indicated for men older than 50 years.*

9. **(3)** The scrotal sac is asymmetric, darker than body skin, and often appears reddened in red-haired men (abnormal finding if found in clients without red hair); it has a surface that may be coarse with small lumps on the skin that are sebaceous or epidermoid cysts that may have an oily discharge.

Disorders

10. **(1)** Gross hematuria in a client older than 40 years should be considered a possible sign of bladder cancer until proven otherwise. Smoking increases the client's risk of bladder cancer.

11. **(2)** Sudden onset of pain with a firm, tender mass in the scrotum is indicative of testicular torsion; pain is not relieved when the involved testicle is elevated to relieve pressure. Prehn's sign, passive elevation of the testes, is associated with epididymitis. The cremasteric reflex is absent. Testicular torsion is most common among neonates and adolescents, with the highest incidence during puberty.

12. **(1)** The lack of pain, increase in size of scrotal contents, and transillumination are characteristic of hydrocele. Orchitis and epididymitis are usually characterized by pain; orchitis is most often associated with parotitis or mumps. There is no history of injury, and in the case of traumatic injury, the scrotum would be tender to palpation.

13. **(1)** Circumcision is helpful in preventing phimosis and paraphimosis, since both are retraction dysfunctions of the prepuce. In phimosis, the foreskin is too tight to be retracted backward over the glans penis. In paraphimosis, once the foreskin has been retracted behind the glans penis, it is too constricted to return to a position of covering the glans penis.

14. **(3)** Acute epididymitis is characterized by acute scrotal pain, dysuria, and unilateral enlargement of the scrotum with abdominal pain. Scrotal pain is relieved when the involved testicle is elevated.

15. **(1)** A male will present with impotence and decreased libido. These same men will often have gynecomastia as a result of the low or absent production of gonadotropin. Klinefelter's syndrome (a chromosomal abnormality with a karyotype of 47,XXY–47,XXXXY) is the most common cause of male hypogonadism, with failure of both spermatic function and virilization.

16. **(1)** Impotence can be caused by antihypertensives such as propranolol (Inderal, Inderal LA). The nonselective β-blockers are believed to decrease vascular resistance and central effect. Erectile dysfunction is reported to begin at doses of 120 mg/day. Other causes include infections, vascular and psychological problems, and traumatic injury.

17. **(1)** Paraphimosis is a retraction disorder related to a constricted prepuce, which can be relieved through circumcision.

18. **(2)** The prostate secretes fluid that is alkaline and helps sperm survive in the acid environment of the female reproductive tract. Androgens are produced by the Leydig's cells of the testes. Sperm are produced in the seminiferous tubules of the testes.

19. **(4)** The findings on the DRE and levels of PSA are the primary indicators of prostatic cancer. These findings should be thoroughly evaluated. The other options listed are directed toward treatment of BPH. Only after prostatic cancer has been ruled out should these be utilized.

20. **(4)** This case involves the differential diagnosis between epididymitis and testicular torsion. Irreversible damage will be done to the testicles if torsion is not released within 3 to 4 hours. Time should not be wasted with other treatments if torsion is strongly suspected.

21. **(1)** Testicular torsion and testicular cancer are considerations that are potentially curable but must be treated early. Hydrocele, epididymitis, and inguinal hernias also require referrals but do not require immediate attention.

22. **(2)** In cases of suspected acute prostatitis, only a rectal exam should be performed, if at all. Vigorous massage must be avoided because of the risk of inducing bacteremia. A urine culture, urethral cultures for gonorrhea and chlamydia, and blood collection for measurement of blood urea nitrogen (BUN) and creatinine levels are indicated to help make the diagnosis.

23. **(3)** BPH is commonly seen in men older than 50 years. Bladder cancer should be ruled out as a diagnosis.

24. **(1)** All of the symptoms listed can be found in the client with prostate cancer, but only the symptoms listed in Option #1 are localized. Many times the client will be asymptomatic.

25. **(1)** Varicocele presents as described, whereas a hernia may transilluminate, and sometimes bowel sounds can be auscultated in the scrotum. Hernias vary in size with Valsalva maneuvers. Tumors do not transilluminate.

26. **(2)** Phimosis is a retraction disorder of the penile foreskin or prepuce and can occur at any age and is usually the result of poor hygiene and chronic infection (the foreskin cannot be retracted over the glans penis). Paraphimosis is the inability to retract the foreskin from behind the glans penis.

27. **(4)** Peyronie's disease is a fibrotic condition that causes lateral curvature of the penis during erection.

28. **(2)** Inflammation of the glans penis and prepuce is usually associated with poor hygiene and is usually found in men with poorly controlled diabetes and candidiasis.

29. **(1)** Candidiasis is the usual cause of balanitis, which is inflammation of the glans penis and prepuce, usually associated with poor hygiene; it is also found in men with poorly controlled diabetes.

30. **(4)** Erection, emission, and ejaculation are sexual impairments with multifactorial causes such as vascular disease, neuropathy, and trauma. Peyronie's disease and priapism are examples of erectile dysfunction.

31. **(3)** Epididymitis presents as described, and on palpation, the epididymis will often feel like a bag of worms, rather than a fairly smooth cord, in the scrotal sac.

32. **(3)** This is the correct definition of erectile dysfunction, and statistics reveal that 40% of 40-year-old males and 70% of 70+-year-old males may experience it. It involves a hemodynamic mechanism of smooth muscle relaxation, which increases the amount of blood flow in the penis and ultimately causes

venous trapping (compression of the subtunical venules) resulting in rigidity.

33. **(1)** Priapism is a condition of prolonged penile erection related to venous obstruction and not related to sexual arousal.

34. **(3)** Males with undescended testicles are more prone to development of prostate cancer. The other conditions listed are not causes of prostate cancer.

35. **(1)** Antihypertensive drugs, such as propranolol (Inderal, Inderal LA), can cause impotence.

36. **(1)** This is the age group (15-35 years) that is affected by testicular cancer, and self-examination can be valuable in securing early diagnosis and treatment. PSA testing is recommended at age 50, and a DRE, at age 40.

37. **(1)** Cirrhosis and diseases of the hepatic system are often causes of gynecomastia. It is thought that cirrhosis and other hepatic disease alter the estrogen/androgen ratio. None of the other diseases has been implicated in gynecomastia.

38. **(2)** Gynecomastia is the result of an increased estrogen-to-androgen ratio in men, and as a result, their breast cancers are estrogen-receptor–positive.

39. **(4)** Prostate cancer is usually found in men older than 50 years and causes rapid onset of urinary obstructive symptoms. On palpation, asymmetric, discrete, hard nodule(s) are located. An increase in size of the prostate of >4 mm is also noted.

40. **(4)** Rapid onset of obstructive symptoms of urinary output would indicate a fast-growing tumor or obstruction of the urinary tract. All of the other symptoms are indicative of BPH, tumor, or stricture of the urinary tract.

41. **(4)** Testicular cancer is primarily found in young men and presents as nonpainful nodules of the involved testicle. Trauma is not a causal factor.

42. **(2)** Acute bacterial prostatitis is caused by an infection in the urinary tract moving up the urethra into the prostate. The most common organisms are *Escherichia coli*, *Pseudomonas* species, and *Streptococcus faecalis*. The condition tends to occur in men between 30

and 50 years of age but can be associated with BPH in older men. Chronic bacterial prostatitis is characterized by recurrent urinary tract infections, with the usual course of antibiotic treatment lasting for 12 weeks (because of blockage of the antibiotics by fibrosis in the prostatic tissue).

43. **(1)** Usually, orchitis presents with a tender unilateral swollen testicle within 7 to 10 days of the onset of mumps (parotitis). An elevated serum amylase level is associated with inflammation of the salivary glands (e.g., as in mumps).

44. **(2)** Nongonococcal urethritis (NGU) is often asymptomatic and as such is difficult to diagnose. NGU commonly produces a clear discharge and is usually caused by chlamydia. Gonococcal urethritis produces a yellow, purulent discharge. If a discharge is present, NGU is hard to differentiate from gonorrhea without a culture. Reiter's syndrome is also associated with untreated chlamydia infections of the urogenital tract.

45. **(1)** *Chlamydia trachomatis* is the most common organism in males with NGU.

46. **(3)** Cryptorchidism is the result of undescended testes, either bilateral or, more often, affecting the right testis. Normally, descent occurs in the seventh to eighth month of gestation.

47. **(1)** AFP (oncofetal antigen) is produced by fetal liver, yolk sac, and intestinal epithelium and disappears from blood soon after birth and is not present in healthy individuals. The AFP level is increased in patients with primary hepatocellular cancer, embryonal cell (nonseminomatous germ cell) cancer, testicular tumors, and other cancers. Prostatic acid phosphatase (PAP) is an enzyme marker. An increased value is the result of increased metabolism and catabolism of cancer cells of the prostate; in three fourths of clients, the cancer arises in the posterior lobe of the prostate. This marker is also used to monitor therapy with antineoplastic drugs and cancer metastatic to bone (osteoblastic lesions). The level of PSA (protein marker), which is more sensitive than PAP, increases in prostate cancer and in BPH. The alkaline phosphatase (ALP) level increases in osteosarcomas and in hepatocellular, metastatic to liver, and primary or secondary bone tumors.

48. **(3)** The mumps virus is responsible for orchitis. Arbovirus and echovirus are implicated in meningitis/encephalitis. Rubeola is associated with complications of otitis media, pneumonia, croup, and encephalitis.

49. **(3)** Obstructive symptoms are common in BPH. Dribbling, hesitancy, loss of normal urine stream, and recurrent urinary tract infections are present in chronic bacterial prostatitis. Dysuria, urgency, frequency, nocturia, and suprapubic heaviness are common symptoms of cystitis. Fever, chills, flank pain, headache, malaise, and costovertebral angle tenderness of acute onset with or without hematuria are indications of pyelonephritis.

50. **(2)** This is considered a urologic emergency because the circulation to the penis may be compromised and because of the inability to void. The client should be referred immediately to a physician.

51. **(2)** The client's age, presentation, and the fact that he is uncircumcised put him at risk for penile cancer. Balanitis does not present with a serosanguineous drainage.

52. **(2)** Diabetes is a common contributor to erectile dysfunction because of the impaired circulation.

Pharmacology

53. **(1)** Doxazosin (Cardura) is also used as an antihypertensive agent; the client may be experiencing orthostatic hypotension. The other answers are directed toward evaluating his BPH, which has already been diagnosed.

54. **(3)** Antifungals (e.g., topical nystatin [Mycostatin] or Ciclopirox [Loprox]) are the treatment of choice. If the infection is recalcitrant, oral fluconazole (Diflucan) 150 mg/day or itraconazole (Sporanox) 100 mg/day can be administered. All the other treatments are inappropriate.

55. **(1)** The client is presenting with classic symptoms of acute bacterial prostatitis. The treatment of choice is trimethoprim-sulfamethoxazole (TMP-SMX). It is important to treat the client for at least 30 days to prevent relapse. Treatment is started pending the results of the culture and sensitivity.

56. **(2)** The client is presenting with classic symptoms of epididymitis. The treatment of choice is TMP-SMX. Nitrofurantoin is a urinary antiseptic, doxazosin is given for BPH, and oxybutynin is indicated for incontinence or enuresis. In differential diagnosis, the gradual onset of pain, voiding problems, urethral discharge, and swelling are more indicative of epididymitis than testicular torsion.

57. **(3)** It is important that women of child-bearing age are not exposed to the sperm of a client taking finasteride. Pregnant women and those of child-bearing age should avoid handling crushed tablets.

58. **(4)** The recommended treatment is for at least 30 days to prevent recurrence. Clients may require continued suppression therapy for an extended period.

59. **(2)** Vitamin E promotes softening of fibrous tissue, and the plaques in Peyronie's disease are composed of fibrous tissue.

Women's Health

Physical Examination & Diagnostic Tests

1. When obtaining a cervical specimen for a Pap smear, the nurse practitioner:

   1. Lubricates the speculum with a water-soluble lubricant to assist in the insertion of the instrument.

   2. Uses a cotton-tipped applicator when obtaining the cervical cells from a prenatal client.

   3. Uses warm water to lubricate the speculum to assist in the insertion of the instrument.

   4. Completes the bimanual portion of the examination first to determine the relative position of the cervix to assist in comfortable insertion of the speculum.

2. To promote client comfort before performing a pelvic exam, the nurse practitioner:

   1. Asks the client to bear down slightly as the speculum is inserted.

   2. Has the client empty her bladder.

   3. Explains each step of the procedure in a calm manner.

   4. Carefully reassures the client that the exam will only take a few minutes.

3. What finding is considered a normal surface characteristic of the cervix?

   1. Small, yellow, raised round area on cervix.

   2. Red patchy areas with occasional white spots.

   3. Friable, bleeding tissue at opening of cervical os.

   4. Irregular, granular surface with red patches.

4. The primary role of a breast ultrasound exam is:

   1. Used as a screening test for breast cancer.

   2. Used for definitive diagnosis of breast cancer.

   3. Used to determine whether a breast lesion is cystic or solid.

   4. Used to locate small lesions before surgery.

5. A screening bone dual-energy x-ray absorptiometry (DEXA) scan is ordered for a 60-year-old postmenopausal woman. The report is returned with a result of −1.5 SD (standard deviation) at the hip. She gives a history of a myocardial infarction 1 year ago and a wrist fracture at age 32. What option would not be considered for this client?

1. Counsel on smoking cessation and alcohol consumption.

2. Initiate therapy with continuous conjugated estrogen 0.625 mg and medroxyprogesterone acetate (MPA) 2.5 mg.

3. Initiate therapy with raloxifene (Evista).

4. Encourage weight-bearing exercises and an increase in calcium intake.

6. When is the optimal time to perform a hysterosalpingogram (HSG)?

1. During menses.

2. Immediately after ovulation.

3. After menses but before ovulation.

4. 3 to 4 days before menses.

7. Which statement about mammography is **false**?

1. Mammography detects all breast cancers.

2. Mammography should be accompanied by breast exam.

3. Negative findings on mammography should not delay biopsy of a clinically suspicious mass.

4. Mammography is a cost-effective method of screening for breast cancer.

8. The use of potassium hydroxide (KOH) when doing a wet mount assists in the diagnosis of:

1. Bacterial vaginosis and candida vaginitis.

2. *Trichomonas* and *Chlamydia* infection.

3. Syphilis and gonorrhea.

4. Herpes and condyloma.

9. The nurse practitioner is reviewing the lab results of an 18-year-old client seen recently for a Pap smear. The results are as follows: Classification—high-grade squamous intraepithelial lesion; endocervical cells seen; adequate smear. The nurse practitioner phones the client and tells her which of the following?

1. "Your Pap smear was normal. Follow up in 1 year, sooner if problems arise."

2. "Your Pap smear shows invasive cancer. I would like you to see a gynecologic oncologist for treatment."

3. "Your Pap smear shows abnormal tissue that needs to be evaluated. Please schedule an appointment for a colposcopy."

4. "Your Pap smear shows a minor abnormality. Sometimes this can signify a disease process just beginning. Please schedule another Pap smear in 4 months for follow-up."

10. A 27-year-old client reports the desire to become pregnant. She and her husband have had regular, unprotected intercourse for more than 1 year. The nurse practitioner completes a thorough history and gynecologic exam and finds no abnormalities. What diagnostic test might he or she order early in the workup?

1. HSG.

2. Tests for anti-sperm antibodies.

3. Semen analysis.

4. Endometrial biopsy.

11. For which woman does the National Osteoporosis Foundation (NOF) recommend a screening bone DEXA scan?

1. A 48-year-old white woman who smokes and has excessive alcohol intake.

2. A 50-year-old woman who has irregular menstrual cycles.

3. A 51-year-old woman receiving long-term corticosteroid therapy for systemic lupus erythematous.

4. A 54-year-old woman who is receiving hormone replacement therapy (HRT).

12. When describing the findings from a normal breast examination, the nurse practitioner documents on the client record:

1. Left nipple everted, several coarse black hairs arising from the areola, enlarged axillary lymph nodes palpated bilaterally, and tender nodes in supraclavicular area.

2. No dimpling or retraction; 1-cm hard, fixed, stellate mass noted next to nipple with

scant nipple discharge; no pain or tenderness on palpation.

3. Right breast slightly larger and denser than left with no nipple discharge, right areola dark pink in color and inverted, left areola dark brown in color and everted, breasts tender to palpation with no axillary nodes noted.

4. Pendulous breasts with no dimpling, retraction, nipple discharge, or areas of discoloration; numerous small nevi near areola with Montgomery's tubercles noted, no supraclavicular or axillary lymph nodes palpated.

13. In an infertility workup, what is the best way to evaluate ovulation?

1. HSG.

2. Postcoital test.

3. Endometrial biopsy.

4. Basal body temperature (BBT) chart.

14. The nurse practitioner is reviewing the lab tests results of a 61-year-old adult client seen recently for a Pap smear. She has been treated for breast cancer with mastectomy and tamoxifen (Nolvadex). She is not receiving and never has received HRT. The results of her Pap smear are as follows: atrophic changes; scant endocervical cells; adequate smear. What is appropriate for the nurse practitioner to tell the client when she phones her with her results?

1. "Your Pap smear is slightly abnormal. I would recommend the use of some estrogen vaginal cream nightly for 3 weeks. Then return to the office to have the Pap smear repeated."

2. "Your Pap smear is normal but shows a mild thinning of the tissue. This is to be expected in someone who is postmenopausal and not taking hormones and does not pose a threat to your health. Please return to the office in 1 year for your annual exam, sooner if needed."

3. "Your Pap smear shows that you don't have enough endocervical cells. Please make an appointment for endocervical curettage."

4. "Your Pap smear is abnormal. This could signify a disease state of the cervix. Please

schedule a colposcopy at your earliest convenience."

15. Which test is the gold standard for the diagnosis of *Chlamydia* infection?

1. Use of KOH wet mount "whiff" test.

2. Presence of inflammatory cells on Pap smear.

3. Direct fluorescent antibody (DFA) test.

4. Culture with special media and collection technique.

16. The nurse practitioner is discussing mammography with a group of women. What is important for the nurse practitioner to tell the women?

1. A mammogram should be done annually for all women of child-bearing age.

2. All women 40 years of age and older should have a mammogram on an annual basis.

3. A mammogram should be done annually after pregnancy, if the woman does not breast-feed.

4. A mammogram should be done only if there is any breast pain or nipple retraction.

17. Which is the most accurate statement regarding a reactive serologic test result for syphilis?

1. All reactive serologic test results require confirmation with a treponemal test.

2. Reactive serologic test results are highly suggestive of active syphilis.

3. A false-positive serologic test result, although rare, can be unnecessarily traumatizing to a client.

4. A reactive serologic test result most likely implies the need for retreatment.

18. In a workup done for a client with secondary amenorrhea, the prolactin serum assay results show a level of 24 ng/ml. Appropriate management includes:

1. Administration of MPA 10 mg bid × 5 days.

2. Referral to a physician.

3. Recording the results as within normal limits.

4. Assessment for nipple discharge.

19. In evaluation of a young adult with amenorrhea and normal secondary sex characteristics, the purpose of the progesterone challenge is to determine the presence of:

    1. Endogenous estrogen.

    2. Thyroxine.

    3. Prolactin.

    4. Adequate body fat.

20. A client comes in complaining of fatigue, breast tenderness, abdominal bloating, fluid retention, and irritability about a week before the onset of her menses. This has been occurring for the past 4 months. What is the most important information for the nurse practitioner to obtain to assist in determining the diagnosis of premenstrual syndrome (PMS)?

    1. The point within the menstrual cycle at which the symptoms occur.

    2. The severity of the symptoms.

    3. Number and frequency of symptoms over past 4 months.

    4. Presence or absence of anxiety or depression.

21. A 65-year-old woman reports to the clinic stating she has been experiencing intermittent vaginal bleeding over the last 2 months. Her last menstrual period (LMP) was >10 years ago. Findings from her last Pap smear, done at the clinic 9 months ago, were within normal limits. She is not taking any hormonal products. She is sexually active with occasional complaints of dyspareunia. What is the most appropriate response of the provider at this time?

    1. Draw blood for a complete blood count (CBC) and thyroid-stimulating hormone (TSH) level and repeat the Pap smear.

    2. Schedule a laparoscopy.

    3. Schedule an endometrial biopsy.

    4. Schedule a pelvic/transvaginal ultrasound exam.

Normal Gynecology

22. The endometrial cycle is often described in three phases. Select the correct phases:

    1. Follicular, menstrual, and luteal.

    2. Proliferative, luteal, and menstrual.

    3. Follicular, secretory, and menstrual.

    4. Proliferative, secretory, and menstrual.

23. The nurse practitioner understands that PMS occurs with greatest frequency and severity in the:

    1. Late luteal phase.

    2. Follicular phase.

    3. Proliferative phase.

    4. Ovulatory phase.

24. Which hormone is **not** released from the anterior pituitary gland?

    1. Follicle-stimulating hormone (FSH).

    2. Luteinizing hormone (LH).

    3. Oxytocin.

    4. Prolactin.

25. What is the primary function of FSH?

    1. Stimulation of maturation of ovarian follicles.

    2. Milk secretion.

    3. Triggering ovulation.

    4. Inhibiting release of LH from the pituitary gland.

26. How is the term *menopause* best defined?

    1. Cessation of ability for natural reproduction.

    2. Completion of 12 months of amenorrhea after the LMP.

    3. An FSH level of 30 mU/ml and estradiol level of 30 pg/ml.

    4. The LMP.

27. In the ovarian cycle, what phase begins with ovulation and ends with the onset of menses?

    1. Follicular phase.

    2. Ovulation.

    3. Proliferative phase.

    4. Luteal phase.

28. Which is **not** a risk factor for heart disease in the postmenopausal female?

    1. Regular exercise.

    2. Cigarette smoking.

    3. HRT.

    4. Diabetes mellitus.

29. An adult client's LMP was 2 months ago. She has had a Periogard T 380 intrauterine device (IUD) in place for the last 4 months. She is complaining of nausea, fatigue, breast tenderness, and abdominal bloating. Her physical exam reveals the following:

    • Abdomen: within normal limits (WNL)
    • Pelvic: cervix—positive Chadwick's sign, IUD strings seen protruding from the cervical os
    • Uterus: enlarged and nontender
    • Adnexa: nontender, without mass, no cervical motion tenderness

    What is the most likely diagnosis?

    1. Uterine fibroid.

    2. Ovarian cancer.

    3. Dislodged IUD.

    4. Pregnancy.

30. What function do the Bartholin's glands have in reproduction?

    1. Prevent vaginitis by maintaining adequate pH.

    2. Prepare the mucous plug that occurs during early pregnancy.

    3. Produce an alkaline secretion that enhances sperm viability.

    4. Produce small amounts of hormones necessary for ovulation.

31. Which is **not** a risk factor for osteoporosis?

    1. Cigarette smoking.

    2. White race.

    3. Alcohol consumption.

    4. Obesity.

32. A young woman complains to the nurse practitioner that she is experiencing headaches, irritability, decreased appetite, and fatigue about 1 week before her menses. Appropriate management includes:

    1. Treating the PMS with increased protein and salt in the diet.

    2. Incorporating daily regular aerobic exercise and dietary changes into her lifestyle.

    3. Ordering a CBC, comprehensive metabolic panel, and urinalysis.

    4. Supplementing the diet with an additional 1 to 2 g of vitamin C.

33. A middle-aged female presents with abnormal uterine bleeding. A hormonal profile reveals increased FSH and LH levels. The most likely cause for these findings is:

    1. Hypothalamic disorder.

    2. Onset of climacteric.

    3. Premature ovarian failure.

    4. Anterior pituitary disorder.

34. While assessing a young adult, the nurse practitioner was asked about douching. What information would be used in the nurse practitioner's teaching plan?

    1. Douching during menstruation is safe.

    2. Since you have a lot of vaginal discharge, daily douching is important.

    3. Hypoallergenic douches include flavored or perfumed types.

    4. Douching removes natural mucus and upsets normal vaginal flora.

35. A 29-year-old female client presents to the family planning clinic for her annual exam. She had a postpartum tubal ligation 6 months ago. She has been feeling tired and nauseated and is slowly gaining weight. She had one menses after delivery, 4 months ago. The nurse practitioner notes the following on physical exam:

    • Abdomen: bowel sounds × 4, soft, no hepatosplenomegaly, palpable mass in lower abdomen, measures 14 cm, no tenderness
    • Pelvic: Bartholin's, urethral, and Skene's glands (BUS) normal; Cervix—os closed, smooth, pink mucosa
    • Bimanual: uterus enlarged, nontender, smooth contours, no cervical motion tenderness
    • Adnexa: not palpable

What is the likely diagnosis?

1. Pregnancy.

2. Uterine fibroid.

3. Premature menopause.

4. Colon cancer.

36. In the Western world, menopause occurs at a mean age of 51 years. Which of the following factors has been linked to influencing the age at which menopause occurs?

    1. Use of oral contraceptives (OCs).

    2. Socioeconomic status.

    3. Age at menarche.

    4. Smoking.

Gynecologic Disorders

37. During a yearly physical examination, a nurse practitioner asks a woman whether she has any problems or questions about sexual function or activity. Initially, the client hesitates, but with further questioning and discussion, she states that she is unsure whether she has ever experienced an orgasm. The nurse practitioner suspects:

    1. Vaginismus.

    2. Primary orgasmic dysfunction.

    3. Secondary orgasmic dysfunction.

    4. Dyspareunia.

38. The nurse practitioner is talking with a young women who has been given a diagnosis of herpes simplex type 2 (genital). In discussing her care, it would be important for the nurse practitioner to include what information?

    1. The initial lesions are usually worse than lesions that occur with outbreaks at a later time.

    2. Her sexual partner will not contract it if she does not have sex when the lesions are present.

    3. This condition can be treated and cured if she takes all of the antibiotics for 2 weeks.

    4. If she becomes pregnant, she will have to have a cesarean delivery.

39. The definition of bacterial vaginosis is:

    1. A syndrome resulting from homeostatic disruption in the vagina.

    2. Vaginitis caused by a flagellated protozoan.

    3. A bacterial sexually transmitted disease (STD) that can be symptomatic or asymptomatic.

    4. A virus characterized by recurrent outbreaks and remissions.

40. A 22-year-old married client complains of severe dysmenorrhea. Findings on the gynecologic exam are normal. Which management protocol is preferred?

    1. Assess for contraceptive interest and, if interested, suggest use of OCs.

    2. Suggest use of prostaglandin synthetase inhibitor.

    3. Suggest over-the-counter use of ibuprofen.

    4. Assess exercise patterns and use of relaxation techniques.

41. Which is **not** a criterion for the diagnosis of bacterial vaginosis?

    1. Positive amine test (whiff test) result.

    2. Presence of clue cells.

    3. Vaginal pH >4.5.

    4. The presence of pseudohyphae.

42. A client with a history of dilatation and curettage (D&C) after a first-trimester spontaneous abortion and subsequent amenorrhea would lead the nurse practitioner to a working diagnosis of which of the following?

    1. Polycystic ovarian syndrome.

    2. Asherman's syndrome.

    3. Hypogonadism.

    4. Premature ovarian failure.

43. The LH/FSH ratio in polycystic ovarian syndrome (Stein-Leventhal syndrome) is:

    1. 1.5:1

    2. 3:1

    3. 6:1

    4. 1:3

44. What are common findings in a client with polycystic ovarian syndrome?

    1. Weight loss, dental caries, and amenorrhea.

    2. Hyperprolactinemia and galactorrhea.

    3. Dysmenorrhea, nodules palpated on bimanual exam, and infertility.

    4. Chronic irregular menses, hirsutism, and increased abdominal girth.

45. The most common cause of dysfunctional uterine bleeding is:

    1. Thyroid disorder.

    2. Blood dyscrasia.

    3. Anovulation.

    4. Uterine tumor.

46. A 30-year-old woman presents with scant pubic hair, minimal breast development, absent cervix, and uterus with a 46,XY karyotype. What is your diagnosis?

    1. Turner's syndrome.

    2. Müllerian agenesis.

    3. Testicular feminization.

    4. Gonadal dysgenesis.

47. The most common cause of a breast mass in clients ages 15 to 25 years is:

    1. Fibroadenoma.

    2. Intraductal papilloma.

    3. Infiltrating lobular carcinoma.

    4. Fibrocystic breast syndrome.

48. An effective treatment for primary dysmenorrhea is:

    1. Nonsteroidal antiinflammatory analgesics.

    2. Tranquilizers.

    3. Progestins.

    4. Steroids.

49. What is a cause of secondary amenorrhea?

    1. Testicular feminization.

    2. Hypogonadotropic hypogonadism.

    3. Congenital absence of uterus.

    4. Extreme exercise.

50. A young woman comes into the clinic for a well-woman checkup. She states that about 3 weeks ago, she had a sore on her labia that went away. It was not particularly painful and did not itch, and there do not seem to be any residual problems from it. The nurse practitioner treats this woman by:

    1. Ordering the treponemal-specific test (FTA-ABS).

    2. Swabbing the area of the lesion for a viral culture.

    3. Advising her to notify her sexual contacts to determine whether they have had any symptoms.

    4. Ordering nystatin (Mycostatin) cream to be applied to the area three to four times a day.

51. A high-school athlete presents to the clinic with concerns regarding her menstrual periods. She states she has not had a period in the past 2 months. She has been in training and running about 3 miles a day for the past 3 months. She has lost approximately 15 lb. Her height is about 63 inches and she currently weights 100 lb. The best response by the nurse practitioner is to:

    1. Determine the client's percentage of body fat and body mass.

    2. Determine FSH serum levels.

    3. Determine serum levels of human chorionic gonadotropin.

    4. Order thyroid function tests.

52. Which is **not** a risk factor for the development of cervical cancer?

    1. Human papillomavirus (HPV).

    2. Virginal status.

    3. Multiple sexual partners.

    4. Previous high-grade squamous intraepithelial lesion.

53. A young woman is complaining of tenderness and burning of her vulva. On examination, the vulva is edematous and excoriated. The nurse practitioner performs a wet mount prep of the vaginal secretions. It reveals pseudo-hyphae and spores. The diagnosis for this client is:

    1. Vulvovaginal candidiasis.
    2. *Chlamydia* infection.
    3. Bacterial vaginosis.
    4. Gonorrhea.

54. The leading cause of death in women with genital cancers, excluding breast cancer, is:

    1. Ovarian cancer.
    2. Endometrial cancer.
    3. Cervical cancer.
    4. Vulvar and/or vaginal cancer.

55. A young woman presents with complaints of an irritation in the vaginal area. This is the first time it has occurred. On vaginal examination, the cervix is inflamed and friable. Flagellated protozoa are seen on the wet prep. The most likely diagnosis is:

    1. Trichomoniasis.
    2. Cervicitis.
    3. *Chlamydia* infection.
    4. Bacterial vaginosis.

56. A 26-year-old female client presents to the emergency department and is seen by the nurse practitioner. The client had a gradual onset of abdominal pain, starting in the periumbilical region and now localized in the right lower quadrant. It is accompanied by nausea, anorexia, constipation, and low-grade fever. The physical exam confirms the diagnosis of acute appendicitis. What diagnostic studies are **least** useful in confirming this diagnosis?

    1. CBC, with differential.
    2. Flat plate of abdomen, kidney-ureters-bladder (KUB).
    3. Pelvic ultrasound exam.
    4. Pregnancy test.

57. Which is **not** a risk factor for endometrial cancer?

    1. Obesity.
    2. Birth control pill use.
    3. Unopposed estrogen use.
    4. Advancing age, >50 years.

58. Which statement is true regarding the diaphragm?

    1. May be inserted up to 24 hours before intercourse.
    2. May be inserted any time up to 6 hours before intercourse.
    3. Should be removed within 1 hour after intercourse.
    4. May only be left in place for 12 hours.

59. A contraceptive method that is associated with an increase in urinary tract infections (UTIs) is:

    1. IUD.
    2. Diaphragm.
    3. Norplant.
    4. Oral contraceptive pills.

60. Which is **not** a risk factor for ovarian cancer?

    1. Family history of ovarian cancer.
    2. Advancing age, >50 years.
    3. Birth control pill use.
    4. Presence of *BRCA 2* gene.

61. What is the most common site of female genital malignancy, excluding the breast?

    1. Ovary.
    2. Endometrium.
    3. Cervix.
    4. Vulva/vagina.

62. A 20-year-old female college student presents to the urgent care center with new onset of painful sores in the vulva. These erupted yesterday and are associated with exquisite pain, fever, and flu-like symptoms of headache, gen-

eral body aches, and mild dysuria. She has a new sexual partner and thinks she saw a sore on his external genitalia after coitus. The examination reveals vesicular lesions covering the labium; extreme tenderness to palpation of the external genitalia; normal Bartholin's, urethral, and Skene's glands (BUS); normal findings on vaginal inspection with a mild leukorrhea; normal cervical mucosa; and slightly tender, minimally enlarged inguinal lymph nodes bilaterally. What is the likely diagnosis?

1. Gonorrhea.

2. *Chlamydia* infection.

3. Herpes simplex virus.

4. Lymphogranuloma venereum.

63. A 21-year-old female client is seen for her annual gynecologic exam. She is sexually active, rarely uses condoms for STD prevention, and has multiple sexual partners. She smokes one pack per day, admits to a sedentary lifestyle, and eats two meals per day, most often at fast food restaurants. Her exam reveals no abnormalities. Her family history and personal medical history are negative for major disease. There are no menstrual abnormalities; her LMP was 1 week ago. The nurse practitioner has done her Pap smear. Which would **not** be appropriate for this client?

1. Cultures for gonorrhea and chlamydia.

2. Lab testing: glucose, cardiac risk profile, and TSH level.

3. Human immunodeficiency virus (HIV) titer and rapid plasma reagin test.

4. Counseling on safe sex practice and contraceptive information.

64. Which is **not** considered to be a risk factor in the development of breast cancer?

1. Early menopause.

2. High-fat diet.

3. Advancing age.

4. Early menarche.

65. A 32-year-old female client, G2 T1 P1 A0 L2, is seen in the clinic by the nurse practitioner for her annual exam and is requesting information on preconception counseling. She has been taking OCs for 3 years without complications. During the past year, she has started an exercise program at a health club 5 days a week and is eating three nutritionally sound meals daily. She has lost 33 lb and is now at her ideal body weight. She quit her job as a postal worker and now stays home with her children. As part of her preconception care, what should the nurse practitioner recommend?

1. Start taking prenatal vitamins with folic acid.

2. Discontinue exercise.

3. Update measles-mumps-rubella (MMR) vaccine.

4. Genetic counseling because of advanced maternal age.

66. The initial workup for abnormal uterine bleeding should include:

1. Referral for diagnostic dilatation and curettage (D&C).

2. Referral for endometrial biopsy to rule out cancer.

3. CBC, pregnancy test, endocrine studies.

4. Coagulation studies, STD cultures.

67. Which is **not** a risk factor for breast cancer?

1. History of maternal breast cancer—premenopausal onset.

2. First pregnancy after age 35.

3. Late menopause, after age 54.

4. Fibrocystic breast disease.

68. A 20-year-old female client presents for her first well-woman exam; she is not sexually active and never has been. Her family history and medical history are negative for any gynecologic diseases. Her menses occur every 28 days and last for 5 days, with a relatively moderate flow and no significant abdominal cramps. Her physical exam/visit today should include which test?

1. Pap smear.

2. Culture for gonorrhea and chlamydia.

3. Stool Hemoccult test.

4. Baseline mammogram.

69. What is the leading cause of death among women in the United States?

    1. Breast cancer.

    2. Colon cancer.

    3. Heart disease.

    4. Stroke.

70. During a gynecologic exam at the family planning clinic, an underweight 17-year-old presents with bruising around her upper torso and genitalia. She is minimally interactive and avoids eye contact as much as possible. Priority intervention should focus on:

    1. Lab work to rule out bleeding disorder.

    2. Nutritional assessment to determine possible anemia.

    3. Determination of possible physical abuse.

    4. Finding out whether she has a support system.

71. Reactive cellular changes noted on a Pap smear are most often associated with:

    1. Inflammation.

    2. Use of estrogen vaginal cream.

    3. Drying artifact.

    4. Use of OCs.

72. Risk factors for cervical cancer include:

    1. Pregnancy after 35 years of age.

    2. Viral exposure.

    3. Low parity.

    4. Prolonged contraceptive use.

73. What is the most common cancer in women in the United States?

    1. Breast cancer.

    2. Colon cancer.

    3. Malignant melanoma.

    4. Lung cancer.

74. A 48-year-old female client presents to the clinic with the following list of complaints: hot flashes, no menses for 14 months, insomnia, crying spells, irritability, decreased libido, and fatigue. At the end of her history and physical exam, she begins to cry and tells the nurse practitioner that she thinks she's going crazy; she then begs the nurse practitioner to tell her what is wrong. Which is **inappropriate** for the nurse practitioner to do at this point?

    1. Obtain blood for lab tests, including FSH and LH levels.

    2. Discuss HRT, including risks and benefits and short-term and long-term treatment strategies.

    3. Provide antidepressant therapy and a referral for counseling sessions for depression.

    4. Provide the client with written information regarding menopause and the options for treatment of symptoms.

75. Care for a client with chancroid should include:

    1. Screening for HIV, as well as syphilis.

    2. Mandatory notification and treatment of all sexual partners.

    3. Screening for lymphogranuloma venereum.

    4. Culture for gonorrhea.

76. During her annual exam, a 39-year-old female complains of recent breast changes. She states that her breasts are painful and frequently feel "lumpy." Because of this, she has stopped doing monthly breast self-examination (BSE), feeling that it is a waste of time. What would be the most appropriate advice to offer her?

    1. Stress the importance of continuing monthly BSE to detect unusual lumps because she knows the feel of her breasts.

    2. Suggest she at least do BSE every 2 months.

    3. Suggest she start getting mammograms to establish some baseline data about her breasts.

    4. Determine when her breasts are nontender and least "lumpy" and change her schedule for BSE.

77. During a breast exam on a young adult female, a 2-cm painless lobular mass in the right breast

that is firm and freely mobile is noted on palpation. Appropriate management includes:

1. Continued observation and rechecking in 3 months.

2. Referral for a mammogram.

3. Referral for probable surgical excision.

4. Obtaining a detailed family history to determine breast cancer risk.

78. A woman with bilateral breast implants asks whether it is really necessary to do monthly BSE because she does not know what to feel for. The most appropriate response would be:

1. Suggest she involve her sexual partner in assessing her breasts on a regular basis.

2. Review the steps in BSE until she feels comfortable with the process.

3. Acknowledge the difficulty in doing BSE after implant surgery.

4. Explain the usefulness of regular mammograms for clients with implants.

79. An adult client comes to the clinic complaining of abnormal vaginal discharge (dark watery brown) along with postcoital bleeding. The nurse practitioner suspects cancer of the cervix. During the vaginal exam, physical findings suggestive of cervical cancer would be:

1. Soft, sill-shaped cervix.

2. Very firm cervix with an ulcer.

3. Vague lower abdominal discomfort.

4. Tender, enlarged lymph nodes.

80. A postmenopausal female is worried about pain in the upper outer quadrant of her left breast. The nurse practitioner should:

1. Do a breast exam and order a mammogram.

2. Explain that pain is related to hormone fluctuations and order laboratory studies.

3. Reassure the client that pain is not a presenting symptom of breast cancer and check for proper fit of the brassiere.

4. Teach the client BSE.

81. A 22-year-old female client comes to the nurse practitioner's office with a complaint of 1 day of fever of 102° F (38.9° C), a diffuse macular rash, vomiting, headache, and decreased urinary output. The history obtained by the nurse practitioner must include:

1. Whether the client's immunizations are up-to-date.

2. Whether the client is currently menstruating.

3. Whether the client has a history of tuberculosis.

4. The type of contraception the client uses.

82. A young female client presents to the nurse practitioner's office with a complaint of abdominal pain. In the United States, this diagnosis results in about 1 death per 1000 and therefore must be considered early in the decision process:

1. Irritable bowel syndrome.

2. Appendicitis.

3. Pyelonephritis.

4. Ectopic pregnancy.

83. A young adult female client presents with a history of vaginal itching and heavy white discharge. The client gives a history of no sexual activity. On exam, the nurse practitioner finds a red, edematous vulva and white patches on the vaginal walls. There is no odor to the discharge. The nurse practitioner expects what factors in the client's history?

1. A vegetarian diet.

2. Recent diarrhea.

3. Early menopause.

4. Recent antibiotic use.

84. A young female client comes to the office complaining of vaginal bleeding. The client states that she has used five tampons in the past 3 hours. She admits to sexual activity and takes OCs. On further questioning, the client states that she started her last pack of contraceptives "about 2 weeks late." The nurse practitioner should:

1. Perform a STAT urine pregnancy test.

2. Perform a STAT CBC.

3. Discuss proper use of OCs.

4. Send the client for a pelvic sonogram.

85. The nurse practitioner knows that the majority of breast cancers occur in which area of the breast?

    1. Upper inner quadrant.

    2. Upper outer quadrant.

    3. Beneath the nipple and areola.

    4. Lower outer quadrant.

86. The client presents with abnormal uterine bleeding and has been found to have endometrial cancer. She returned to the nurse practitioner because she does not understand how this is possible when the result of the Pap smear 6 months ago was negative. The best response is:

    1. Uterine cancer develops quickly.

    2. Pap smears are difficult to read and mistakes can happen.

    3. Pap smears are not useful in detecting uterine cancers in most cases.

    4. The previous Pap smear did not have an adequate sample.

87. A postmenopausal woman is seen in the office with complaints of frequent urination, stress incontinence, vaginal dryness, and dyspareunia. Her last menstrual cycle was 6 years ago and she elected to not take HRT. She has increased her intake of soy products. What is the most common cause of her symptoms?

    1. UTI.

    2. Cystocele.

    3. Bacterial vaginitis.

    4. Atrophic vaginitis.

Pharmacology

88. A 42-year-old female client presents to the office with complaints of dysuria, urinary frequency, and urgency. These symptoms began early this morning. She leaves a clean-catch midstream urine specimen, which shows the following: white blood cells (WBCs) too numerous to count (TNTC)/high-power field (HPF), 4 to 5 red blood cells / HPF, positive nitrites. A urine culture is set up and will be ready in 3 days. Which is NOT a correct treatment for an uncomplicated lower UTI?

    1. Phenazopyridine (Pyridium) 200 mg 1 tablet PO tid × 2 days.

    2. Trimethoprim-sulfamethoxazole (Bactrim DS) 1 tablet PO bid × 5 days.

    3. Ceftriaxone (Rocephin) 1 g IM.

    4. Nitrofurantoin (Macrobid) 1 tablet PO bid × 5 days.

89. The results of the Women's Health Initiative (WHI) provided evidence-based data that have led to new guidelines in assessing the risk/benefit ratio for initiation of HRT in postmenopausal women. Which statement is NOT correct?

    1. HRT is indicated for the treatment of menopausal symptoms such as vasomotor and urogenital symptoms.

    2. HRT should be continued for primary prevention of coronary heart disease.

    3. HRT can be continued for the prevention of postmenopausal fractures caused by osteoporosis.

    4. HRT should be limited to the shortest duration consistent with treatment goals and benefits in consideration of risks for the individual woman.

90. A 46-year-old female client is being seen in the clinic by the nurse practitioner. She was last seen 2 weeks ago for an upper respiratory tract infection and was treated with amoxicillin (Amoxil) 250 mg PO tid × 10 days. She completed her medication last week but now is aware of vaginal itching and a cottage cheese–like vaginal discharge. She states that she has never experienced such intense itching before. She is in a mutually monogamous relationship. Her LMP was 2 weeks ago. Her partner had a vasectomy 2 years ago. Wet mount with KOH shows negative whiff test result, rare clue cells, positive lactobacilli, positive hyphae and spores, few WBCs, and no trichomonads. She is leaving tomorrow for a week-long cruise. She is not taking any medications and has no known drug allergies. The nurse practitioner knows that the best treatment for this problem is:

    1. Metronidazole (Flagyl) 500 mg PO bid × 7 days.

    2. Clindamycin (Cleocin) vaginal cream, one applicator full vaginally qhs × 7 days.

3. Fluconazole (Diflucan) 150 mg, 1 tablet PO one time.

4. Hydrocortisone (Cortaid) 1% cream, apply sparingly bid × 7 days.

91. A 25-year-old female client presents with complaints of a malodorous vaginal discharge, described as white and watery. She douches with vinegar and water every 2 weeks. She uses a diaphragm for contraception. She and her boyfriend have been sexually active for 2 years, using condoms for STD prevention with every act of coitus. She denies any dyspareunia. Her LMP was 1 week ago, and there are no noted changes in her normal menstrual pattern. Her wet mount with KOH shows a positive whiff test result, TNTC clue cells/ HPF, no lactobacilli, no hyphae or spores, no trichomonads, and few WBCs. What is the diagnosis and treatment for this client?

1. *Chlamydia* infection: doxycycline (Vibra tabs) 100 mg PO bid × 10 days.

2. *Candida albicans* infection: terconazole (Terazol 7 cream) 1 applicator full per vagina qhs × 7 days.

3. Herpes simplex type 2: acyclovir (Zovirax) 200 mg 1 PO q4h × 5 days.

4. Bacterial vaginosis: metronidazole (Metrogel) vaginal gel 1 applicator full per vagina qhs × 5 days.

92. A 55-year-old female client is being seen in the clinic for her annual exam. She went through a natural menopause 5 years ago and has never been interested in hormonal therapy. She smokes one pack per day and does no formal exercise. She is a G2 T2 P0 A0 L2. Her family history is positive for osteoporosis in her mother and negative for myocardial infarction and cancer in her parents. Findings of her physical exam today were normal, and a mammogram performed yesterday revealed no abnormalities. She is now interested in hormonal therapy but wants to know what her alternatives are. Which choice **has not** been clinically proven for prevention of osteoporosis?

1. Estradiol (Estrace) 0.5 mg 1 tablet PO qd and micronized progesterone (Prometrium) 100 mg, 1 tablet PO qd.

2. Weight-bearing exercise three times weekly.

3. Discontinue cigarette smoking.

4. Wild Mexican yam cream applied to skin three times daily.

93. A young female is seen in the STD clinic. She noticed some itchy bumps in the vulvar area and is concerned that they could be cancer. On careful inspection, the nurse practitioner notes the following: five cauliflower-like, warty, pinkish lesions in the lower introitus; two smaller lesions nestled anterior to the hymeneal ring of the vagina. There are no cervical abnormalities. The result of a wet mount with KOH is negative. A specimen was obtained for culture for gonorrhea and chlamydia, a Pap smear was done, and blood was drawn for an HIV titer and rapid plasma reagin test. Which is **not** an appropriate treatment for this client?

1. Podofilox (Condylox) application q12h × 3 days.

2. Trichloroacetic acid application; do not wash off.

3. Cryotherapy with liquid nitrogen applied to lesions.

4. Benzathine penicillin 2.4 million units IM weekly × 3 weeks.

94. A young adult female client is being seen in the urgent care unit by the nurse practitioner. She is complaining of vaginal itching, thick yellow mucus discharge, and urinary discomfort. She is sexually active and uses condoms with one of her partners, but not both. On physical exam, no abnormalities are detected in the abdomen; the pelvic exam reveals BUS to be within normal limits; cervix has a mucopurulent discharge exuding from the os; the mucosa is friable to palpation; and results of the bimanual exam are negative. Specimens were obtained for culture but results are not yet available. Wet mount with KOH reveals a negative whiff test result, few clue cells, TNTC WBCs/HPF, no yeast, and no trichomonads. What is the likely diagnosis and appropriate treatment?

1. *Chlamydia* infection; give azithromycin (Zithromax) 1 g PO single dose.

2. *Chlamydia* infection; give ceftriaxone (Rocephin) 125 mg IM.

3. Herpes simplex virus; give acyclovir (Zovirax) 200 mg 1 capsule PO q4h × 5 days.

4. Trichomoniasis; give metronidazole (Flagyl) 2 g PO single dose.

95. A 52-year-old woman is being seen for her annual gynecologic exam. She had a hysterectomy with ovarian conservation at age 40 because of uterine fibroids and dysfunctional uterine bleeding. She has been taking oral estrogen (conjugated equine estrogen, 0.625 mg) replacement therapy for 1 year. Although estrogen replacement therapy has definitely reduced the discomfort of hot flashes, vaginal dryness, mood swings, and insomnia, she still experiences flushes and some night sweats. Her diagnostic evaluation shows the following lipid panel: total cholesterol level = 180 mg/dl; low-density lipoprotein (LDL) level = 112 mg/dl; high-density lipoprotein (HDL) level = 52 mg/dl; triglyceride level = 325 mg/dl. What, if any, change might be considered in her medication regimen?

1. No change should be considered at this time.

2. Decrease dosage of conjugated equine estrogen to 0.3 mg daily.

3. Recommend stopping conjugated equine estrogen.

4. Suggest changing route of administration to transdermal.

96. An adult female client is seen in the family planning clinic for a consultation on contraception. She is using birth control pills but forgets to take them because her work schedule changes every week. She is looking for an effective method that will be easy to remember. She has been married for 14 years, is G2 T2 P0 A0 L2, and is a nonsmoker. She has no history of any major diseases and no history of gynecologic abnormalities. She has never been treated for an STD and is in a mutually monogamous relationship. She is needle-phobic and faints when she has to have blood drawn. What contraceptive method would be a good choice for this client?

1. Depo-Provera injection every 3 months.

2. Norplant implantation system for 5 years.

3. IUD.

4. Diaphragm.

97. A young adult female client is being seen at the family planning clinic by the nurse practitioner. The client wants birth control pills but has heard that they are dangerous to one's health. When asked for clarification, she lists the following: weight gain, ovarian cancer, heavy or irregular periods, and infertility. The nurse practitioner tells her: "I can see that you are concerned about your health . . ."

1. "There are a lot of fallacies about birth control pills. They actually are believed to reduce the risk of ovarian cancers, help to regulate the bleeding, and are not associated with causing infertility. There can be a minor increase in body weight of 3 to 5 lb."

2. "Perhaps you would be better off trying the Norplant system or Depo-Provera."

3. "What you have heard is true. They can be dangerous to your health and many people experience these problems."

4. "There are a lot of fallacies about birth control pills. While ovarian cancer and infertility are risks that are taken with the use of the birth control pill, they do not cause weight gain or bleeding changes in periods. Pap smears done every year will detect such things as ovarian cancer."

98. A 41-year-old female client is seen in the family planning clinic. She is seeking information about contraceptive methods because her Norplant system is due for removal next month. She is in a new sexual relationship and plans to use condoms for STD prevention. She is in excellent health, is a nonsmoker, and is nulliparous. Her menses are every 28 days, with light flow. Which is **inappropriate** for the nurse practitioner to recommend?

1. OCs.

2. IUD.

3. Norplant system.

4. Depo-Provera injections.

99. An adult female client is taking oral contraceptive agents. She calls the clinic with complaints of bleeding through the first 2 weeks of every package of pills. She has been using this pill for 4 months and takes it at the same time every day. Her present pill is a low-dose monophasic pill. She is not taking any other medications and she denies any adverse effects of the birth control pills. She would like to con-

tinue taking OCs, if possible. The nurse practitioner's advice should include:

1. Discontinue the pills and do not restart them. An alternative contraceptive method should be used.

2. Change to a higher dosage, higher progestational agent.

3. Try taking the pills first thing in the morning on an empty stomach to improve metabolism of the agents.

4. There is no cause for concern; breakthrough bleeding is a normal side effect of OCs.

100. An adult female client is seen by the nurse practitioner at the family planning clinic. The client mentions that she has heavy, irregular menses. There has been an increase in facial acne and facial/abdominal hair growth over the past few years. She is G1 T1 P0 A0 L1 and is not planning future pregnancies. After a pelvic exam during which findings are normal, the client decides she wants OCs. Which OC would the nurse practitioner prescribe for this client?

1. Loestrin 1/20.

2. Triphasil.

3. Demulen 1/35.

4. Birth control pills are inappropriate for this client.

101. A 41-year-old female client is seen for her 6-week-postpartum exam by the nurse practitioner. She is breast-feeding without difficulty and plans to continue for a year. She wants to begin using a contraceptive and plans no further pregnancies. Which is an **inappropriate** choice for this client?

1. Depo-Provera 150 mg IM injection every 3 months.

2. IUD.

3. Progestin-only oral contraceptive.

4. Combined oral contraceptive.

102. A 38-year-old female client is seen for her 6-week-postpartum exam by the nurse practitioner. The client was breast-feeding for a short time but discontinued 4 weeks ago. Her menses have resumed. She is contemplating another pregnancy in a year or so, but if she

became pregnant before that she wouldn't mind. She is seeking contraception. She smokes one pack per day. Findings on examination are normal, with the uterus being well involuted. Which is **contraindicated** in this client?

1. Progestasert IUD.

2. Oral contraceptive agents.

3. Depo-Provera injection.

4. Condoms and spermicide.

103. A 25-year-old female client is seen by the nurse practitioner for her annual exam. The client is interested in contraceptive choices. She just quit smoking and is well motivated to remain a nonsmoker. She is taking phenobarbital and phenytoin (Dilantin) for seizure control. She is G3 T2 P0 A1 L1. She may be planning future pregnancies but is unsure at this time. She is in good health other than the seizure disorder, and exam findings are normal. What contraceptive method is contraindicated in this client?

1. Diaphragm.

2. Depo-Provera injection.

3. IUD.

4. Norplant implantation system.

104. A 22-year-old female client presents to the urgent care department and is seen by the nurse practitioner. She is complaining of abdominal pain, low-grade fever, and mucopurulent vaginal discharge. Her symptoms began 3 days ago and are getting worse. She has a new sexual partner and has not used condoms with him yet. Her menses just ended; she is taking OCs. She denies nausea, vomiting, or anorexia. Her exam reveals findings consistent with pelvic inflammatory disease (PID). Specimens were obtained for gonorrhea and chlamydia culture. Which represents an **inappropriate** treatment plan for the nurse practitioner to follow?

1. Administration of ceftriaxone (Rocephin) 250 mg IM.

2. Administration of doxycycline (Vibra tabs) 100 mg PO bid × 10 days.

3. Ordering a CBC and erythrocyte sedimentation rate.

4. Hospitalization.

105. What is the primary role of progestins in post-menopausal HRT?

    1. Reduce side effects of estrogen-related breast tenderness.

    2. Provide endometrial protection against hyperplasia

    3. Stabilize mood swings and reduce hot flashes.

    4. Reduce occurrence of breakthrough bleeding.

106. An older female client is seen by the nurse practitioner for her annual exam. She has been receiving HRT for 6 months, having started herself on the pills left over by her deceased mother. She brings the pills with her, because she wants to continue taking these and requests a prescription for Estrace 1 mg daily. She has an intact uterus, is in excellent health, and denies any complaints. She does not have any contraindications to the use of HRT. Exam findings are normal. Which represents an **incorrect** and potentially dangerous plan for the nurse practitioner to follow?

    1. Endometrial biopsy.

    2. Prescription for Estrace 1 mg daily plus MPA (Provera) 2.5 mg daily.

    3. Prescription for Estrace 1 mg daily.

    4. Instruct the client on the risks and benefits of HRT.

107. An older adult female client is seen for follow-up to discuss the HRT that she began 3 months ago. She needs a refill of her HRT but is not sure it is working right. She continues to experience hot flashes, moodiness, and decreased libido and has many sleep disturbances. She is taking Premarin 0.625 mg daily and Provera 2.5 mg daily. She denies any vaginal bleeding. Which is **not** an acceptable choice for the client?

    1. Premarin 0.9 mg, 1 tablet PO qd, and Provera 5 mg, 1 tablet PO qd days 1 to 12.

    2. Premarin 0.9 mg, 1 tablet PO qd, and Provera 5 mg, 1 tablet PO qd days 16 to 25.

    3. Premarin 0.3 mg, 1 tablet PO qd, and Provera 2.5 mg, 1 tablet PO qd.

    4. Premarin 1.25 mg, 1 tablet PO qd, and Provera 10 mg, 1 tablet PO qd days 1 to 12.

108. Which is **not** a contraindication to the use of HRT in the postmenopausal female?

    1. Recent deep venous thrombosis.

    2. Chronic active hepatitis.

    3. Controlled hypertension.

    4. Undiagnosed abnormal genital bleeding.

109. A young adult female client presents to the clinic with complaints of a malodorous, yellowish vaginal discharge and vulvovaginal itching. She has never had a gynecologic exam and is extremely apprehensive. She is sexually active and has had a new sexual partner for 2 months. She states that they use condoms most of the time and are not interested in alternate forms of contraception at this time. Her LMP was 1 week ago. Her wet mount with KOH shows few clue cells, moderate lactobacilli, few WBCs, no yeast, and TNTC mobile trichomonads. Appropriate treatment for this client would include:

    1. Metronidazole (Flagyl) 2 g PO, single dose.

    2. Metronidazole (Metrogel) vaginal cream, 1 applicator full per vagina qhs × 5 days.

    3. Fluconazole (Diflucan) 150 mg PO, single dose.

    4. Terconazole (Terazol) vaginal cream, 1 applicator full per vagina qhs × 7 days.

110. Which dose of conjugated equine estrogen (Premarin) is the minimal effective dose for prevention of osteoporosis?

    1. 0.3 mg.

    2. 0.625 mg.

    3. 0.9 mg.

    4. Premarin is inappropriate.

111. A single woman presents for contraceptive counseling and expresses a preference for a diaphragm. Which factor in her history would make a diaphragm a poor choice?

    1. Three UTIs in the past year.

    2. Strong desire to avoid pregnancy.

    3. Last two Pap smears showed atypical cells.

    4. Nulliparous cervix.

112. Combination oral contraceptive pills prevent pregnancy primarily by:

    1. Decreasing fallopian tube motility.

    2. Thinning of cervical mucus.

    3. Suppressing ovulation.

    4. Causing inflammation of the endometrium.

113. A young adult client is hesitant to be fitted for an IUD because of strong antiabortion views and asks your opinion. Which explanation least accurately describes the probable action of an IUD?

    1. Slows transport of ovum through the fallopian tube, causing it to age and die in transit.

    2. Prevents effective implantation of a fertilized ovum.

    3. Action is no different from that of spermicide.

    4. Slows transport of sperm.

114. What is a unique advantage of a Progesterone T IUD?

    1. Lowest failure rate of IUDs.

    2. May be left in place for up to 10 years.

    3. Decreases menstrual blood loss and dysmenorrhea.

    4. Must be replaced annually.

115. An older female client is seen by the nurse practitioner for her annual exam and needs a refill of her HRT. She is feeling well and has not voiced concerns. The client had a total abdominal hysterectomy and bilateral salpingo-oophorectomy as treatment for benign fibroids 2 years ago. Exam findings are normal. She takes conjugated estrogen (Premarin) 0.625 mg from days 1 to 25 and MPA (Provera) 10 mg from days 16 to 25. What changes would be appropriate for the nurse practitioner to make in the HRT regimen?

    1. No changes needed; the client is doing well with the present regimen.

    2. Premarin 0.625 mg daily and discontinue the Provera.

    3. Premarin 0.625 mg daily and Provera 2.5 mg daily.

    4. Premarin 0.625 mg days 1 to 25 and Provera 5 mg days 16 to 25.

116. Which statement about progestin-only pills is true?

    1. Women who are breast-feeding should not use progestin-only pills.

    2. Ovulation suppression is as effective with progestin-only pills as with combined oral contraception pills.

    3. There is an increased incidence of functional ovarian cysts.

    4. The risk of ectopic pregnancy is lower for women using progestin-only pills.

117. Before HRT is prescribed, which clinical approach should have the highest priority?

    1. The decision about use should rest primarily with the client after appropriate education and counseling have been provided.

    2. For most women the benefits of HRT far outweigh any possible side effects, so HRT should be actively encouraged.

    3. Involving the sexual partner in the counseling session is likely to lead to a higher rate of compliance with HRT.

    4. Education regarding HRT should include a thorough review of risk factors and possible side effects in order to avoid liability issues.

118. The most common side effect associated with depomedroxyprogesterone (DMPA; Depo-Provera) is:

    1. Nausea.

    2. Acne.

    3. Menstrual cycle changes.

    4. Increased menstrual cramps.

119. The nurse practitioner is teaching a client about taking alendronate (Fosamax); her information includes:

    1. Take it midmorning.

    2. Take with food.

    3. Take with a full glass of orange juice.

    4. Remain upright after taking medication.

120. The addition of a progesterone to an estrogen regimen for a postmenopausal woman with a uterus reduces the risk of:

    1. Endometrial cancer.

    2. Cervical cancer.

    3. Gallbladder disease.

    4. Breast cancer.

121. The treatment of choice for trichomoniasis is:

    1. Azithromycin (Zithromax) 1 g PO, single dose.

    2. Ofloxacin (Floxin) 500 mg PO, single dose.

    3. Metronidazole (Flagyl) 2 g PO, single dose.

    4. Clindamycin (Cleocin) 300 mg PO, single dose.

122. A 25-year-old woman comes into the office with complaints of profuse malodorous discharge. The nurse practitioner's diagnosis is bacterial vaginosis. The nurse practitioner would:

    1. Advise the client to notify her sexual contacts regarding the diagnosis.

    2. Treat the problem with metronidazole (Flagyl) 2 g, one dose.

    3. Initiate treatment with doxycycline (Vibramycin) 100 mg PO bid × 7 days.

    4. Determine whether the woman is pregnant before initiating a course of treatment.

123. A young woman who is taking a low-dose OC calls the clinic in a panic, stating that she forgot her pill 2 days ago. She is taking phenytoin (Dilantin) for seizure activity and has been seizure-free for more than a year. She asks, "What should I do about my pills?" The most appropriate response is:

    1. Advise her to take the forgotten dose today along with the regular dose.

    2. Refer her to her physician for advice about the Dilantin.

    3. Advise her to continue taking the pills but to use another contraceptive through the rest of this cycle.

    4. Advise her to come to the clinic for a "morning-after" pill.

124. A vaginal culture has confirmed the presence of chancroid in a homeless woman who presented with a painful genital ulcer. The treatment regimen of choice should be:

    1. Ceftriaxone (Rocephin) 250 mg IM in a single dose.

    2. Erythromycin (E-Mycin) 500 mg PO qid × 7 days.

    3. Metronidazole (Flagyl) 2 mg PO in a single dose.

    4. Clindamycin (Cleocin) cream 2%, 1 full applicator (intravaginally) × 5 days.

125. The nurse practitioner is counseling a 49-year-old woman who had her LMP 10 months ago. She is experiencing some hot flashes and night sweats and is not sleeping as well as she would like. These symptoms are affecting her ability to work effectively because she finds herself tired and "cranky." She tells the nurse practitioner that HRT is not an option for her. Which statement about an evidence-based alternative measure is the most accurate?

    1. Venlafaxine HCL (Effexor SR) has been effective in reducing hot flashes in randomized control trials.

    2. Raloxifene HCL (Evista) has been demonstrated to cause a significant reduction in hot flashes when compared with placebo in clinical trials.

    3. Black cohosh is efficacious in treating menopausal symptoms according to many large, controlled trials.

    4. Isoflavones, specifically soy, have been shown in studies to be significantly more effective in reducing hot flashes than placebo.

126. A young adult female presents to the office for evaluation of abdominal pain. The client admits to recent sexual activity and states that she does not have her partner use condoms. On exam, the nurse practitioner finds vaginal discharge and cervical motion tenderness. In addition to sending cultures to the lab, the nurse practitioner would treat this client with:

    1. Penicillin G, 2.4 million units IM.

    2. Metronidazole (Flagyl), 500 mg PO bid × 7 days.

    3. Ceftriaxone (Rocephin), 125 mg IM and azithromycin (Zithromax) 1 g PO.

    4. Acyclovir (Zovirax) 400 mg PO bid × 7 days.

16 Answers & Rationales

Physical Examination & Diagnostic Tests

1. **(3)** Lubricants, other than water, should not be used if a cervical specimen is being obtained for Pap smear analysis; certain ones can alter the appearance of the cells and affect cytologic accuracy. Endocervical cell retrieval is diminished with the use of a cotton-tipped applicator, and such an applicator is not recommended for use in any female, regardless of pregnancy status. The bimanual exam is performed after the internal vaginal exam.

2. **(2)** An empty bladder will provide for client comfort and will assist the nurse practitioner in making a more accurate assessment during the bimanual portion of the exam. Options #1 and #3 help reduce the client's anxiety, which ultimately may assist in the achievement of comfort.

3. **(1)** A nabothian cyst is a small, white or yellow, raised, round area on the cervix and is considered to be a normal variant. The surface of the cervix should be smooth and may have a symmetric, reddened circle around the os (squamocolumnar epithelium, or ectropion). The other options are all unexpected, abnormal findings.

4. **(3)** A breast ultrasound exam is used to determine whether a lesion is solid or cystic. Sonography misses 50% of lesions <2 cm. The test is not sensitive enough to be used for routine screening and cannot replace mammography. The definitive diagnosis of breast cancer is breast biopsy.

5. **(2)** The World Health Organization defines osteoporosis as a bone mineral density T-score below −2.5 SD and osteopenia as a T-score between −1 and −2.5. This woman has early signs of osteopenia. She is not a candidate for HRT (conjugated equine estrogen + medroxyprogesterone acetate [MPA]) because of her cardiovascular history. Evista has been shown to prevent the progression of osteoporosis and, as a selective estrogen-receptor modulator (SERM), may be a good alternative to HRT. Certainly, the other two lifestyle modifications are important in reducing the risk of developing osteoporosis.

6. **(3)** The hysterosalpingogram (HSG) is used to document the presence of a normal uterine cavity and the patency of the fallopian tubes. A contrast dye is injected into the uterus and x-ray films are taken to assess anatomy. The best time to do this test is 2 to 5 days after menses but before ovulation.

7. **(1)** Approximately 10% of breast cancers are not seen on mammograms.

8. **(1)** Potassium hydroxide (KOH) lyses epithelial and white blood cells, making it easier to visualize *Candida* (yeast) cells. *Candida* cells are resistant and remain intact. KOH also assists in the diagnosis of bacterial vaginosis by alkalinizing vaginal discharge, causing a distinct fishy odor. This is a positive amine or whiff test result.

9. **(3)** The Pap smear is a screening test for cervical cancer and precancerous states. The diagnostic test needed to confirm the diagnosis of a high-grade lesion is the colposcopy with guided biopsies. The results of this test are clearly abnormal and must be acted upon. Waiting a year could be deleterious to the client's health. This is not a Pap smear report that one would choose to redo in 4 months; the client needs a diagnostic test, not another screening test. The Pap smear does not indicate a diagnosis of cervical cancer; therefore a referral to a gynecologic oncologist is premature at this time.

10. **(3)** All of the tests may be included in the workup for infertility. Because male factors account for 35% to 40% of infertility, a semen analysis should be done early in the workup. HSG and endometrial biopsy are tests that require scheduling at specific times of the menstrual cycle. Tests for anti-sperm antibodies would be done if the postcoital test revealed abnormalities.

11. **(3)** The National Osteoporosis Foundation (NOF) has conducted cost analyses on the value of a screening bone dual-energy x-ray absorptiometry (DEXA) scan for evaluation of bone mineral density. The NOF reports that BMD testing is cost-effective for postmenopausal women between the ages of 50 and 60 who have other risk factors for the development of osteoporosis. Those risk factors include lifestyle factors of minimal exercise, smoking, excessive alcohol intake, and low calcium intake. Other risk factors include genetic history of disease, slender physical frame, premature menopause, hyperthyroidism, multiple myeloma, rheumatoid arthritis, chronic renal disease, use of corticosteroids, and long-term use of anticonvulsants. The woman with the history given in Option #3 would meet the NOF criteria.

12. **(4)** Longstanding nevi and Montgomery tubercles are normal findings; "pendulous breast" is just a description of size, which is important to note. Enlarged lymph nodes and tender supraclavicular nodes are potential causes for concern. A fixed stellate mass with nipple discharge is not normal, and although asymmetry might be normal, the different colors of the areolae and unilateral nipple inversion could represent a problem.

13. **(4)** The basal body temperature (BBT) chart is an easy and inexpensive tool with which to evaluate for ovulation. Clients should be taught, on the first visit, how to use a BBT thermometer and record the findings on a BBT chart. The remaining answers are usually included in an infertility workup but do not indicate whether ovulation has occurred.

14. **(2)** Atrophic changes on the cervix of a postmenopausal female are to be expected, as is the paucity of endocervical cells. Because of her medical history of breast cancer, she is not a candidate for the use of estrogen vaginal cream, nor are findings from the Pap smear abnormal. Endocervical curettage is used as a biopsy technique for sampling tissue from the endocervical canal; however, it is not appropriate to recommend this invasive procedure for a client with scant endocervical cells, but rather for one with abnormal endocervical cells. Since this Pap smear report really is not classified as abnormal, there is no need to recommend a diagnostic procedure for the client.

15. **(4)** Culture is the only certain or definitive method of diagnosis. A cervical specimen is collected and cultured, and the results take about 2 to 6 days to obtain. The direct fluorescent antibody (DFA) test is fast and has good sensitivity and specificity.

16. **(2)** Mammography is recommended annually by the American Cancer Society for all women 40 years of age and older. There is no need for annual mammograms for all women of child-bearing age; breast-feeding does not preclude the use of mammography, and screening is not done only for breast symptoms.

17. **(1)** Serologic tests are good screening tests, but positive results require follow-up with a treponemal test to detect specific antibodies.

18. **(2)** Serum prolactin assay levels >20 ng/ml indicate the need for medical referral, usually to an endocrinologist. The most common cause of hyperprolactinemia and galactorrhea (milky breast discharge) is a pituitary tumor or lesion of the hypothalamus. Other causes may be hypothyroidism, medications (narcotics, tranquilizers, antihypertensives), and OCs.

19. **(1)** A positive withdrawal bleed after a progesterone challenge indicates adequate levels of endogenous estrogen. A serum prolactin level should be obtained as part of the amenorrhea workup in addition to a serum pregnancy test. A diagnosis of anovulation can be made on the basis of the successful withdrawal bleed and normal prolactin levels. Low body fat and abnormal thyroxine levels can also lead to amenorrhea but do not affect results of the progesterone challenge test.

20. **(1)** The occurrence of the symptoms during the luteal phase of the cycle, that is, after ovulation, will assist the nurse practitioner in making the diagnosis of premenstrual syndrome (PMS). Having the client keep a calendar to track her symptoms for three cycles is very helpful for both diagnosis and measurement of successful treatment. The severity of the symptoms, while important, is not the most important information.

21. **(3)** If bleeding resumes after 1 year of amenorrhea in a postmenopausal woman or persists longer than 6 months after initiation of HRT, further evaluation is necessary. The most common cause of this abnormal finding is endometrial atrophy, but more serious pathologic conditions must be definitively ruled out. An endometrial biopsy should be scheduled to further evaluate the cause of bleeding.

Normal Gynecology

22. **(4)** Inside the uterus, the lining first proliferates and begins preparation for implantation of the fertilized egg. During the secretory phase, glandular epithelium develops, further enhancing the lining. If no fertilized egg arrives for implantation, the lining sloughs off; this is the menstrual phase.

23. **(1)** PMS occurs approximately 5 to 11 days before the onset of menses (late luteal phase) and is gone within 1 to 2 days of the onset of menses. This phase is progesterone dominant. The follicular phase is estrogen dominant.

24. **(3)** Oxytocin is released from the posterior pituitary gland. Follicle-stimulating hormone (FSH), luteinizing hormone (LH), and prolactin are all released from the anterior pituitary gland. The other hormones released from the anterior pituitary are thyroid-stimulating hormone (TSH), adrenocorticotropic hormone (ACTH), and growth hormone.

25. **(1)** FSH stimulates the maturation of ovarian follicles, resulting in a dominant follicle. Milk secretion is dependent on prolactin. The production and release of LH is regulated by estrogen. LH is responsible for ovulation.

26. **(2)** In 2001, the Stages of Reproductive Aging Workshop (STRAW) developed standardized definitions for menopause events. The phrases "in menopause" or "going through menopause" are misnomers and actually refer to the period before menopause termed appropriately *menopause transition* or *perimenopause*. Menopause is one point in time and is defined after 12 months of amenorrhea following the final menstrual period. Although after menopause FSH levels rise 10-fold to 15-fold with marked reductions in estradiol, other menstrual irregularities can create a variation in these levels. Therefore these levels are not considered as the best definition for menopause.

27. **(4)** The ovarian cycle is divided into three phases. The follicular phase begins on the first day of menses and continues until day 14, when ovulation usually occurs. Immediately after ovulation, the empty follicle begins to enlarge and develops into a corpus luteum, which releases increasing amounts of progesterone. If implantation does not occur, the corpus luteum regresses, causing the onset of menses. This phase, from ovulation to menses, is the luteal phase.

28. **(1)** As many as 30% of all coronary events are associated with tobacco use. HRT increases the risk of cardiovascular disease. The rate of mortality from cardiovascular disease in patients with diabetes is two to four times higher than that in nondiabetic patients.

29. **(4)** Pregnancy is the most likely diagnosis for this client, given the list of symptoms and physical findings. She certainly could have a uterine fibroid; however, it is not contributing to the symptoms listed. Ovarian cancer could present with nausea, fatigue, and abdominal bloating; however, it would cause neither the enlarged uterus nor the positive Chadwick's

sign. A dislodged intrauterine device (IUD) will usually change its position, thereby causing the strings to be less visible or causing the IUD itself to be expelled into the vagina or endocervical canal.

30. **(3)** Maintaining an alkaline pH is important to promote viability of sperm that are deposited into the vaginal vault.

31. **(4)** Obesity is not a risk factor for osteoporosis. Cigarette use, white race, and alcohol consumption, in addition to others not listed here, are considered to be risk factors for osteoporosis.

32. **(2)** Conservative management for PMS including daily exercise, stress reduction, dietary changes, and reassurance that her symptoms are valid should help the client gain more control. A low-salt diet is encouraged; when necessary, a diuretic may be used to reduce fluid retention. The use of vitamins B_6, A, and E may be helpful as well. Laboratory studies are not indicated here but might be helpful if the symptoms were sustained throughout the menstrual cycle.

33. **(2)** As the function of the ovaries declines and the amount of circulating estrogen begins to fall, the middle-aged female may begin to experience the symptoms commonly associated with menopause. The body's feedback system will attempt to stimulate the ovaries and increase the estrogen level. FSH and LH levels rise in response to these efforts.

34. **(4)** Douching is never necessary. It changes the normal pH and upsets the normal vaginal flora. Douching during menstruation could cause "retrograde menstruation," a potential precursor to endometriosis. Copious vaginal discharge can be a symptom of infection and warrants workup.

35. **(1)** Pregnancy is the most likely diagnosis, requiring a pregnancy test and pelvic ultrasound exam to confirm it. Even though she has had a tubal ligation, failure rates of 1 in 300 have been reported. This client could have uterine fibroids; however, they do not generally present with this symptom complex and are not associated with amenorrhea, although they do cause uterine enlargement. Premature menopause could cause all these symptoms, including amenorrhea, but not the enlarged uterus. Colon cancer can present with these symptoms and could certainly be responsible for an abdominal mass, but not uterine enlargement or amenorrhea.

36. **(4)** The age at onset of menopause has fluctuated very little over the past several centuries, even though life expectancy has increased. Of the options, only smoking has been found to cause an earlier menopause (on average, 1.5 years earlier). Research has indicated that there is a direct correlation between the number of cigarettes smoked, number of years of smoking, and age at menopause. Nulliparity and epilepsy have also been associated with an earlier age at onset of menopause.

Gynecologic Disorders

37. **(2)** Dyspareunia is painful intercourse and vaginismus is painful vaginal spasms on penetration. Primary orgasmic disorder is when an individual has never achieved orgasm, usually a lifelong problem. Secondary orgasmic dysfunction refers to an acquired problem of loss of orgasmic function after an individual has experienced orgasm.

38. **(1)** The initial outbreak is usually the worst. Herpes can be transmitted even when there is no lesion present, and it cannot be cured. Vaginal delivery is allowed, if there are no genital lesions at the time of labor.

39. **(1)** Bacterial vaginosis results when the normal environment in the vagina is disrupted. The normal vaginal lactobacilli are decreased or absent, and there is an overgrowth of many different types of anaerobic bacteria. Trichomoniasis is caused by a flagellated protozoan, and gonorrhea is caused by bacteria and may be asymptomatic. The virus that causes recurrent outbreaks of genital lesions is herpes genitalis type 2 (HSV-II).

40. **(1)** OCs will reduce prostaglandin production, which is thought to be the primary cause of dysmenorrhea.

41. **(4)** The criteria for the diagnosis of bacterial vaginosis are characteristic milky homogeneous discharge, pH >4.5, amine odor (positive whiff test result) with addition of KOH, and the

presence of epithelial cells studded with coccobacilli that obscure the borders (clue cells). Pseudohyphae are present in candidiasis.

42. **(2)** In Asherman's syndrome, a normally functioning uterus has been damaged and scarred as a result of instrumentation, usually a dilatation and curettage (D&C). Ovulation may be occurring normally, but there is no endometrium built up; therefore no endometrium is shed (menstruation does not occur). Of course, pregnancy, as well as the other diseases listed, should be ruled out in this client.

43. **(2)** The LH/FSH ratio in polycystic ovarian syndrome is 3:1. The normal LH/FSH ratio is 1.5:1.

44. **(4)** The criteria for the diagnosis of polycystic ovarian syndrome include menstrual irregularity, increased body weight, hirsutism, androgen excess evidenced by results of lab studies and physical findings, chronic anovulation, and multiple bilateral ovarian cysts. The findings listed in Option #1 are associated with anorexia nervosa or bulimia; those listed in Option #2, with a prolactin-secreting pituitary tumor; and those listed in Option #3, with endometriosis.

45. **(3)** Ninety percent of dysfunctional uterine bleeding is caused by anovulation. The lack of progesterone allows asynchronous, excessive proliferation of the endometrium. This tissue is fragile, and the normal hemostatic mechanism is altered. Thyroid disease, blood dyscrasias, and uterine tumors can mimic dysfunctional uterine bleeding and must be ruled out.

46. **(3)** A female-appearing person with a 46,XY karyotype is referred to as having androgen insensitivity syndrome, or testicular feminization. This maternal X-linked recessive disorder accounts for approximately 10% of all cases of amenorrhea, and persons with this karyotype do not appear different until puberty. These clients present with amenorrhea, scant or absent pubic hair, and abnormal or no breast development. Persons with müllerian abnormalities have a normal XX karyotype with abnormalities of the fallopian tubes, uterus, and upper vagina occurring in fetal development. In Turner's syndrome, there is congenital absence of ovaries because of the loss of one X chromosome.

47. **(1)** The most common breast mass in young women <30 years old is the fibroadenoma. This benign breast mass is the third most common breast mass, after fibrocystic changes and carcinoma. Fibrocystic breast changes are seen most commonly in women 30 to 50 years old. Intraductal papilloma is a wart-like growth located in the mammary duct and occurs in women 40 to 50 years old. Malignant breast neoplasms occur most frequently in women older than 40 and are rarely seen in women 15 to 25 years old.

48. **(1)** Nonsteroidal antiinflammatory analgesics inhibit prostaglandin synthesis and are effective in the treatment of primary dysmenorrhea. The other agents listed have no demonstrated effectiveness in primary dysmenorrhea. Other measures to decrease discomfort are exercise, relaxation techniques, heat application, and low-dose oral contraceptives (OCs).

49. **(4)** Secondary amenorrhea is defined as no menses for three cycle lengths or 6 months in a woman with previously established menses. Exercise can cause an increase in estrogen and endorphin levels, which influences the release of gonadotropin-releasing hormone (GnRH). Without appropriate GnRH release, FSH and LH are not released appropriately, resulting in anovulation, which may lead to amenorrhea. The other conditions listed are causes of primary amenorrhea.

50. **(1)** This has the characteristics of a syphilitic lesion and needs to be evaluated. Only after determining the presence or type of the sexually transmitted disease (STD) can it be treated effectively. The herpes viral culture should be done while the lesion is present and the fluid from the vesicles can be obtained.

51. **(3)** Pregnancy is the most common cause of amenorrhea in young women. It is important to rule out pregnancy in a female client with a problem of amenorrhea, even if she is very athletic. Interviewing the client regarding her sexual practices is unreliable. The presence or absence of pregnancy should be determined before other diagnostic studies are done.

52. **(2)** A person who has never engaged in coital activity is not considered to be at risk for cervical cancer because of the unlikelihood of exposure to human papillomavirus (HPV). In addition to others not listed here, the

presence of HPV, multiple sexual partners, and/or previous high-grade squamous intraepithelial lesion are considered to be risk factors in the development of cervical cancer.

53. **(1)** The pseudohyphae and spores on the wet mount with KOH are diagnostic of candidiasis. *Chlamydia trachomatis* infection is diagnosed by direct immunofluorescence assay (DFA) or by culture for chlamydia. Gonorrhea is diagnosed by cervical culture, and bacterial vaginosis has microscopic findings of clue cells and positive amine odor.

54. **(1)** Ovarian cancer is the leading cause of death in women with genital cancers, excluding breast cancer, in the United States.

55. **(1)** The presence of flagellated protozoa confirms the diagnosis of trichomoniasis. *Chlamydia* infection is best diagnosed by DFA or culture. Bacterial vaginosis is diagnosed by a wet mount revealing clue cells and a positive amine test result. Inflammatory cervicitis is generally asymptomatic and will not cause vaginal irritation.

56. **(3)** The pelvic ultrasound exam is not a useful test for the diagnosis of appendicitis, because it will not allow for adequate examination of the appendix. The complete blood count (CBC) with differential is useful because of the expected rise in white blood cells (WBCs) in this inflammatory state. The flat plate of the abdomen and kidney-ureters-bladder (KUB) is very helpful in determining the extent of the problem and in ruling out other diagnoses. Since ectopic pregnancy can cause these symptoms, the practitioner should consider it as part of the differential diagnosis.

57. **(2)** Birth control pills have been shown to reduce the risk of endometrial cancer. Obesity, unopposed estrogen use, and advanced age—in addition to other factors not listed here—are considered to be risk factors for development of endometrial cancer.

58. **(2)** The diaphragm may be inserted up to 2 hours before intercourse and should be removed no sooner than 6 hours after intercourse has ended. It should not be left in place longer than 24 hours.

59. **(2)** Urethral discomfort and recurrent urinary tract infections (UTIs) are associated with diaphragm use and are the most common

reasons for discontinuing use and changing birth control methods.

60. **(3)** Birth control pill use has been shown to reduce the risk of ovarian cancer. Family history of ovarian cancer, advancing age, and the presence of the *BRCA 2* gene—in addition to others not listed here—are considered to be risk factors for development of ovarian cancer.

61. **(2)** The endometrium is the most common site of female genital malignancy.

62. **(3)** Herpes simplex virus type 2 commonly presents dramatically in the primary outbreak. Gonorrhea is generally associated with a mucopurulent vaginal discharge and is not accompanied by vesicular lesions. *Chlamydia* infection can be associated with dysuria and, unless accompanied by PID, is not generally accompanied by fever or body aches, nor is it associated with vesicular lesions. Lymphogranuloma venereum is a rare disease classically accompanied by pustular enlargement of the lymph nodes, particularly the inguinal nodes. It is associated not with vesicles, but with buboes.

63. **(2)** Screening lab blood work for glucose, cardiac risk profile, and TSH level in this age group without any stated risk factors is not cost-effective and is of little value. The client can be better served with a discussion regarding diet and exercise. Since this client is at risk for STDs, counseling and testing for these is a reasonable approach. Contraceptive information educates the client and allows her to make wiser choices about family planning.

64. **(1)** Early menopause has not been associated with the development of breast cancer. High-fat diet, advancing age, early menarche, and others not listed here have been identified as risk factors in the development of breast cancer.

65. **(1)** The use of prenatal vitamins with folic acid before conception has been found to reduce the risk of neural tube defects in the fetus. It is important for the client to continue her exercise program, although some discussion about the type of exercise and any limitations is important once pregnancy is achieved. Since the client has had two previous pregnancies, it is likely that her rubella immune status has been determined;

if she is found to not be immune to rubella, then a measles-mumps-rubella (MMR) vaccine should be recommended. This client is not of advanced maternal age and therefore does not require genetic counseling.

66. **(3)** Baseline lab work should be performed to determine the presence of anemia, possible pregnancy, and/or endocrine dysfunction.

67. **(4)** Fibrocystic breast disease is not a risk factor for breast cancer. In addition to others, those listed in Options #1, #2, and #3 are considered to be risk factors for breast cancer.

68. **(1)** The recommended age for a female to begin having Pap smears performed is at the onset of sexual activity or at 18 years of age. Since this client is 20 years old and has not had her first Pap smear, this would be the most appropriate test to perform. It is not necessary to perform STD screening for clients who have not been sexually active. Stool Hemoccult testing and mammography are not recommended as screening procedures in the young adult.

69. **(3)** Heart disease remains the leading cause of death among women in the United States.

70. **(3)** The presence of bruising, particularly on genitalia, suggests abuse. Combined with her nonverbal behavior, the bruising should prompt the nurse practitioner to explore the possibility of abuse.

71. **(1)** Reactive cellular changes are most commonly associated with inflammation, including typical repair. Other causes include atrophy with inflammation (atrophic vaginitis), IUD use, radiation, and diethylstilbestrol exposure in utero. OCs do not cause reactive changes, and estrogen vaginal cream may be used to treat atrophy.

72. **(2)** Cervical cancer has been directly linked with exposure to high-risk types of human papilloma virus (HPV). Pregnancy after 35, low parity, and prolonged contraceptive use are not risk factors for cervical cancer.

73. **(1)** Breast cancer is the most common cancer in women in the United States. The number of deaths caused by lung cancer is higher than the number of deaths caused by breast cancer in the United States.

74. **(3)** These symptoms are classic for menopausal syndrome, although it is true that there are some depressive symptoms listed. Antidepressant therapy and counseling for depression at this stage of treatment is not appropriate. Testing, teaching, and treatment in this case should be aimed at the menopause. The depressive symptoms will undoubtedly improve with greater understanding and treatment of the menopausal symptoms.

75. **(1)** Chancroid is well established as a cofactor for human immunodeficiency virus (HIV) transmission.

76. **(4)** Monthly breast self-examination (BSE) is an important method of detecting early breast changes.

77. **(2)** Symptoms are most likely indicative of benign fibroadenoma. Mammography is indicated. Surgical excision is unlikely to be necessary for a young woman.

78. **(2)** She needs to become more knowledgeable about the normal feel of implants, as well as her own breast tissue. Mammography is not a substitute for BSE.

79. **(2)** A very firm cervix, along with a cervical lesion or ulcer, is suggestive of cancer of the cervix, which can be confirmed with a Pap smear.

80. **(1)** This complaint is an indication for clinical breast exam and mammography. Although breast pain is not a common presenting symptom for breast cancer, it can be. Teaching SBE is important, but not the most important action at this point; hormonal fluctuations can explain breast pain, as can excessive caffeine intake, but should be a diagnosis of exclusion after malignancy is ruled out.

81. **(2)** Toxic shock syndrome occurs primarily in menstruating women ages 12 to 24 who use tampons. The diagnosis is made when the following symptoms are present: fever >102° F (38.9° C), macular rash, hypotension, and involvement of three or more organ systems.

82. **(4)** More than 16% of ectopic pregnancies present as surgical emergencies. In the United States, 1 in 1000 deaths associated with ectopic pregnancies occur as a result of blood loss.

83. **(4)** Almost half of all vaginal infections are due to candidiasis. The majority of women who have candidiasis have recently taken antibiotics. It is not an STD.

84. **(1)** It is important to evaluate the client for threatened abortion as soon as possible. It is most likely too soon for the CBC to reflect blood loss. A pelvic sonogram will take longer than a urine pregnancy test, and it is imperative that the client be immediately referred for a D&C, if her pregnancy test result is positive.

85. **(2)** The most common site for breast cancer occurrence is the upper outer quadrant, followed by the area beneath the nipple.

86. **(3)** Pap smears are crucial for the detection of cervical cancer but do not diagnose uterine cancer. In the early stages uterine cancer can be asymptomatic and would not be detectable even on bimanual examination.

87. **(4)** Vulvovaginal changes, such as atrophic vaginitis, often become apparent and bothersome several years after the last menstrual period (LMP) in women not receiving estrogen therapy. Inadequate data exist to demonstrate that isoflavones have a positive effect on vaginal symptoms. Vaginal lubricants have been found to be therapeutic in relieving symptoms of vaginal dryness. If nonprescription remedies do not provide relief and if no contraindications exist, estrogen, often topically applied, is the treatment of choice.

Pharmacology

88. **(3)** Rocephin is a very effective drug for treatment of complicated UTI but is unnecessary in the treatment of uncomplicated lower UTI. Bactrim DS and Macrobid are both very effective for UTI treatment. Pyridium will help to make the client more comfortable until the antibiotic reaches effective levels for treatment.

89. **(2)** The Women's Health Initiative (WHI) study was stopped early because after 5.2 years, in the opinion of the Safety/Data Monitoring Board, the health risks for the women in the study (mean age = 63 years) taking estrogen plus progestin exceeded the benefits. The study indicated that in the women who were taking estrogen plus progestin, the risk for myocardial infarctions, strokes, and thromboemboli, as well as the risk for breast cancer, was higher than that in women receiving placebo. The study did show benefits also. Women taking HRT were less likely to have a fracture caused by osteoporosis and less likely to have colorectal cancer. Additionally, the study did not address the shorter-term use of HRT for treatment of menopausal symptoms, which is the primary indication for initiating the therapy. This landmark study stresses the need for providers to discuss the risks and benefits of initiating or continuing HRT with postmenopausal women.

90. **(3)** Fluconazole is now approved for single-dose oral treatment of uncomplicated vulvovaginal candidiasis. It is most convenient for this client, who is unlikely to be extremely compliant with vaginal creams, given the upcoming travel. She does not have any contraindications to its use. Metronidazole and clindamycin are treatments for bacterial vaginosis and not for *Candida* infections. Hydrocortisone is a topical steroid used for inflammatory dermatologic conditions, and although it may help relieve the itching, it would not treat the candidiasis.

91. **(4)** Metronidazole vaginal gel is the treatment of choice for bacterial vaginosis in the nonpregnant female. The presence of the clue cells, absence of lactobacilli, and the malodorous discharge associated with the positive clue cells are markers for the diagnosis of bacterial vaginosis.

92. **(4)** Although some authors may recommend herbal treatments for menopausal symptoms, there have not been any controlled studies regarding prevention of disease with this substance. Traditional allopathic Western medicine supports the use of HRT for the prevention of osteoporosis. The use of weight-bearing exercise and increased calcium intake have been shown to help maintain bone health. Cigarette smoking increases the risk of bone loss. This client can reduce her risk by quitting smoking.

93. **(4)** Benzathine penicillin 2.4 million units IM is the treatment of choice for syphilis, but this

client has condyloma acuminatum, not condyloma latum. Topical use of podophyllin, trichloroacetic acid, and cryotherapy are all accepted treatment modalities for condyloma acuminatum.

94. **(1)** *Chlamydia* infection will often present this way; the dysuria, mucopurulent discharge, and cervical friability should be noted. The treatment of choice in ambulatory care settings is single-dose therapy with azithromycin 1 g PO. The treatment listed in Option #2 is for gonorrhea, not *Chlamydia* infection. Herpes simplex virus will present with painful vesicles in the vulvovaginal region, and recurrences are treated with acyclovir 200 mg, 1 capsule PO q4h × 5 days. Trichomoniasis can present this way; however, the absence of trichomonads on the wet mount is the key; the suggested treatment for trichomoniasis is metronidazole 2 g PO in a single dose.

95. **(4)** A hepatic effect caused by the first-pass metabolism in the liver occurs with oral estrogen products. A 25% increase in triglycerides has been associated with this route of administration. Because transdermal estrogen is not dependent on gastrointestinal absorption and is not affected by the first-pass metabolic effect, this option should be considered. A discussion regarding risks/benefits of continuing estrogen replacement therapy is appropriate. Because she is only 52 and is still experiencing menopausal symptoms, reducing the most common dosage or stopping the medication unless significant risks are apparent will probably not be the most therapeutic option.

96. **(3)** The IUD would be a good choice for this client because it is extremely effective (>99%). There is not much she has to do to maintain it, and there are no injections involved for insertion or removal. The Depo-Provera injections, although extremely effective (>99%), require an injection every 3 months, which could lead to decreased compliance by the client. The Norplant system of implants is also very effective (>99%), but it too requires injections for insertion and removal, and she is trying to avoid that. The diaphragm is a noninvasive contraceptive that is effective (88%), but it requires her to be a more active a participant in its use. None of these methods are contraindicated for this client, but an attempt should be made to help her

choose one with which she is likely to be comfortable.

97. **(1)** The nurse practitioner should try to find out what the client has heard and dispel the fallacies, if possible. Recent research supports the benefits of OCs in terms of protection from ovarian and endometrial cancer. There is generally a reduction in the amount of menstrual bleeding and a regulation of the cycle. Minimal weight fluctuations are reported. Infertility is not associated with OC use. To suggest either Norplant or Depo-Provera injections to someone who voices concerns about irregular menses or weight gain is sure to lead to an unhappy client, for these are quite common side effects of both methods. Options #3 and #4 are incorrect and misleading; Pap smears do not screen for ovarian cancer.

98. **(2)** The IUD is not recommended for use by an individual who is nulliparous or for one who is not in a stable, mutually monogamous relationship because of the increased risk of complications. The use of OCs in a 41-year-old nonsmoker in good health is acceptable without concern. The client is already familiar with Norplant and may not be aware that she could have a new set of implants inserted when she has the others removed. Depo-Provera would be equally appropriate for this client.

99. **(2)** Very often, changing to a pill with a stronger or different progestational agent will resolve the problem of bleeding irregularities associated with OCs. There are so many choices one can make in the dosage or strength of a birth control pill that it is likely that the client's problem can be resolved with a different pill. Taking the pill at a different time of day or on an empty stomach will do nothing to resolve the stated problem. The problem stated is not breakthrough bleeding, but rather prolonged bleeding likely associated with poor endometrial support. If a change is not made in the pills, the client will continue to bleed in this fashion, and anemia may eventually develop as a consequence.

100. **(3)** A pill such as Demulen 1/35 is a good choice for a client with more androgenic characteristics because of the ability of this pill to exhibit a strong estrogenic effect with a moderate progestational effect. Loestrin 1/20 is a poor choice for several reasons: the

weaker doses of estrogen and progestin may not be adequate to support her endometrium, nor will this pill have a positive effect on the androgenic characteristics displayed by this client. Triphasil is a triphasic pill and does have a positive progestational effect that should support the endometrium well; however, the progestin in this pill tends to be slightly more androgenic, which is undesirable for this client.

101. **(4)** The use of combined OCs is not recommended for breast-feeding mothers because combined OCs can decrease the amount of milk produced and affect its quality. Progestin-only OCs are cleared for use in breast-feeding mothers because there has not been any proven deleterious effect on either milk quantity or quality. Depo-Provera and the IUD are also accepted contraceptive methods for use by lactating females.

102. **(2)** OCs are contraindicated for use in a cigarette smoker who is 35 years of age or older. There is no contraindication to the use of Depo-Provera injection in the cigarette smoker. The Progestasert IUD would probably be a good IUD choice for this client because it is only approved for 1 year's use, and it is safe for use by a cigarette smoker as well. The only contraindication to the use of condoms and spermicide is allergy to either substance.

103. **(4)** The Norplant implantation system is contraindicated in the person with seizure disorder taking phenobarbital or Dilantin because there is a potential for either reduced anticonvulsant effect or reduced contraceptive effect. This does not occur with Depo-Provera, allowing the client to use this method freely without concern. The IUD is not contraindicated for use with anticonvulsant medications, and the client is a good candidate for its use. The diaphragm is not contraindicated with the use of anticonvulsant therapy.

104. **(4)** It is not necessary to hospitalize the client with acute PID who is not vomiting or pregnant. If she does not respond well to outpatient treatment, then hospitalization can be recommended. The medications listed are the accepted treatment of choice for outpatient management of PID, and administration should be started before the results of the lab tests are available, on the

basis of the client's clinical presentation. The CBC and sedimentation rate are helpful to track the WBC count and inflammatory response of the body.

105. **(2)** Unopposed estrogen use by a woman with an intact uterus increases her risk for endometrial hyperplasia and progression to endometrial cancer. Women who have taken unopposed estrogen for more than 3 years have a fivefold increased risk of endometrial cancer compared with women not treated with this regimen. The addition of progesterone to the regimen provides uterine protection. It is, however, the progestin component of HRT that is responsible for the breakthrough bleeding, about which many women complain at the initiation of therapy, and this leads to discontinuation of the drug. Some women are also intolerant of progestins, which have been linked to irritability.

106. **(3)** The use of unopposed estrogen in the client with an intact uterus could put her at risk for endometrial hyperplasia or cancer. The addition of a progestin protects the endometrium adequately. The client is an excellent candidate for endometrial biopsy to document the status of the endometrium. This client also needs to be educated about the risks and benefits of HRT.

107. **(3)** Lowering the dosage of the estrogen would not help the client's symptoms. The other dosage regimens listed are all acceptable choices for this client, proving that there are many effective ways for one to use HRT, allowing for individualization of the regimen to the client.

108. **(3)** Well-controlled hypertension is not a contraindication to the use of HRT.

109. **(1)** Metronidazole 2 g PO in a single dose is the treatment of choice for trichomoniasis. Metronidazole vaginal cream does not effectively treat vaginal trichomoniasis. Fluconazole and terconazole are treatments for vaginal candidiasis.

110. **(4)** A dose of 0.625 mg of conjugated equine estrogen (Premarin) is the minimal effective dose for the prevention of osteoporosis. HRT helps to maintain bones, but this effect only lasts as long as HRT is taken. Because of the risks for cardiovascular disease from using

HRT, it is no longer recommended for osteoporosis prevention. Other methods of osteoporosis prevention include regular exercise, smoking cessation, and sufficient intake of calcium (1200 mg to 1500 mg of elemental calcium) and vitamin D (400 to 800 IU) daily.

111. **(1)** The diaphragm predisposes many women to UTIs. Some women are sensitive to contraceptive cream or jelly. The diaphragm has been associated with toxic shock syndrome; hence, its use should be avoided during menses and it should not be left in place longer than 24 hours.

112. **(3)** The primary mechanism of action of OCs is suppression of ovulation. Ovulation is suppressed in 95% to 98% of clients. Should ovulation occur, the other mechanisms of action likely to prevent conception are thickening of cervical mucus, causing the endometrium to become atrophic, making the uterine environment unfavorable for implantation.

113. **(3)** Though still unproven conclusively, the mechanisms of action for IUDs include preventing blastocyst implantation by inducing a low-grade endometritis, the copper's effects on enzymes, progesterone's actions on the endometrium, and inhibition of sperm/ovum migration.

114. **(3)** A progesterone-releasing IUD acts to decrease blood loss and cramping.

115. **(2)** The client no longer requires the use of Provera to protect the endometrium from the potential effects of estrogen; therefore the progestin can be discontinued and the client can be given continuous estrogen therapy without concern. The other dosage regimens listed are appropriate for a client with an intact uterus who is receiving HRT.

116. **(3)** The progestin-only pill does not consistently suppress ovulation. This suppression only occurs in 40% to 60% of cycles. This makes the progestin-only pill less effective than combined contraceptive pills. Mechanisms of action that contribute to the progestin-only pill's effectiveness are creating an atrophic endometrium and possibly altering tubal physiology by decreasing ovum transport. Progestin-only pills contain no

estrogen and are a good choice for the breast-feeding woman.

117. **(1)** Informed consent is essential. The pros and cons of HRT should be explained, but the choice is the client's.

118. **(3)** Depo-Provera is frequently associated with menstrual cycle changes. In fact, this irregular bleeding is the most commonly cited reason for discontinuation. These menstrual cycle changes range from heavy, irregular bleeding to spotting and even amenorrhea. Nausea and acne are usually effects of estrogen and are not seen with Depo-Provera.

119. **(4)** Clients taking alendronate (Fosamax) are instructed to take the medication on arising, 30 minutes before eating, with a full glass of water. Clients should be instructed to remain erect after taking the medication to prevent esophageal irritation. Taking medication with food reduces bioavailability by 40%; taking it with coffee or orange juice decreases bioavailability by 60%; and taking it after eating significantly reduces absorption.

120. **(1)** Women with a uterus taking unopposed exogenous estrogen have an increased risk of endometrial cancer. The addition of progesterone decreases this risk. The addition of progesterone may prompt bleeding, which many women view unfavorably. Progesterone does not affect cervical cancer, breast cancer, or gallbladder disease.

121. **(3)** Metronidazole (Flagyl) in a single 2-g dose is the treatment of choice for trichomoniasis. An alternative is giving the 2 g in divided doses on the same day. This regimen causes less nausea and may improve compliance.

122. **(4)** Metronidazole (Flagyl) is the treatment of choice for bacterial vaginosis. However, pregnancy should be ruled out before treatment is begun because metronidazole should not be used if there is any possibility that the woman is pregnant. The sexual partners do not have to be treated, and doxycycline is not the drug of choice.

123. **(3)** She requires added protection through this cycle because of the low-dose OC. Dilantin may also decrease effectiveness of OCs, especially low-dose OCs.

124. **(1)** Because of homeless status, the nurse practitioner needs to use a single-dose treatment. Erythromycin, although a correct medication, is a poor dosing choice for this client.

125. **(1)** The most accurate answer is Effexor SR. A combined serotonin and norepinephrine reuptake inhibitor, this drug has been found to reduce hot flashes at a dose of 25 to 150 mg/day in several clinical trials. Many individuals consider the "natural," over-the-counter products to be safer than prescription drugs. However, these products can have pharmacologic effects and side effects. Clients should be questioned about use of these drugs at the time of the exam. Critics argue that the trials of the use of black cohosh have been too small, uncontrolled, and not randomized to provide evidence-based information on the herb's efficacy and safety. Soy has been found to be moderately effective in reducing hot flashes, but comparable results have been seen in placebo groups as well. A side effect of Evista, a drug used to prevent postmenopausal osteoporosis, is the occurrence of hot flashes.

126. **(3)** The most common cause of PID in sexually active women is gonococcal infections. Gonococcal infections are often accompanied by *Chlamydia* infection, and they are usually both treated.

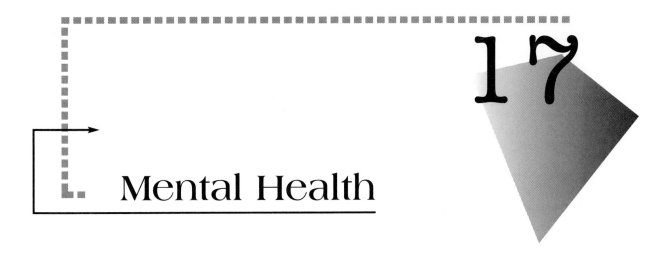

Mental Health

Psychosocial Examination & Diagnostic Tests

1. The mental status examination enables the nurse practitioner to identify:

   1. Intelligence quotient (IQ) and reasoning.

   2. Abstract thinking and memory functioning.

   3. Reasoning and psychomotor skills.

   4. Memory functioning and IQ.

2. A client with a history of psychiatric problems arrives at the clinic shouting that he is a messenger of God and knows the meaning of the prophecies in Revelations. This behavior is assessed as:

   1. A delusion.

   2. A hallucination.

   3. Magical thinking.

   4. An illusion.

3. An assessment of a client experiencing auditory hallucinations would most likely reveal:

   1. Client mumbling to self, tilted head, eyes darting back and forth.

   2. Performance of obsessive-compulsive rituals such as a radio turning off and on and talking to self.

   3. Hyperactivity, expansive mood, easy distractibility.

   4. Cool, aloof, unapproachable, avoiding enclosed areas.

4. The MAST and the CAGE are screening instruments for which disease process?

   1. Glaucoma.

   2. Depression.

   3. Alcoholism.

   4. Diabetes.

5. When receiving the records from another agency, the nurse practitioner notes on the summary sheet that the client has a dual diagnosis. This means the client has:

   1. Both manic and depressive symptoms of bipolar affective disorder.

   2. Two closely related psychiatric disorders (e.g., panic disorder and bulimia nervosa).

   3. Coexistence of both a psychiatric disorder (e.g., depression) and a substance abuse disorder (e.g., alcohol dependence).

   4. Coexistence of a personality disorder (e.g., borderline personality) and a psychiatric disorder (e.g., panic disorder).

6. In obtaining a history from an older adult, the nurse practitioner understands that when a client "makes up stories or answers" to the questions, this is known as:

   1. Perseveration.

   2. Confabulation.

   3. Echolalia.

   4. Alcoholic encephalopathy.

7. In taking a history from a client with depression, which is the most important question for the nurse practitioner to ask?

   1. Have you ever experienced hallucinations, delusions, or illusions?

   2. Have you ever been hospitalized in a psychiatric facility?

   3. Do you regularly take antidepressants or other medications?

   4. Have you thought about or attempted suicide?

8. A common laboratory finding associated with bulimia nervosa is:

   1. Hyperkalemia.

   2. Hypochloremia.

   3. Elevated liver enzyme levels.

   4. Platelet abnormalities.

9. The nurse practitioner knows that habituation is likely when a client gives a history of:

   1. The same dose of the drug having reduced effects.

   2. Less of the medication producing the desired effects.

   3. No withdrawal symptoms when the drug is stopped.

   4. Increasing side effects with an increase in the dosage of drug.

10. Which statement is correct about mental health in the older adult and supports research findings in the literature?

   1. Self-esteem does not decline as a person ages.

   2. Older adults are consistently concerned about their physical appearance.

   3. Older adults have a negative self-image in comparison with younger adults.

   4. Learning ability is not maintained because of loss of short-term memory.

11. During a mental status examination, which question would be helpful in assessing a client's abstract thinking ability?

   1. Can you repeat the following numbers: 1, 3, 5, 7, 9?

   2. What is today's date?

   3. How are a carpet and a hardwood floor alike?

   4. Can you tell me the name of three past US presidents?

Psychiatric Disorders

12. An elderly client is experiencing a recent onset of confusion. The nurse practitioner is trying to determine whether the confusion is related to depression or dementia. In evaluating this client, what specific finding would be helpful in making this distinction?

   1. Whether confusion worsens in the evening.

   2. Early morning agitation, hyperactivity, and insomnia.

3. Signs of anger, hostility, and loss of control.

4. Reality distortions and preoccupation with family matters.

13. A client calls the clinic and asks to speak to the nurse practitioner. When he or she answers the telephone, the client states that he is going to commit suicide. The priority goal is to:

    1. Refer the client to an appropriate treatment facility.

    2. Encourage ventilation of angry and depressed feelings.

    3. Assess the lethality of the suicide plan.

    4. Establish rapport with the client.

14. During an intake interview with a 26-year-old man given a diagnosis of generalized anxiety disorder, the nurse practitioner might observe what type of behaviors?

    1. An inflated sense of self.

    2. Constant relation to future events.

    3. Inability to concentrate and irritability when questioned.

    4. Nervousness and fear of the nurse practitioner during the interview.

15. An elderly woman answers the nurse practitioner's questions by mumbling in low tones with answers that seem inappropriate. What would be initial findings associated with a diagnosis of dementia?

    1. Sees people floating across the ceiling of her room.

    2. Has problems with cognition and confusion.

    3. Hears voices at night telling her to change her clothes.

    4. Shows fear when the nurse makes any movement toward her.

16. An older client comes to the office with the complaint of confusion. The daughter is concerned that her mother has Alzheimer's disease. Which of these assessments would indicate that this client is experiencing delirium versus dementia?

    1. The confusion has been slowly developing.

    2. The confusion started after the client started taking cimetidine (Tagamet).

3. The client's attention span has not been affected.

4. The client's memory has been impaired.

17. While talking with a nurse practitioner about his chemical dependency, a client states, "I wish I had never used cocaine. It has ruined my life!" What would be the most appropriate response by the nurse practitioner?

    1. "You should think before you do something."

    2. "Things will work out; don't worry."

    3. "It sounds like you've thought a lot about your cocaine use."

    4. "You shouldn't be so hard on yourself. You can change."

18. The nurse would expect which symptoms in a client with a diagnosis of schizophrenia?

    1. High energy with varying sleep patterns and nonstop conversation.

    2. Extreme and frequent mood swings with hyperactivity and difficulty concentrating.

    3. Paranoia, delusions, hallucinations, and diminished self-care.

    4. Antisocial behavior, manipulativeness, charisma, and ability to lie convincingly.

19. Dementia can be distinguished from delirium by:

    1. Dementia lasts days to weeks compared with delirium, which lasts months to years.

    2. Dementia is often associated with medications or systemic illness.

    3. Dementia exhibits a disturbance in attention that is not present in delirium.

    4. Dementia does not include altered perception, such as hallucinations.

20. An elderly client is brought to the nurse practitioner by his family for evaluation of increasing confusion over the past few days. The client has a history of dementia; however, the family states that this is a definite change. What course of action would the nurse practitioner consider?

    1. Help the family look for a nursing home.

    2. Order an immediate magnetic resonance imaging (MRI) scan.

    3. Perform a comprehensive medication review.

    4. Order a urinalysis (UA).

21. A middle-aged, upper-middle-class, married woman presents to your clinic for the third time in 2 months with a complaint of headache, gastrointestinal upset with abdominal pain, and difficulty sleeping. Results of previous exams have been essentially negative. You suspect the client has depression, but she has been reluctant to complete even the briefest of screenings for this. Today, the client requests "something for sleep," again stating she "doesn't have time to take a bunch of tests." Which tentative diagnosis seems most likely?

    1. Hypochondriasis.

    2. Domestic violence.

    3. Addiction.

    4. Irritable bowel syndrome.

22. An elderly client was taken to the clinic in a confused state that began suddenly 24 hours ago. She fails to be oriented to person, time, or place. She was incontinent of urine because of her confusion. She looks apathetic and is drowsy. The nurse practitioner would suspect:

    1. Delirium.

    2. Dementia.

    3. Depression.

    4. A psychotic disorder.

23. The nurse practitioner is examining a young adult who has been a long-term intravenous cocaine user. What other findings would alert the nurse practitioner to a frequent complication?

    1. Epistaxis and chronic rhinorrhea.

    2. Cardiac arrhythmias and hypertension.

    3. Chest congestion and wheezing.

    4. Hepatitis and cellulitis.

24. An adult client has a history of irritability, loss of appetite, inability to concentrate, and feelings of depression and "burnout" at work. He mentions that he recently missed several days of work. He is doing and taking everything he can to relax. What would be an appropriate question to ask this client?

    1. "Do you drink alcohol or take drugs?"

    2. "Have you ever felt this way before?"

    3. "When you feel depressed, do you talk to your wife?"

    4. "Have you lost your job?"

25. Physical findings of cocaine abuse include:

    1. Bradycardia, miosis, hypertension.

    2. Hypertension, tachycardia, tremor.

    3. Hypotension, bradycardia, abdominal cramps.

    4. Decreased level of consciousness, tachycardia, excessive salivation.

26. Which neurotransmitters are associated with the etiology of acute mania in bipolar affective disorder?

    1. Epinephrine and norepinephrine.

    2. Serotonin and dopamine.

    3. Dopamine and norepinephrine.

    4. γ-Aminobutyric acid (GABA) and renin-angiotensin.

27. All of the following behaviors meet the criteria for substance abuse in the *Diagnostic and Statistical Manual of Mental Disorders, Fourth Edition* (DSM-IV) **except**:

    1. Repeated arrests for drunk driving.

    2. Multiple absences from work because of substance use.

    3. Chronic anxiety attacks.

    4. Recurrent arguments with spouse about his or her drinking behavior.

28. An elderly client's wife is concerned about her husband's increasing confusion and agitation. Not only has he exhibited symptoms of increased confusion, but he also is unable to care for his physical needs. He has been incontinent of urine and feces and sometimes is totally unaware of other people. What would be an assessment priority for this client?

    1. Evaluate changes in social habits.

    2. Assess for hallucinations and impaired reality testing.

    3. Evaluate his orientation to person, place, and time.

    4. Determine whether he is experiencing a problem with impaired judgment.

29. A client is transferred to the alcohol treatment unit from the emergency department. What is important to include in the therapeutic milieu during detoxification?

    1. Keep the environment adequately lit to diminish illusions.

    2. Keep a radio or television on in the room to assist to maintain orientation.

    3. Speak quietly when in the room to avoid overstimulation.

    4. Keep the suction equipment available in case of seizures.

Pharmacology

30. A client has been receiving fluphenazine (Prolixin) for the past 3 weeks. The nurse practitioner's assessment notes include the following: temperature elevated (105.8° F [41° C]), marked muscle rigidity, agitation, and confusion. The nurse practitioner understands these findings are often associated with the diagnosis of:

    1. Acute dystonia.

    2. Tardive dyskinesia.

    3. Neuroleptic malignant syndrome.

    4. Extrapyramidal disorder.

31. The preferred antidepressant for an elderly client is:

    1. Amitriptyline (Elavil).

    2. Citalopram (Celexa).

    3. Trazodone (Desyrel).

    4. Haloperidol (Haldol).

32. A client has been referred to the nurse practitioner. The client's medical history reveals long-term use of antianxiety agents that the client considers harmless. The nurse practitioner understands that antianxiety agents can:

    1. Cause drug dependency.

    2. Produce hepatotoxicity and nephrotoxicity.

    3. Lead to functional damage of the cardiopulmonary system.

    4. Cause profound dissociative personality problems.

33. An older female has a diagnosis of dementia and is taking haloperidol (Haldol) 2 mg HS. The nurse practitioner observes her engaging in a restless, repetitive movement with her legs. She states that not only does she have ongoing movement, but she also feels jittery. The nurse practitioner would interpret this activity to be:

    1. Ataxia.

    2. Akathisia.

    3. Agitation.

    4. Dyskinesia.

34. What is the best initial treatment plan for a sleep disorder in the elderly client?

    1. Medicate with amitriptyline (Elavil).

    2. Medicate with trazodone (Desyrel).

    3. Discuss the importance of naps daily.

    4. Decrease noise and light in the environment.

35. An elderly client presents with a new symptom of acute confusion over the last 24 hours. Which should the nurse practitioner do first during the examination?

    1. Drug history.

    2. Electrocardiogram.

    3. Mini mental status exam.

    4. Thyroid profile.

36. The nurse practitioner is aware that the following class of drugs is most likely to precipitate a hypertensive crisis in the elderly.

    1. Narcotic analgesics.

    2. Monoamine oxidase (MAO) inhibitors.

    3. Barbiturates.

    4. Phenothiazines.

37. The nurse practitioner knows that the following class of drugs would have the greatest effect on memory in the elderly client:

    1. Phenothiazines.

    2. Tricyclic antidepressants.

    3. Benzodiazepines.

    4. MAO inhibitors.

38. The nurse practitioner understands that adolescents who use lysergic acid diethylamide (LSD):

    1. Experience withdrawal symptoms within 24 hours.

    2. Develop tolerance quickly and need increased amounts.

    3. Experience flashbacks and depression.

    4. Experience disorientation and delusional feelings.

39. Of the following antidepressants, which one has the most sedating effects, making it a good sleep aid?

    1. Fluoxetine (Prozac).

    2. Doxepin (Sinequan).

    3. Trazodone (Desyrel).

    4. Paroxetine (Paxil).

40. In the management of acute alcohol withdrawal delirium, a nurse practitioner may want to use all of the following drugs **except**:

    1. Chlordiazepoxide (Librium).

    2. Lorazepam (Ativan).

    3. Thiamine.

    4. Chlorpromazine (Thorazine).

41. The nurse practitioner's findings on physical examination of an adolescent are as follows: disheveled appearance, 5-lb weight loss since last visit 2 months ago, pulse strong and regular at 128 bpm, +4 deep tendon reflexes, nasal mucosa erythematous and ulcerated. His mother relates that he has been getting in trouble at school, avoids the family, has no appetite, and is not sleeping much at night. The nurse practitioner suspects use of:

    1. Heroin.

    2. Marijuana.

    3. LSD.

    4. Crack cocaine.

42. Which laboratory results would be **least** important to obtain before prescribing lithium for a client?

    1. Thyroid-stimulating hormone, triiodothyronine, thyroxine.

    2. Blood urea nitrogen, creatinine.

    3. UA, electrolytes.

    4. Alanine aminotransferase, aspartate aminotransferase, lactate dehydrogenase.

43. A client comes to the rural clinic having taken an undetermined amount of heroin. Before transferring the client to a psychiatric treatment facility, the nurse practitioner anticipates that the drug of choice for an opioid overdose is:

    1. Clonidine (Catapres).

    2. Methadone (Dolophine).

    3. Naloxone (Narcan).

    4. Naltrexone HCl (ReVia).

44. Benzodiazepines are useful in the treatment of all the disorders below, **except**:

    1. Alcohol withdrawal.

    2. Anxiety.

    3. Obsessive-compulsive disorder.

    4. Seizures.

45. When starting administration of a psychotropic medication in the elderly, a good rule of thumb is:

    1. Start low; go slow.

    2. Higher doses are almost always needed.

    3. Side effects of psychotropic medications will usually not affect other medications.

    4. Adult dosages can be used initially without any problems.

46. A client is a 20-year, 2-pack-a-day smoker with a history of chronic bronchitis. What is the prescription to give to this client who wishes to stop smoking?

   1. Nicotine polacrilex (Nicorette) gum 2-mg piece, chew for 30 minutes, q1-2h × 6 weeks, then q2-4h × 3 weeks, then q4-8h × 3 weeks, then discontinue.

   2. Nicotine patch (Nicoderm) 21 mg/24 hr qd × 6 weeks, then 14 mg/24 hr qd × 2 weeks, then 7 mg/24 hr qd × 2 weeks, then discontinue.

   3. Bupropion HCl (Zyban) 150 mg qd × 3 days, then 150 mg bid for 7 to 12 weeks and to stop smoking when medication is started.

   4. Nicotine patch (Nicoderm) 14 mg/24 hr qd × 6 weeks, then 7 mg/24 hr qd × 6 weeks, then discontinue.

47. The nurse practitioner understands the following about the use of benzodiazepines in the older adult:

   1. Withdrawal symptoms may occur within 24 hours of abruptly stopping the medication.

   2. Adverse side effects are minimal and tend to minimize the incidence of falls and other injuries.

   3. Long-acting medications (e.g., chlordiazepoxide [Librium]) are preferred over the shorter-acting medications (e.g., lorazepam [Ativan]).

   4. Larger doses are needed to maintain therapeutic levels for the anxious or agitated client.

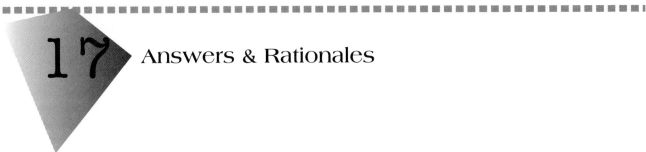

17 Answers & Rationales

Psychosocial Examination & Diagnostic Tests

1. **(2)** The mental status examination provides a basic assessment of the client's intellectual functioning (reasoning, abstract thinking, memory). The intelligence quotient (IQ) is determined by psychological testing. Psychomotor skill assessment is part of a neurologic examination.

2. **(1)** Delusions are false, fixed beliefs that can be of a persecutory or grandiose nature. In this instance, the client is experiencing a delusion of grandeur. Often, elderly clients with a diagnosis of dementia will have delusions, which worsen with acute illnesses. A hallucination is a false sensory experience. An illusion is a misinterpretation of reality. Magical thinking is when the client feels that his/her thoughts or wishes can control other people.

3. **(1)** The client experiencing the auditory hallucination will often look out into space and act as if he/she is listening to someone talking. This is associated with behaviors such as tilting the head, mumbling, and eye movement.

4. **(3)** The Michigan Alcoholism Screening Test (MAST) and the CAGE (Cut down, Annoyed, Guilty, Eye opener) are used to alert providers to the possibility of alcoholism.

5. **(3)** Dual diagnosis involves both a psychiatric diagnosis and a substance abuse diagnosis.

6. **(2)** Clients who experience confabulation are fabricating events or situations to fill in gaps in their memory, usually in a plausible way, are exhibiting signs and symptoms of dementia from chronic alcohol abuse. Confabulation is a common symptom of alcohol amnesic disorder, or Korsakoff's syndrome. Echolalia is the parroting or automatic, meaningless repeating of another's words. Perseveration is the involuntary persistent repetition of an idea or response (e.g., client keeps repeating the same phrase over and over).

7. **(4)** Although it is important to know whether the client has ever experienced hallucinations, delusions, or illusions and whether the client has ever been hospitalized in a psychiatric facility, the single most important factor to ascertain is whether the client has contemplated suicide. In addition, determination of a specific plan and the means to do it are also involved in the questioning about suicidal ideation. It is also important for the nurse practitioner to determine whether the client regularly takes antidepressants or other medications. The client may have stopped taking his/her antidepressant, causing an acute exacerbation of depression, or another medication that he/she may be taking may be causing an increase in depression.

8. **(2)** The other abnormalities are not usually associated with bulimia. The hypochloremia is associated with purging (self-induced vomiting).

9. **(1)** Habituation exists when the same dose of the drug produces reduced effects, and it is usually seen with the development of physical dependence on any medication. Addiction occurs when there is a deep-seated psychological need for the drug/medication.

10. **(1)** According to research, self-esteem, along with attitude and morals, is maintained as a client ages. Older adults tend to have a more positive self-image and are more confident when compared with younger adults. Learning ability is maintained, although more time is often needed for the early phases of the learning process. Retrieval of information in long-term memory is slower, and short-term memory is diminished.

11. **(3)** This question requires the client to compare and tell how two things are alike or different; it is used to evaluate the thought process oriented toward development of an idea without application to a particular object; and it is independent of space and time. Asking for today's date assists in determining orientation; requesting the names of past presidents assists in evaluating long-term memory; and asking the client to repeat numbers assists in evaluating short-term memory.

Psychiatric Disorders

12. **(1)** Confusion can occur in both dementia and depression. However, with dementia, symptoms worsen at night and are commonly referred to as *sundowning*. Additionally, the nurse practitioner must also ensure that the increased confusion is not a result of an acute illness. Often, the only sign or symptom the elderly client with dementia may have is confusion. Usually, the culprit is a urinary tract infection (UTI). The nurse practitioner should order a urinalysis (UA) to ensure that the confusion is not the result of an acute illness and is reversible.

13. **(4)** The nurse practitioner must first establish trust and rapport with the caller before an assessment can be made. If rapport is not established, the client will hang up the phone. The nurse practitioner understands that by keeping the client talking, the client is prevented from acting out the suicidal threat.

14. **(3)** Impaired concentration and irritability are major characteristics of generalized anxiety disorder. Clients with generalized anxiety disorder often pace within the exam room because of their irritability, and they are more focused on the here and now and have low self-esteem.

15. **(2)** Confusion and cognitive function problems (e.g., short-term memory loss) are initial signs of dementia. The severity of the symptoms is dependent on what stage of cognitive degeneration the client is manifesting. The other options are characteristic of hallucinatory experiences and usually occur later. This client may also be exhibiting signs and symptoms of an acute illness. The culprit is usually a UTI, and the nurse practitioner should order a UA to ensure that that cause of the confusion is not related to a reversible cause.

16. **(2)** Cimetidine (Tagamet) is not tolerated well in the elderly client, and one of the major side effects in the elderly client is confusion. Anytime a new medication is added to an elderly client's medication regimen, an abrupt onset of confusion must be reviewed closely because it may be caused by the new medication or a drug-drug interaction with an existing medication. Another possibility is the onset of an acute illness that often manifests as acute confusion in the elderly client; most often the culprit is a UTI. In addition to a careful medication review, UA should be done to rule out a UTI. When a patient has true dementia, the onset of confusion develops slowly, over a longer period, not acutely, which is an indication that another underlying problem is causing the acute confusion. The attention span and memory may be affected in each diagnosis.

17. **(3)** The nurse's statement acknowledges the client's feelings and is open-ended, which promotes open discussion and helps the client clarify his or her feelings and thoughts. Option #1 is condescending and punitive. Option #2 offers false reassurance. Option #4 tends to discount the client's feelings.

18. **(3)** The characteristics of schizophrenia are delusions, tangential thought, suspiciousness, disorganized behavior, and hallucinations.

19. **(4)** Although clients with a diagnosis of dementia do not usually have altered perception that include hallucinations and illusions, it is occasionally seen in those with underlying psychiatric disorders. Dementia normally last for months to years and the client never recovers. Delirium is an acute process and is often associated with medications or a systemic illness and is reversible, once the acute problem is addressed and resolved.

20. **(4)** One of the most common reasons for an acute change in mental status in the elderly client with dementia is an acute infection. This is usually a UTI. Usually, the elderly client with dementia is incontinent, and because of the changes of aging, does not recognize the normal signs and symptoms of a UTI (burning, urgency, frequency, suprapubic tenderness); and elderly clients do not typically have elevated temperatures with UTIs. The nurse practitioner should order a UA to ensure that an acute infectious process is not the cause of the acute confusion. While waiting for the results of the UA, the nurse practitioner should conduct a medication review to ensure that no new prescribed, over-the-counter, or herbal medications have been added because this is the second most common reason for acute confusion in the elderly client.

21. **(2)** The indicators of domestic violence in this case are the multiple vague physical complaints without supporting objective data, the suspected depression, and the reluctance to wait around in the clinic for extended periods. This client is on the verge of disclosing the abuse, if a provider would only ask her about domestic violence.

22. **(1)** On the basis of the acute confusion state and the incontinence, the client is experiencing delirium. This is most likely caused by sepsis, with the source being a UTI. The fact that she has mental status changes (disoriented to person, place, or time, in addition to the acute confusion, delirium, and incontinence) provides clues to the diagnosis of sepsis. Dementia is more insidious than acute. Depression and psychosis are not consistent with the assessments. The major symptoms of depression include loss of interest in regular activities, sleep disorder, decreased appetite, loss of concentration, inactivity, guilt, lack of energy, and suicidal thoughts. Symptoms of psychotic disorders include thoughts and behavior indicating that the client is not in touch with reality (e.g., auditory and visual hallucinations and talking to self).

23. **(4)** More than 50% of intravenous cocaine users have hepatitis, phlebitis, endocarditis, and acquired immunodeficiency syndrome (AIDS). Epistaxis, rhinorrhea, and nasal congestion are seen most often in intranasal users of cocaine. Chest congestion, wheezing, and eventual emphysema occur in long-term crack smokers. Although cardiac arrhythmias, hypertension, and respiratory arrest can occur, they are not the common complications.

24. **(1)** The nurse practitioner should suspect this client to have a mood disorder and/or chemical dependency. It would be appropriate to determine exactly how much, how long, and how often he consumes alcohol or any other drugs. The key points in the situation are the occupational burnout, depressive symptoms, and ineffective coping measures (taking and doing everything to relax, but with no relief).

25. **(2)** Bradycardia and excessive salivation are not found with cocaine abuse. There are no drug antagonists that can be used for cocaine overdose, although naloxone is given to reduce the concurrent toxic effects of other narcotic drugs that may be in the client's system.

26. **(3)** Dopamine and norepinephrine (drugs that stimulate the noradrenergic and dopaminergic receptors) can precipitate mania or hypomania in clients. γ-Aminobutyric acid (GABA) and acetylcholine may also be neurotransmitters involved in the process. In addition, stimulants such as amphetamines and cocaine can also cause manic-like symptoms.

27. **(3)** Chronic anxiety attacks are not part of the *Diagnostic and Statistical Manual of Mental Disorders, Fourth Edition* (DSM-IV) criteria for substance abuse.

28. **(4)** While all of the items listed are appropriate to assess in this patient, it is most important to determine judgment. If he cannot make safe judgments, he is at high risk for behaviors considered to be unsafe in his condition, such as driving, walking alone, and running bath water.

29. **(1)** The patient needs to be able to easily interpret his surroundings. Shadows or areas of poor lighting will increase the illusions. When the nurse practitioner is in the room, it is important for him or her to speak in clear tones and make sure to include the client in the conversations to decrease the paranoia and feelings that people are talking about him. Radio and television may be too much stimuli and may not be of any assistance in maintaining orientation. Suction equipment is for physical safety and is not part of the therapeutic milieu.

Pharmacology

30. **(3)** The client is experiencing a rare problem called *neuroleptic malignant syndrome*. This client would require immediate referral and hospitalization. This can also occur with the medication prochlorperazine (Compazine). Acute dystonia, parkinsonism, and akathisia are associated with extrapyramidal disorder or acute movement disorder. Tardive dyskinesia occurs late in therapy and is often irreversible. Slow worm-like movements of the tongue are the earliest symptom, followed by grimacing, lip smacking, and involuntary limb movements.

31. **(2)** Citalopram's (Celexa's) favorable side effect profile makes it a useful alternative to the traditional tricyclic antidepressants. It has the shortest half-life of the currently marketed serotonin reuptake inhibitors. Amitriptyline (Elavil) has the most anticholinergic and sedating effects of the antidepressants. There may be pronounced effects on the cardiovascular system (hypotension). Geropsychiatrists agree it is best to avoid amitriptyline in the elderly; however, "low dose" (10, mg, PO, qhs) means low cost and can be effective in controlling neuropathic pain. Trazodone (Desyrel) is very sedating for the elderly client. Haloperidol (Haldol) is an antipsychotic medication and is not to be used at all in long-term care facilities.

32. **(1)** Physical dependence can occur, even with low doses of the medication. This is a particular problem in the elderly, who are sensitive to low-dose ranges. If possible, it is better to slowly taper the patient's dose of the antianxiety medication; often, the patient can receive a much lower dose.

33. **(2)** Akathisia is a feeling of restlessness. The nurse practitioner should slowly taper the client's dose of haloperidol (Haldol) 2 mg HS. It is possible that the client may not need the medication or that one of the newer atypical antipsychotics would be more effective with fewer side effects. Clients may complain of a feeling of muscular quivering. Ataxia is a disorder wherein muscular incoordination occurs with voluntary muscular movements. Agitation is a general finding that may be part of the psychotic behavior. Dyskinesia is a defect in voluntary movement.

34. **(4)** Correction of environmental factors and treatment of underlying iatrogenic and medical problems should be addressed initially. Amitriptyline (Elavil) can cause excessive somnolence. Trazodone (Desyrel) may be of particular use when sleep disturbance is prominent; however, it does not represent the best initial plan. The goal is to begin with good sleep hygiene before starting pharmacologic therapy. Eliminating naps during the day may be useful in facilitating sleep.

35. **(1)** Drug-drug interactions are a common cause of acute confusion in the elderly client. Assessment of the client's drug history can minimize the need to do further costly interventions if the client only needs medication adjustment. The other options would be included in the plan after the drug history had been completed and had been ruled out as a potential problem. The nurse practitioner must always consider that an acute illness, such as a UTI, may be the cause of acute confusion. A UA should also be obtained, because a UTI can quickly progress to sepsis.

36. **(2)** In combination with tyramine-rich foods that have undergone an aging process such as cheese, wine, beer, salami, and yogurt, catecholamines are released from the nerve endings, causing a hypertensive crisis. The other drugs listed cause hypotension.

37. **(3)** The benzodiazepines cause sedation and decreased attention, which in turn affect the memory. Although phenothiazines and antidepressants may also cause sedation, they don't affect memory.

38. **(3)** Flashbacks, depression, and psychotic behavior can occur with lysergic acid diethylamide (LSD) use. There are no withdrawal symptoms or physical dependence associated with use. Commonly, the adolescent remains oriented but experiences hallucinations and altered bodily sensations.

39. **(3)** Trazodone (Desyrel) has sedation as a side effect, which has made it less popular as an antidepressant; however, it is commonly prescribed for insomnia.

40. **(4)** All of the drugs listed may be used in management of acute alcohol withdrawal delirium except chlorpromazine (Librium), which is an antipsychotic that has no use in the management plan.

41. **(4)** Often, some of the first indications of drug use in adolescents are related to a sudden change in behavior or school performance. Heroin use symptoms are constricted pupils, respiratory depression, needle tracks, and poor nutrition. Marijuana use symptoms are slow reflexes, tachycardia, conjunctival injection, nasal congestion, and increased appetite. LSD use symptoms are dilated pupils, reddened eyes, hypertension, increased appetite, and hallucinations. The use of central nervous system stimulants, such as crack cocaine, leads to hypertension, weight loss, anorexia, insomnia, hyperreflexia, and a perforated or ulcerated nasal septum.

42. **(4)** It is **not** important to evaluate liver function before initiating treatment with lithium. The adverse side effects of lithium affect renal, cardiac, and thyroid function. Baseline electrolyte values are also important to obtain.

43. **(3)** Naloxone (Narcan) is a narcotic antagonist and is used for the reversal of narcotic depression, including respiratory depression. Clonidine (Catapres) is a central α_2-adrenergic agonist and is indicated for treatment of hypertension. Methadone is used in the treatment of opioid addiction. The Food and Drug Administration (FDA) has placed methadone in a special drug category that allows medically supervised administration of the drug to addicts with long-term, intractable addictions to heroin. Naltrexone's (ReVia's) therapeutic classification is narcotic detoxification adjunct.

44. **(3)** Seizures, alcohol withdrawal, and anxiety are commonly treated with benzodiazepines. They are **not** the drug of choice for obsessive-compulsive disorder; selective serotonin reuptake inhibitors are usually used.

45. **(1)** The rule of thumb for starting medications in the elderly client is to start low and go slow; therefore dosages should be reduced by 30% to 50% to start therapy and gradually increased as necessary. Adverse effects are likely to occur because of slowed drug metabolism, which occurs with aging. These effects include hypotension, arrhythmias, and sedative and anticholinergic effects.

46. **(2)** A highly nicotine-dependent client benefits from intense counseling and prescription of alternative nicotine delivery during the smoking cessation process. The nicotine patch is usually the preferred form of replacement, since the gum is noncontinuous and withdrawal symptoms may occur during nonchewing times. The nicotine patch delivers a fixed dose of nicotine on a continual basis, is applied once daily, and eliminates the gastrointestinal upset that often occurs with the gum. If this client insisted on using the gum, the dose should be 4 mg, not 2 mg. Option #4 is too low a dose with which to start treatment for this client and is not the correct dosing schedule. Zyban (bupropion HCl) would be used in conjunction with the nicotine patch, and clients are to quit smoking 1 to 2 weeks after starting treatment with Zyban (bupropion HCl), not immediately.

47. **(1)** The dose of benzodiazepines should be tapered slowly in the older adult. Withdrawal symptoms occur within 24 hours in clients taking the shorter-acting medications and may not occur for several days in clients taking long-acting medications. The adverse effects of oversedation, dizziness, confusion, and sometimes hypotension contribute to falls and other injuries in the elderly. In Option #3, short-acting medications are preferred. Typically, larger doses are not needed, but rather small initial doses with gradual increases.

18

Research & Theory

Research

1. When one is designing a research project that will involve clients, from the options presented, the most important point to be included in the written consent to participate is:

   1. The directions regarding the use of a black pen.

   2. The anticipated date for publication of the completed research report.

   3. The assurance of privacy and confidentiality.

   4. The number of previously published research studies about this topic.

2. When determining whether to incorporate a new procedure into your clinical practice based on the findings of a recent study, which of the following should you consider?

   1. The statistical significance of the findings.

   2. The statistical relevance of the findings.

   3. The statistical software program used.

   4. The statistical background of the researcher.

3. The research process is similar to the process nurse practitioners use to provide client care in that both are decision-making processes that include the steps (in the order presented here) of:

   1. Assessing, teaching, evaluating, and discussing.

   2. Defining, planning, implementing, and charting.

   3. Questioning, evaluating, diagnosing, and teaching.

   4. Assessing, planning, implementing, and evaluating.

4. Both descriptive and inferential statistics are used in research. However, their purposes are different in that:

   1. Inferential statistics are used for assigning participant code numbers.

   2. Descriptive statistics are used for assigning participant code numbers.

   3. Inferential statistics are used for hypothesis testing.

   4. Descriptive statistics are used for hypothesis testing.

241

5. In an ambulatory care setting, the nurse practitioner might find it difficult to utilize nursing research because:

   1. The demands of providing primary care leave little time for research utilization.

   2. Procedures for research utilization have not been well defined in the literature.

   3. Research published in professional journals is too difficult for clinicians to access.

   4. Ambulatory care settings have little in common with the settings used for most research.

6. The scientific method for conducting research uses the null hypothesis, which is statistically based. The correct format for the null hypothesis is:

   1. There **is** no significant difference between two groups.

   2. Group A is greater than group B.

   3. Group A is less than group B.

   4. There is a 95% probability that group A is different from group B.

7. When evaluating claims made on advertisements, such as "Drug X has been used for 5 years with over 1 million doses administered in the United States, Canada, and Great Britain. Drug X stops heartburn, aids in digestion, and prevents esophageal reflux and is the 'treatment of choice' to relieve GERD," the nurse practitioner realizes that the claim is:

   1. Invalid, because there is no control or comparison group and no statistics are stated.

   2. Valid, because there are sufficient numbers of users who have had success.

   3. Invalid, because the level of significance is not mentioned to be at the 0.05 level.

   4. Valid, because the cohort and Hawthorne effects are operating.

8. In your practice, you have noticed that female clients who are pregnant and still in their teens generally seem to go into labor before their due date (as determined by ultrasound exam), while the women who are in their mid-twenties usually go into labor at or after their due date. Which statistical analysis would answer the research question, "Among pregnant women in a nurse practitioner's practice, is there a statistically significant difference between the length of gestation for women age 16 to 19 when compared with women age 23 to 26?"

   1. Multiple regression.

   2. Chronbach's alpha.

   3. The two-tailed t test.

   4. Pearson's correlation.

9. The utilization of research in nursing practice can be equated with:

   1. The nursing process.

   2. The change process.

   3. Discharge planning.

   4. Family planning.

10. You are compiling monthly statistics for your practice, and one of the elements of your analysis is the cultural background of your clients. What level of data is "cultural background"?

   1. Nominal level data.

   2. Ordinal level data.

   3. Interval level data.

   4. Ratio level data.

11. A nurse practitioner practicing with a physician in general practice is compiling the practice statistics at the end of the month. The clients who received care range from infants to the elderly. Of the following data from the monthly report, which are most likely to be normally distributed?

   1. The lab tests scheduled for the clients.

   2. The gender of the clients.

   3. The primary diagnoses of the clients.

   4. The ages of the clients.

12. A nurse practitioner practicing with a physician in general practice is compiling the practice statistics at the end of the month. The clients who received care range from infants to the elderly. The nurse practitioner and the physician want to know the average monthly income of their clients. Which would be the most appropriate statistical measure of the "average income,"

assuming that income is exact in dollars and cents?

1. The mean.

2. The median.

3. The mode.

4. The range.

13. A nurse practitioner is evaluating research articles for a research utilization project. The majority of the articles indicate that either random selection or random assignment was used to select the sample for that study. Because certain procedures in research are used across disciplines, what can be assumed for studies in which randomization has been used?

1. The ages of the research subjects in these studies will be negatively skewed.

2. The research subjects in these studies will automatically be 50% male and 50% female.

3. The ages of the research subjects in these studies will be positively skewed.

4. The researchers were attempting to obtain the most representative sample.

14. The ability to predict outcomes of care is desirable both in research and in practice. If a nurse practitioner wanted to create a theoretical model for a specific aspect of his/her practice to predict the client outcomes, which statistical method would be used to analyze the clinical data?

1. Descriptive statistics.

2. Repeated measures *t* test.

3. Multiple regression.

4. Chi-square test for independent samples.

15. Research articles are being evaluated for a utilization project. What can the nurse practitioner do if he/she does not understand the statistical procedures that were used for the analysis of data in an article?

1. Assume that the correct procedure was used and read about the method or consult a statistician for an explanation of the statistics.

2. Assume that the article is beyond his/her ability to understand, so set that one aside and go on to the next article.

3. Assume that the correct procedure was used and, instead of reading the results section, read the discussion of the findings section.

4. Assume that the article is beyond his/her ability to understand and use someone else's critique of the reported study.

16. The nurse practitioner has determined that the office procedures for diagnosis and stabilization of new cases of diabetes need to be evaluated and possibly changed. Which would be the best choice for the first phase of the evaluation?

1. Design and conduct a double-blind clinical trial.

2. Design and conduct a research utilization project.

3. Design and conduct a research project in which men and women are compared.

4. Design and conduct a study to test Callista Roy's theoretical model.

17. A nurse practitioner was reading a nursing research article in which there were no statistically significant findings. The most appropriate response would be:

1. "Reading this article was a waste of my time."

2. "Because of reading this article, there is no reason to conduct similar studies."

3. "Reading this article raises new questions for my practice."

4. "Because of reading this article, I will immediately change my practice."

18. In a recently published study, the researcher reported "The statistical analysis used to identify the differences between the two variables was Pearson's correlation." Which most specifically tells what is wrong with this statement?

1. Pearson's correlation can be used only with three or more variables.

2. Pearson's correlation actually identifies the common factors between variables.

3. Pearson's correlation can be used only when there is a single variable.

4. Pearson's correlation actually identifies the relationship between variables.

19. Qualitative research studies are conducted by nurse researchers because:

    1. Qualitative studies help to identify and define nursing concepts.

    2. With qualitative methods, there are no concerns about the rights of research subjects.

    3. Qualitative approaches provide precise measures for statistical analysis.

    4. Nurse researchers find qualitative research designs easier to use.

20. The normal ranges of blood chemistry values are most like which statistical concept?

    1. The standard error.

    2. The mean.

    3. The standard deviation.

    4. The median.

21. The five major sequential steps of research utilization are:

    1. Establish a client relationship, perform a health assessment, make a diagnosis, devise a plan of care, evaluate the treatment.

    2. Identify the problem, assess published research, design the innovation, evaluate, decide whether to adopt the innovation.

    3. Review the popular literature, review the practice's clients, summarize the findings, evaluate, do client teaching.

    4. Review the client's lab test results, complete a thorough health assessment, make a diagnosis, implement the treatment, evaluate.

22. Both *qualitative* and *quantitative* research methods are used in nursing research because:

    1. Master's-prepared nurses conduct quantitative studies, while doctorally prepared nurses conduct qualitative studies.

    2. Master's-prepared nurses conduct qualitative studies, while doctorally prepared nurses conduct quantitative studies.

    3. They complement each other because they produce different types of findings about the same concepts.

    4. They complement each other because they produce the same types of findings about different concepts.

23. Nursing research subscribes to the scientific method for the design of research studies. The advantage of this is that:

    1. Nursing research is based on logically constructed arguments.

    2. Nursing research is designed to answer any research question.

    3. Nursing research findings are precise and need not be duplicated.

    4. Nursing research findings are generalizable to all client populations.

24. With the restructuring of health care delivery and a shift in the provision of nonacute care from the hospital to ambulatory care settings and the home, previous nursing research that was conducted in hospitals:

    1. Now becomes applicable to all in-hospital providers of care.

    2. Remains relevant in the new settings; client care is unchanged.

    3. Should be applied directly to client care provided in the new settings.

    4. May no longer be applicable to the delivery of client care.

25. Nurse researchers strive to substantiate causality so that client outcomes can be consistently predicted. For the nurse practitioner, the ability to predict the outcomes for every client could mean that:

    1. The appropriate treatment would be prescribed for each client.

    2. No further studies would need to be conducted about treatments.

    3. The client's individual qualities would not need to be considered.

    4. Treatments would not need to be individualized for each client.

26. The reason that quantitative research articles always have a section containing descriptive findings is that descriptive data analysis:

    1. Provides the basis for making inferences about the findings.
    2. May yield statistically significant findings that were unexpected.
    3. Is conducted for predicting client outcomes in nursing settings.
    4. Organizes the data for clearer understanding of subjects and variables.

27. The difference between univariate and multivariate studies is:

    1. The number of subjects in the sample.
    2. The number of variables being studied.
    3. The number of sites for collecting data.
    4. The number of statistical hypotheses.

28. The independent variable and the dependent variable of a research study might be thought of as:

    1. The cause (the independent variable) and the effect (the dependent variable).
    2. The median (the independent variable) and the mode (the dependent variable).
    3. The outcome (the independent variable) and the treatment (the dependent variable).
    4. The sample (the independent variable) and the population (the dependent variable).

29. *Variance* is a key statistical concept. How would current research methods change if there were no variance?

    1. We would need to increase the sample size in all of our research studies to 100 research subjects or greater.
    2. Since our current research methods do not depend on the presence of variance, we would not need to change our current methods.
    3. We would need to decrease the sample size of all our research studies to 15 research subjects.
    4. Since our current research methods are based on the presence of variance, we would not be able to use our current methods.

Theory

30. While nursing theories vary greatly in their perspectives on nursing care, all nursing theorists explicitly incorporate three key concepts. These three concepts, which are basic to nursing care, are:

    1. Individuals, families, and communities.
    2. Primary, secondary, and tertiary prevention.
    3. Past, present, and future well-being.
    4. Person, health, and environment.

31. The theoretical basis for nursing practice is:

    1. A relatively new approach to nursing care.
    2. Borrowed from other professions such as medicine.
    3. As old as formal nursing and began with Florence Nightingale.
    4. Unrelated to the conduct of nursing research studies.

32. The verification of the more abstract nursing theories (e.g., that of Martha Rogers) is often hampered by:

    1. The lack of adequate measures for the theoretical concepts.
    2. Prior studies that did not support the theory.
    3. The lack of adequate laboratory settings for conducting experiments.
    4. Prior studies that were conducted in other countries.

33. Basing nursing practice on nursing theory contributes to the professionalization of nursing practice by:

    1. Adapting the medical model to nursing care.
    2. Limiting the choice of treatments for clients.
    3. Determining what type of clients will be seen by the nurse.
    4. Providing a consistent perspective for providing care to clients.

34. A nurse practitioner has decided to incorporate a nursing theoretical model into his/her ambulatory care practice where there is a strong emphasis on the clients doing as much as possible to maintain their own health. Of the choices below, which nursing model is most applicable to this setting?

    1. Orem's Self-Care Model, also known as *The Self-Care Deficit Theory of Nursing*.
    2. Roy's Adaptation Model.
    3. Roger's Science of Unitary Human Beings.
    4. King's Interacting Systems Model.

35. Of the following choices, which nursing theorist is considered to have general systems theory as philosophical orientation to her model?

    1. Sister Callista Roy.
    2. Martha Rogers.
    3. Rosemarie Parse.
    4. Betty Neuman.

36. Which nursing theory addresses nursing outcomes in terms of primary, secondary, and tertiary prevention?

    1. Roy's Adaptation Model.
    2. Neuman's Health Care Systems Model.
    3. King's Interacting Systems Framework.
    4. Watson's Human Caring Theory.

37. Which nursing model primarily addresses health promotion?

    1. Watson's Human Caring Model.
    2. Neuman's Health Care Systems Model.
    3. Pender's Health Promotion Model.
    4. Roy's Adaptation Model.

18 Answers & Rationales

Research

1. **(3)** By federal law, clients must be assured of their privacy and confidentiality. The other information is interesting and may be included but is not required by federal law.

2. **(1)** In published research reports, of the choices listed, only the first choice is consistently reported by researchers. The clinical relevance is considered, not the statistical relevance. The specific program used does not make a difference, since all are based on the same statistical formulas. Researchers frequently work with statistical consultants, so a researcher's background is not a limitation to a published study.

3. **(4)** Only the last choice contains those elements common to both processes: assessing, planning, implementing, and evaluating.

4. **(3)** Neither type of statistics is used to assign participant code numbers. Descriptive statistics are used to describe the sample.

5. **(1)** Inadequate time can be a barrier to research utilization in any setting. The process of research utilization is well delineated by researchers. With the ever-increasing availability of professional journals via the Internet, access is rarely a problem. A considerable body of research has been conducted in ambulatory care settings.

6. **(1)** The correct format for the null hypothesis is, "There is no significant difference between the two groups." The alternate, or research, hypothesis may take the other forms.

7. **(1)** Even though the claims detail extensive use of "Drug X," there must be statistical evidence as demonstrated through the use of control or comparison groups that will render a level of significance.

8. **(3)** Only the t test compares two independent groups with respect to a variable.

9. **(2)** Incorporating research findings into practice often results in a change in practice. The nursing process is most like conducting research.

10. **(1)** The variable of "cultural background" is categorical data or nominal level data.

11. **(4)** The gender and primary diagnosis are nominal level data, and the lab tests would be skewed, while the age would approximate the normal curve.

12. **(2)** The median income would be most representative of the average because the income of 50% of clients is above and the income of 50% of clients is below the median. The mean could be influenced by one client with a very high or very low income, and the mode only identifies the income that is reported most often. The range only identifies the lowest and the highest income and does not present an average.

13. **(4)** Randomization is a research technique used to increase the amount of control in any research design. The other three options are false; they do not occur because of randomization.

14. **(3)** Of the choices, only multiple regression examines the relationship between two or more variables in a way that permits prediction.

15. **(1)** In reviewing research, it is necessary to understand the statistical methods that the researcher used to determine the value of the study findings for the practice setting. The researcher's discussion may not provide the full extent of the findings, and someone else's critique may reflect a specific point of view that does not apply in every situation.

16. **(2)** As a first step, a research utilization project would include a thorough review of the published literature on which to base a change. A full study may not be needed, and testing a theoretical model is not appropriate for this situation.

17. **(3)** The lack of significant findings is an important piece of information about the topic of the research and definitely is not a waste of time. Particularly when findings are nonsignificant, more studies need to be conducted about this topic. Ideally, changes in practice are based on the findings of more than one study.

18. **(4)** Correlations identify the relationships between variables. Two or more variables may be used. Factor analysis is used to identify common factors.

19. **(1)** The purpose of qualitative designs is to identify and define nursing concepts. Qualitative designs do not yield precise measures, are usually not analyzed statistically, are more difficult to use, and carry the same concerns about the rights of subjects as all other research designs.

20. **(3)** The normal ranges of blood chemistry values are based on studies that identified the standard deviation for each blood chemical. The mean and the median are averages, and the standard error is not applicable to this situation.

21. **(2)** This option contains the published steps. All other options are nursing actions taken on behalf of the client (in no particular order).

22. **(3)** The two methods complement each other because they produce different types of findings about the same concepts. The educational preparation of the researcher does not dictate the research method used.

23. **(1)** The scientific method is highly organized and is based on logical reasoning. Findings are rarely precise, and studies do need to be duplicated. Some questions are not answerable by our current research methods. Because of small samples and other limitations, many findings from nursing research are **not** generalizable.

24. **(4)** Such a drastic change in health care delivery may make previous studies no longer applicable to nursing care. Health care restructuring has changed the way client care is provided.

25. **(1)** The ability to always predict client outcomes would mean that each client would receive the appropriate, individualized treatment. Treatments would still have to be individualized, and individual qualities would need to be considered. Because new treatments are always being devised, there would be a need for ongoing research.

26. **(4)** Descriptive data analysis organizes the data, and it facilitates understanding. Descriptive statistics cannot be used for significance testing or for making inferences; inferential statistics are used. Predictions are made from studies that use inferential statistics.

27. **(2)** "Variate" refers to the number of variables in the study.

28. **(1)** The independent variable may be considered the cause or the treatment, and the dependent variable may be considered the effect or the outcome. The median, mode, sample, and population are not designations for independent or dependent variables.

29. **(4)** All of our current research and statistical analysis methods depend on the presence of variance or variation; if variance is no longer present, our current methods could no longer be used. If there is no variance, a sample of one would be adequate.

Theory

30. **(4)** All current theories incorporate person, health, and environment. Other concepts may or may not be explicitly included in nursing theories.

31. **(3)** The theoretical basis for nursing practice began with Florence Nightingale and has been used for practice and for research for more than a century. Nursing theories are specifically developed for nursing.

32. **(1)** The lack of adequate measures for theoretical concepts is a major roadblock in many areas of research, and particularly so with the more abstract theories. Prior studies always provide information about the theory, even when they were conducted in other countries. More abstract concepts tend not to be studied in lab settings.

33. **(4)** Theory-based practice contributes the consistent perspective that permits the comparison of care across settings. Theory-based practice does not necessarily limit treatments or determine client types. Theory-based practice specifically eliminates reliance on the medical model.

34. **(1)** Orem's Self-Care Model focuses on the client participating in and being in control of his/her own health care. Roy's Adaptation Model is most appropriate for acute care settings; Roger's Science of Unitary Human Beings, for holistic health settings; and King's Interacting Systems Model, for a mental health setting.

35. **(4)** Betty Neuman's Health Care Systems Model, Imogene King's Systems Interaction Model, and Dorothy Johnson's Behavioral Systems are based on general systems theory. Roy's Adaptation Model has stress and adaptation as the framework. Martha Roger's Science of Unitary Human Beings and Rosemarie Parse's Human Becoming Model are based on a humanistic developmental framework.

36. **(2)** Betty Neuman identified the need to implement nursing interventions through use of one or more of three prevention modalities (primary, secondary, and tertiary prevention).

37. **(3)** Pender's Health Promotion Model is an excellent nursing model that readily fits into a nurse practitioner's scope of practice. The other theorists' models—Neuman's Health Care Systems Model, Watson's Human Caring Model, and Roy's Adaptation Model—are useful models for professional nursing practice.

19

Issues & Trends

1. The nurse practitioner understands the following about the Health Insurance Portability and Accountability Act of 1996 (HIPAA).

   1. Allows health insurance providers to deny insurance because of preexisting medical conditions.

   2. Provides for easier access to all providers to obtain secure and private health information.

   3. A National Provider Identifier and Employer Identifier, which is part of HIPAA, was designed to help speed enrollment, determination of eligibility, and claims processing through a national set of identification numbers that provides a mechanism to identify a specific provider, insurer, or patient.

   4. The compliance date for the HIPAA rule, which requires health care organizations, insurers, and payers that have been using any electronic means of storing patient data and performing claims submission (Final Rule for National Standards for Electronic Transactions) was initiated April 14, 2003.

2. Considering the four advanced practice roles of clinical nurse specialist, nurse practitioner, certified nurse midwife, and nurse anesthetist,

which role became accepted by and included into the practice arena without significant controversy?

   1. Clinical nurse specialist.

   2. Nurse practitioner.

   3. Certified nurse midwife.

   4. Nurse anesthetist.

3. Historically, who was one of the most outspoken opponents of the nurse practitioner role?

   1. Loretta Ford.

   2. Hildegard Peplau.

   3. Martha Rogers.

   4. Dorothea Orem.

4. Who started the first nurse practitioner program?

   1. Hildegard Peplau.

   2. Mary Breckenridge.

   3. Agnes McGee.

   4. Loretta Ford.

5. Which is the most important action in developing health policy skills in the nurse practitioner?

   1. Acquire political allies in Congress.

   2. Work on a campaign.

   3. Support causes such as prevention of teen pregnancy or acquired immunodeficiency syndrome.

   4. Write letters and editorials.

6. Which is the least important barrier to collaborative advanced nursing practice?

   1. Prescriptive authority.

   2. Reimbursement privileges.

   3. Legal scope of practice.

   4. Political activism.

7. For the nurse practitioner to obtain reimbursement, an understanding of which is important?

   1. Minimum Nursing Data Set (MNDS).

   2. *ICD-9-CM*, *CPT*, and HCPC codes.

   3. HCPC codes and NANDA diagnoses.

   4. Medicare and Medicaid numbers.

8. Steps of the change process according to Kurt Lewin are:

   1. Unsolving, mobilizing, recruiting, finalizing.

   2. Building relationships, acquiring resources, choosing solution, stabilizing.

   3. Unfreezing, moving, refreezing.

   4. Forming, storming, norming.

9. What was the major impetus for nurse practitioner development?

   1. Need for an expert nurse clinician.

   2. Shortage of primary care physicians.

   3. Trend for specialized nurses to diagnose and manage unstable acute and chronic conditions.

   4. Movement of graduate nursing education to diagnosis and treatment of major illness.

10. The nurse practitioner understands that Medicare B provides:

    1. Hospitalization costs for the insured.

    2. Health insurance benefits for low-income families.

    3. Benefits that cover physicians, nurse practitioners, medical equipment, and outpatient services.

    4. Outpatient laboratory services, radiography services, and skilled nursing care in appropriate facilities.

11. What is the impact of the Balanced Budget Act of 1997 on nurse practitioner practice?

    1. Authorizes all states to provide nurse practitioners with prescriptive authority.

    2. Provides for only wellness visits and primary care services.

    3. Prevents a physician from billing 100% for a nurse practitioner's services.

    4. Allows direct Medicare payments to nurse practitioners in both rural and urban settings.

12. In the clinic, you have observed the following: one medical assistant is usually pleasant and helpful; the other is often abrasive and angry. The most important basic guideline to be observed by the nurse practitioner who must resolve a conflict between two medical assistants is:

    1. Require the medical assistants to reach a compromise.

    2. Weigh the consequences of each possible solution.

    3. Encourage ventilation of anger and use humor to minimize the conflict.

    4. Deal with issues, not personalities.

13. A male nurse practitioner approaches another nurse practitioner who is his friend and tells him that one of the female physicians at the clinic often follows him into the supply room and tells him how good-looking he is. Yesterday, she patted his hand and said, "I wish we would get to know each other better. I would make it worth your while—better benefits at the clinic, more money." The male staff nurse asks his friend, "What do I do? I don't want to date her,

but I don't want to lose my job. I just want her to leave me alone!" The best reply for the friend would be:

1. "Tell her that her behavior makes you feel uncomfortable and that you want her to stop."

2. "Go for it! Date her and see if you get what she promises."

3. "Go to the human relations office at the agency right away and relate to them the entire situation."

4. "Contact your lawyer and get advice as soon as possible, in case she decides to turn the tables and accuse you of advances."

14. The nurse practitioner understands that "incident to" services are reimbursed at which percentage?

1. 75%.

2. 80%.

3. 85%.

4. 100%.

19 Answers & Rationales

1. **(4)** The four major goals of HIPAA are: ensure health insurance portability by eliminating job-lock because of preexisting medical conditions, reduce health care fraud and abuse, enforce standards for health information, and guarantee security and privacy of health information. Because of protests from civil libertarians and individuals concerned about Big Brother having the ability to identify, track, and gain information about anyone in the country by means of a single identification number, the National Individual Identifier has been put on the sidelines until some type of reasonable compromise can be worked out that would assure all sides that there would be no abuses of such an identifier system. The first compliance HIPPA rule went into effect on April 14, 2003, and it relates to national standards for electronic transactions.

2. **(1)** According to the National Commission on Nursing (1983) and the Task Force on Nursing Practice in Hospitals (1983), the clinical nurse specialist (CNS) role was accepted quite rapidly. The psychiatric CNS role is considered the oldest and most highly developed of the CNS specialties and helped initiate the growth of other CNS specialties.

3. **(3)** Martha Rogers argued that the development of the nurse practitioner role was a ploy to lure nurses out of nursing and into medicine, hence weakening and undermining nursing's unique role in health care. This led to a major division within nursing, which led to barriers to the establishment of nurse practitioner educational programs within the mainstream of graduate nursing education.

4. **(4)** Loretta Ford, RN, PhD, and Henry Silver, MD, established the first pediatric nurse practitioner program at the University of Colorado. Mary Breckenridge established the Frontier Nursing Service in the depressed rural mountain area of Kentucky, which led to training nurse midwives. Agnes McGee is credited with offering the first postgraduate program for nurse anesthetists at St. Vincent's Hospital in Portland, Oregon. Hildegard Peplau started the first psychiatric CNS program at Rutgers University.

5. **(1)** Although all of these actions are important for the nurse practitioner in development of policy skills, the most important is acquiring political allies. Having political allies in decision-making places (legislature) will enable the nurse practitioner to be active and informed regarding issues surrounding regulation, limitations on admitting privileges and prescriptive authority, and managed care.

6. **(4)** There are three major issues that are central to the expansion of the nurse practitioner role—prescriptive authority, reimbursement privileges, and legal scope of practice. Although political activism is important, it is not specific to collaborative practice.

7. **(2)** The *ICD-9-CM* (*International Classification of Diseases, 9th Edition*) codes are diagnostic codes that identify the condition, illness, or injury to be treated and are used for billing insurance carriers. *CPT* (*Current Procedural Terminology*) codes specify the procedure or medical service given (more than 7000 terms). Medicare and state Medicaid carriers are required by law to use *CPT* codes. The Health Care Financing Administration Common Procedure Coding System (HCPC) is used for reporting supplies and medical equipment.

8. **(3)** Lewin described three processes of change: unfreezing—involves breaking the habit, disturbing the equilibrium; moving—development of new responses based on new information with a change in attitudes, feelings, behaviors, or values; and refreezing—reaching a new status quo, stabilizing and integrating new behaviors with appropriate support that is available to maintain the change. Forming, storming, and norming refer to the stages of group process development. Option #2 lists Havelock's change theory steps.

9. **(2)** According to most sources, the nurse practitioner role developed because of a shortage of primary care physicians in the 1960s and 1970s, when medical specialization was the trend.

10. **(3)** Medicare is regulated by the federal government and includes the services described, plus outpatient laboratory and radiography services. Hospitalization costs are covered under Medicare A.

11. **(4)** The Balanced Budget Act is a crucial and significant piece of legislation that allows direct payments to nurse practitioners at "80% of the lesser of either the actual charge or 85% of the fee schedule amount of the same service if provided by a physician." This does not change the "incident to" rule, which allows a physician to bill for 100% for a nurse practitioner's services (i.e., provided the physician is in the suite at the time of the service and readily available to provide assistance).

12. **(4)** Conflict must be addressed directly by the nurse practitioner. The personal characteristics of each of the medical assistants must not enter into the conflict resolution process. Determine the issue of conflict and then work on possible solutions to resolve the issue. Compromise is just one method of conflict resolution wherein both parties must be willing to give up something.

13. **(1)** There are two ways to deal with sexual harassment at work: informally and formally through a grievance procedure. Always start with the direct approach; ask the person to STOP! Tell the harasser in clear terms that the behavior makes you uncomfortable and that you want it to stop immediately.

14. **(4)** The nurse practitioner is reimbursed at 100% of "incident to" services. Medicare services provided entirely by the nurse practitioner are reimbursed at 80% of the lesser of the actual charge or 85% of the fee schedule amount of physicians, while Medicaid services are reimbursed at 75%.

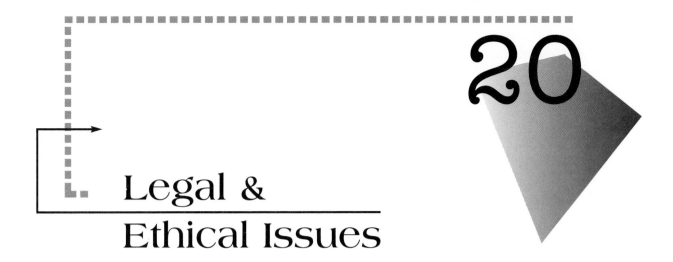

Legal & Ethical Issues

1. An occurrence-form professional liability insurance policy is preferred because:

   1. The amount of insurance money available to pay a claim increases with each renewal of the policy.

   2. The policy proceeds are available to pay claims regardless of when the claim is reported to the carrier.

   3. The carrier will be notified of a potential claim during the policy period.

   4. The coverage is broader than that provided by a claims-made policy form.

2. Early reporting of a potential professional liability claim is advantageous because:

   1. Insurance carriers have a 10-day reporting window after which the coverage is canceled.

   2. Documents and witnesses needed to defend the claim are more likely to be available at the time of the event.

3. Insurance premiums will be reduced upon a good-faith showing of cooperation with the carrier.

4. Risk management personnel require such reporting in order to comply with Joint Commission on the Accreditation of Healthcare Organizations (JCAHO) mandates.

3. Your nursing license may be in jeopardy if:

   1. You appropriately delegate medication administration to a trusted RN employee, who administers a fatal dose.

   2. You delegate client assessment tasks to an LPN who has been floated to your outpatient clinic for the day.

   3. You provide nursing care services consistent with established standards of practice in your jurisdiction.

   4. The medical assistant in your supervising physician's office exceeds the scope of her authority, but you take prompt action to correct the problem.

4. Your client is a 46-year-old mentally challenged man who has been given a diagnosis of colon cancer. Consent for his corrective surgery should be obtained from:

   1. The client himself.

   2. The client's 84-year-old mother, who is his closest relative.

   3. The client's court-appointed guardian.

   4. The administrator of the group home where the client lives.

5. Your client is a 75-year-old woman with metastatic cancer. Her affairs are in order; she has arranged all her finances and her own funeral rites. She has systematically secured enough barbiturates to successfully end her life; she asks you to mix the drugs for her in some pudding to make them palatable for ingestion. Your best course of action would be to:

   1. Mix the medications as requested and stay with her while she consumes the preparation.

   2. Consult with family and attending physician to warn them about the client's proposed course of action.

   3. Seek an immediate order for an antidepressant.

   4. Sit down with the client and conduct a physical and psychological needs assessment.

6. The Patient Self-Determination Act (PSDA), passed by Congress in 1990, resulted in which of the following policy changes?

   1. Hospitals are mandated to assist every client to create a "living will."

   2. Federally funded managed care organizations (MCOs) are required to inform subscribers about their rights under state law to create advance directives.

   3. Home health agencies are required to have do not resuscitate (DNR) orders on file for all terminally ill clients.

   4. Hospitalized clients are obligated to select a surrogate decision maker to make health care decisions for them if they become incapacitated.

7. Both the Food and Drug Administration (FDA) and the Department of Health and Human Services (DHHS) have regulations governing research activities involving human subjects. The principal investigator is responsible for:

   1. Securing a signed special research consent form.

   2. Reporting back to the institutional review board if a subject is injured during the course of the study.

   3. Appearing before the institutional review board to present the study and secure approval to proceed with subject recruitment at the facility.

   4. All of the above.

8. If you are served with a summons and complaint (i.e., lawsuit documents), the first step you should take is to:

   1. Call the client to determine the basis for the action and what you allegedly did wrong.

   2. Call the client's lawyer (listed on the first page of the lawsuit) to get more information about the case.

   3. Call your insurance company for instructions on how to proceed.

   4. Confer with your colleagues and review the chart to see whether you need to clarify your notes.

9. As a nurse practitioner in an impoverished rural area, you frequently encounter a female client in a situation of domestic violence with few community options for referral. Participating in community education forums and fund-raising for a safe house is an example of applying the ethical principle of:

   1. Autonomy.

   2. Nonmaleficence.

   3. Justice.

   4. Veracity.

10. Nurses practicing in expanded roles should carry professional liability insurance for which of the following reasons?

    1. Premiums are often modest and are a tax-deductible business expense.

    2. Even if the employer insures the nurse practitioner, there may be situations of conflict

between employer and nurse necessitating separate legal counsel.

3. As roles expand, so does the liability potential.

4. All of the above.

11. The confidentiality of medical records is always a valid concern, especially in this age of computerization, "smart cards," and fax machines. Release of medical information to third parties is:

1. A creature of state law, meaning that state statutes control the processing of such requests.

2. Prohibited without the informed consent of the client.

3. Automatic when the requesting party is a third-party payer or insurer.

4. Disallowed if the records contain proof of a diagnosis of acquired immunodeficiency syndrome (AIDS).

12. Which categories of persons are **not** included in the definition of disability under the Americans with Disabilities Act (ADA)?

1. Profoundly deaf employees.

2. Persons who are wheelchair-bound.

3. Current users of illegal drugs.

4. Persons with mental retardation.

13. If your client is having a problem with a managed care plan, you can offer to assist in the following ways:

1. Suggest that the client contact the customer service department (may be called "member services") at the plan to resolve the issue; filing a formal grievance may be necessary.

2. Remind the client, who is a member of the "senior" plan for Medicare recipients, that he/she may complain to the federal Office of Personnel Management (OPM).

3. Remind the client that the state's insurance department also investigates complaints against health plans.

4. All of the above.

14. If a piece of equipment malfunctions while being used on a hospitalized client, the risk manager would probably recommend the following course of action:

1. Return the item to the manufacturer with a description of the problem and a request for analysis.

2. Tag and sequester the item at the facility and defer analysis pending risk management review of the litigation potential.

3. Send the item to the biomedical engineering department with a request for immediate equipment breakdown and troubleshooting.

4. Repair the item, either in-house or by contracting with an outside firm, and return it to service as soon as possible.

15. Nurse expert witnesses are essential in the adjudication of most professional negligence claims against nurses. The following criteria for nurse experts are sought by attorneys:

1. Appropriate professional education, preferably at the technical level.

2. Relevant and recent professional work experience.

3. Ability to understand and articulate the legal issues involved in the claim.

4. Authorship of medical texts in the clinical subject areas.

16. Which federal law mandates the tracking of implantable medical devices?

1. The Administrative Procedures Act (APA).

2. The PSDA.

3. The Safe Medical Devices Act (SMDA).

4. The Omnibus Budget Reconciliation Act (OBRA) of 1987.

17. Which of the following are elements of a broad-based risk management program?

1. A hazardous materials compliance program as part of a comprehensive safety and security system.

2. An early-warning/incident reporting program to identify elements of risk.

3. A system of contract review to avoid assuming liabilities that should be borne by others.

4. All of the above.

18. The type of insurance coverage that is purchased (or self-insured) by an organization to handle employee job-related injuries is:

    1. Professional liability insurance.

    2. Business interruption insurance.

    3. Directors and officers insurance.

    4. Workers' compensation insurance.

19. A nurse practitioner is driving her personal vehicle on a job-related errand and is struck by a semitrailer on the interstate. The car is totaled, and she is severely injured. Which insurance policies will respond to these losses?

    1. The nurse practitioner's personal auto policy and her employer's workers' compensation policy.

    2. The employer's business auto policy and workers' compensation policy.

    3. The nurse practitioner's homeowner's policy.

    4. The semitrailer driver's personal auto policy.

20. Nurse practitioners with hospital privileges may be affected by the part of the Health Care Quality Improvement Act known as *the National Practitioner Data Bank (NPDB)*. Which of the following statements about the Data Bank is **not** true?

    1. Professional liability insurance claims payments made on behalf of nurse practitioners must be reported to the NPDB.

    2. The facility granting medical staff privileges must query the NPDB before approving a practitioner's privileges.

    3. The purpose of the NPDB is to be a nationwide flagging system that provides information about malpractice claims, licensure actions, and restrictions on privileges so that practitioners may not easily move from one jurisdiction to another to escape quality review.

    4. Insurance companies report all malpractice payments made on behalf of affected nurse practitioners within 30 days of the date the payment was made, if the amount of the claim is in excess of $11,000 and no matter how it was settled.

21. In 1985 Congress took action against a phenomenon known as *patient dumping* by enacting what was known at the time as *the COBRA law*, now referred to as *EMTALA, the Emergency Medical Treatment and Active Labor Act*. Which statement about EMTALA is **not true**?

    1. The original purpose of the statute was to prohibit the transfer of uninsured and untreated clients from the emergency department of one hospital to another (usually the county hospital).

    2. Subsequent rules and case law have expanded the statute so that almost any unauthorized transfer of a client from one facility to another is potentially problematic.

    3. To effect a proper transfer, the forwarding facility need not notify or secure the acquiescence of the receiving facility.

    4. The transferring facility must use appropriate transport methods and send copies of clients' medical records.

22. You are a nurse practitioner wishing to effect change in the state's laws regarding the dispensing of prescription medications by nurse practitioners. You would take your case to:

    1. The state legislature.

    2. The state board of nursing.

    3. The state board of pharmacy.

    4. The nursing specialty organization.

23. The common meaning of "gag clauses" or "gag orders" in the managed care arena is:

    1. The MCO declines to publish, in its subscriber contracts, the treatments that are excluded from coverage under the plan.

    2. The MCO refuses to allow its member services personnel to answer certain subscriber questions about covered benefits.

    3. MCO contracts with providers to disallow providers' offering treatment alternatives that the providers know are not covered by clients' plans.

    4. Providers are prohibited from offering experimental treatment to clients.

24. Under the Safe Medical Devices Act of 1990, which of the following health care providers or organizations are required to report the death of a client to the FDA if the death is related to the use of a medical device?

    1. Physicians' office staff.

    2. Hospitals, home health agencies, and ambulance companies.

    3. Nurse family members treating clients without compensation.

    4. Physicians making home visits.

25. A client receives a medication that was intended for another person. An appropriate way to document this event in the medical record would be:

    1. "Client was given x mg of y drug in error."

    2. "X mg y drug administered to client. No adverse effects noted. Physician notified."

    3. "Client received wrong medication. Incident report filed. Practitioner disciplined."

    4. "Practitioner inadvertently administered y drug to wrong client. Supervisor notified. Family threatening litigation."

26. The one reason that clients offer, above all others, for suing practitioners for medical negligence is:

    1. The care they received was substandard.

    2. The provider made an honest mistake.

    3. The client wasn't "heard" when he/she attempted to communicate with the provider.

    4. The client participated fully in all aspects of medical decision making, but the results were disappointing.

27. Informed consent is based on the ethical principle of:

    1. Beneficence.

    2. Respect for persons.

    3. Nonmaleficence.

    4. Autonomy.

28. The four elements of a professional negligence claim are:

    1. Duty, fulfillment of duty, professional relationship, and wrongful act.

    2. Professional responsibility, fault, harm to the client, and wrongful act.

    3. Duty, breach of duty, causal connection between the act and the harm, and harm to the client.

    4. Professional relationship, intentional wrongful act, proximate cause, and damage to the client.

29. You are making an initial home health care visit to an elderly lady whose spouse tells you that she is often confused. He answers all your questions and dominates the discussion. You proceed to do your initial assessment; the wife does seem to be oriented to time, place, and person. Who is the proper party to sign the written form to request/consent for services?

    1. The husband.

    2. The wife (client).

    3. The attending physician.

    4. The home health aide who will be providing continuing care.

30. An expert witness is usually required in a nursing negligence case because:

    1. Knowledge of medical or nursing facts is not considered intuitive to a lay jury.

    2. Jurors are allowed to use their "sixth sense" regarding the facts presented to them.

    3. Fact witnesses are not able to present an unbiased account of the circumstances in dispute.

    4. Appropriately credentialed experts have more credibility in the eyes of lay jurors.

31. The standard of care for a nurse practitioner, in a trial, will be established by expert witness(es). The expert opinion will be based on:

    1. National norms for the specialty.

    2. Facility policies and procedures.

    3. Professional literature.

    4. All of the above.

32. Alternative dispute resolution is a process wherein the parties to a dispute resolve their differences outside of a court trial. Advantages to this system of problem solving include all **except**:

    1. The parties usually prefer the process because they have an opportunity to be heard in a less formal and less intimidating environment.

    2. The process is often less time-consuming and less costly than traditional litigation.

    3. Damage awards are less likely to include nonfinancial compensation.

    4. Insurers are amenable to working with mediators with a track record of fairness and successful case resolution.

33. The statute of limitations is:

    1. The state law that prescribes the time frames within which a nursing negligence action may be filed.

    2. The law that states that minors have no legal authority to sue nurses for malpractice.

    3. The law that limits the right of clients to sue nurse practitioners for negligent acts.

    4. The federal law that limits a nurse practitioner's right to countersue a client for malicious prosecution.

34. A family nurse practitioner is driving along the interstate on the way to a nursing seminar. The practitioner observes a head-on collision and decides to stop to render aid. Which statement is **false** with respect to the practitioner's potential liability for malpractice?

    1. There is no legal obligation to stop to render assistance; if the practitioner had driven by the accident, there would be no liability on his/her part.

    2. If appropriate nursing care is provided, gratuitously, the practitioner will be protected from liability under that state's Good Samaritan Law.

    3. Even if the practitioner acts in a grossly negligent manner, the Good Samaritan Law will shield him/her from liability.

    4. The protections afforded by the Good Samaritan Law may differ from state to state;

the practitioner should research his/her state's law on the subject.

35. If a practitioner is subpoenaed to appear for a deposition in a nursing negligence case, appropriate preparation is prudent. One of the following tips would not be suggested by the practitioner's attorney. Which piece of advice is **not** appropriate?

    1. Discreetly chew gum to calm your nerves and dress for dinner because depositions usually take all day and you won't have time to change.

    2. Review the client's medical record and any other materials suggested by the attorney before the appearance for questioning.

    3. Take as much time as needed to think about responses before answering; don't let an attorney put words in your mouth.

    4. Be straightforward and truthful; remember that "I don't know" and "I don't remember" are acceptable responses.

36. Which of the following documentation tips is **not** a good idea?

    1. Carefully document your criticism of a fellow provider's clinical decision in the client's medical record. This will protect you if your treatment decisions need to be defended later.

    2. Use standard abbreviations in the medical record so that subsequent readers will have no doubt as to your meaning and intent.

    3. Document telephone conversations with the client and/or the family in the medical record. Be particularly vigilant about recording changes in the client's medications.

    4. Document noncompliant client behaviors in the medical record; be thorough, yet factual.

37. If a client is under the age of majority for the state in which he/she is seeking health care, what factors would be considered to determine whether the client is "emancipated" and able to consent to medical treatment?

    1. Whether the client is married.

    2. Whether the client is in the military.

3. Whether the client is living outside the "care, custody, and control" of a parent or guardian.

4. All of the above.

38. In 1987, and again in 1994, Congress acted to update many of the regulations that govern the provision of long-term care services. What is important for an employer or nurse manager in this environment to know?

    1. Nursing assistants working in long-term care facilities must be formally trained and certified.

    2. Clients or residents have specific rights, such as the right to information about their physical condition, medical benefits, and associated costs.

    3. New and swifter sanctions are available for reviewers to impose on facilities with deficiencies.

    4. All of the above.

39. A nurse practitioner is employed in a private medical office. There is a lot of activity at the front desk where some clients are checking in for appointments, staff are scheduling tests, and telephone advice triage is in progress. What changes should be implemented to preserve client confidentiality?

    1. Orient the fax machine and computer monitor such that incoming reports or other data cannot be read by nonstaff members.

    2. Do all telephone scheduling from a more secure location, such as a conference room in the back office.

    3. Create a more private space to confer with clients who need follow-up information or explanations of tests or treatments.

    4. All of the above.

40. A nurse-employer would be well advised to have procedures in place to appropriately terminate an employee. To avoid a charge of discrimination or a claim for wrongful termination, the employer should be particularly sensitive to the protections afforded to select groups. Which of

the following is **not** a protected class under the antidiscrimination statues?

    1. Pregnant women.
    2. Gay men.
    3. Those age 40 and older.
    4. The handicapped.

41. Which activity could be considered grounds for a sexual harassment claim?

    1. A male employee tells an off-color joke to another man. The joke is overheard by a female co-worker who seems to appreciate the humor in it. The joke-telling is an isolated incident.

    2. A nurse-supervisor conducts an employee performance review. The supervisor does not mention a prior social relationship with the employee; the ratings are appropriate for the level of performance; the employee receives a salary increase.

    3. A co-ed locker room is decorated with multiple centerfold photos from a popular men's magazine. The female employees find this offensive and have filed several complaints.

    4. A nurse is complimented on her appearance and asked on a date by her boss. She informs the boss that she is married and not seeking another relationship. The incident is forgotten.

42. The client is a comatose lady who needs a feeding tube inserted for long-term nutritional needs. Her husband presents the nurse practitioner with a document that he says is his wife's living will. It is signed by him and sets out, so he says, the wishes of his wife with respect to the feeding tube. The living will is not a legally binding document because:

    1. The wife did not sign the document.

    2. The husband is not authorized to execute a living will on behalf of his wife.

    3. This type of advance directive must be signed by the individual while he/she is legally competent to execute documents.

    4. All of the above.

43. A nurse practitioner is helping out at a clinic for homeless women. A client with diabetes, in her third trimester of pregnancy, has been reasonably compliant with respect to insulin therapy. Now, however, she has announced her intent to abandon her insulin regimen because she has heard on the streets that some drugs are harmful to fetuses. Which option is **not** legally appropriate for the nurse practitioner, as her health care provider, to consider?

    1. Seek the support of the clinic's attorney to file a petition for court-ordered treatment for the client.

    2. Attempt to engage the client in dialogue to provide her with accurate medical information.

    3. Detain the client in the homeless shelter and administer the insulin, with or without her consent.

    4. Confer with social services to find an appropriate interim placement for the client until her medical and legal issues can be sorted out.

44. The purpose of the ADA is:

    1. To level the playing field with respect to employment and other opportunities for disabled people.

    2. To create a federal entitlement program for people with AIDS.

    3. To guarantee wheelchair access to every residential and commercial building.

    4. To authorize interpreters for deaf employees at all private businesses.

45. As a result of the US Supreme Court's ruling on assisted suicide, the current state of the law on this topic is:

    1. Assisted suicide is still a criminal offense in most jurisdictions.

    2. A physician may prescribe a fatal dose of medication with the concurrence of the ethics committee.

    3. A nurse practitioner may prescribe a fatal dose of medication with the concurrence of the supervising physician.

    4. A pharmacist may instruct a client how to mix and ingest a fatal dose of prescription medication.

46. A professional negligence or medical malpractice case is a civil action. The difference between a civil lawsuit and a criminal lawsuit is:

    1. The damages sought in a civil suit are monetary; one private party sues another for money.

    2. If you are convicted in a criminal case, you are still covered by your professional liability insurer.

    3. In a criminal case, your state sues you for money; other penalties do not apply.

    4. In a civil suit, if you do not prevail, you could be incarcerated.

47. Which of the following is **not** a form of alternative dispute resolution?

    1. Mediation.

    2. Binding and nonbinding arbitration.

    3. Settlement conference.

    4. A jury trial.

48. It is particularly important for nurses who care for children to have adequate professional liability insurance coverage because:

    1. Damages are always higher when a child is the injured party.

    2. Juries tend to award fewer dollars to injured children because the children are eligible for a variety of social programs that cover their medical expenses.

    3. The statute of limitations is often tolled (put on hold) until the minor reaches majority, so the time frame within which the child can file a lawsuit is extended.

    4. Insurers are sensitive to the increased risk posed by minor claimants so the coverage is difficult to obtain.

49. A health care provider has a duty to disclose certain information to the client as part of the informed consent process. Exceptions to this duty would include all of the following **except**:

    1. The client has waived the right to receive the data.

    2. It is a bona fide emergency situation.

3. The provider believes that the information would be harmful to the client and invokes the therapeutic privilege.

4. The client is 80 years old and the elderly are unable to comprehend complex medical facts.

50. When the nurse practitioner is contemplating providing a detailed reference on a former employee, it is important to consider which of the following?

    1. The requirements of the human resources department of the nurse practitioner's employer.

    2. If the comments are perceived as negative and the former employee becomes aware of them, the nurse practitioner could subject himself or herself to suit for defamation.

    3. If the employee exhibits unsafe client care practices, it may be wiser to risk legal action from the employee than to subject future clients to this unsafe practitioner.

    4. All of the above.

51. The primary purpose of a pre-employment physical exam is to:

    1. Identify existing health problems that might adversely affect the company's insurance rates.

    2. Determine the mental status of the applicant.

    3. Determine whether the applicant is physically capable of doing the job.

    4. Document any existing disabilities and recommend accommodations.

52. A nurse practitioner involved in work-related surveillance knows that the records related to this activity must be held for how many years after employment?

    1. 5 years.

    2. 25 years.

    3. 30 years.

    4. Can be destroyed only after the employee's death.

53. The nurse practitioner knows that when treating a work-related injury it is required that he/she:

    1. Document thoroughly because of the high probability of legal action.

2. Communicate directly with the client's employer.

3. File a report that documents the injury and treatment with the industrial commission.

4. Notify the Occupational Safety and Health Administration (OSHA).

54. Which situation would be considered reportable under the Occupational and Safety Health Act?

    1. A 3-cm abrasion of the forearm.

    2. A warehouse worker with back strain reassigned to office work for a week.

    3. A twisted ankle that responded to ice and Ace wrap.

    4. A minor closed head injury with no loss of consciousness.

55. The purpose of an OSHA 200 log is to record:

    1. Occupational injuries and illnesses.

    2. Only work-related deaths.

    3. Dangerous workplace situations.

    4. Lost work days.

56. The ADA regulates how employers treat the disabled. Under the ADA, disability is defined as a physical or mental impairment that substantially limits one or more major life activities of an individual or a record of a situation in which an individual is regarded as having such an impairment. This would include:

    1. A history of addiction.

    2. Paralysis.

    3. Bipolar disorder.

    4. All of the above.

57. Bioethical practice dilemmas are best described as situations in which proposed treatment alternatives are:

    1. Ranked from most to least acceptable.

    2. Not appealing to involved parties.

    3. Lacking acceptance by anyone.

    4. Less than perfect approaches to the situation.

20 Answers & Rationales

1. **(2)** The most important advantage of an occurrence policy is that the coverage is available regardless of how long it takes to become aware of a claim (the long "tail" of a medical malpractice claim). The limits do not automatically increase. The carrier need not be notified during the policy period, as is required with claims-made coverage. The coverage under each policy may be as broad as the carrier allows.

2. **(2)** Fact witnesses and necessary paperwork are always easier to discover the closer in time you seek them after a medical misadventure. Memories are fresh and documents are less likely to be misplaced or destroyed. There is no rigid reporting window required by insurance carriers, but they do want to be notified in a timely manner. Insurance premiums may be reduced if an insured's track record is clean (i.e., no claims), but not because of mere compliance with policy requirements. Risk management employees prefer early notification so that damage control efforts may be implemented promptly, not for regulatory reasons.

3. **(2)** Assessment skills are presumed to be within the purview of the professional nurse, not those with fewer years of nursing education. Also, in this scenario, the LPN is an unknown entity to the delegator. Delegating to the LPN should be done cautiously after determining that person's skill level. Your license is not in jeopardy if you delegated appropriately, as in Option #1, but an error was made and is attributed to the delegatee. Actions in Options #3 and #4 are appropriate for the role.

4. **(3)** The client's capacity to consent is questionable; therefore alternatives must be sought. If the client has a court-appointed guardian, as set out in Option #3, then that person is the decision maker. The court has already made a determination of the client's legal incapacity and appointed the person to whom you will look for consent. If there were no guardian, you would determine whether the client himself could provide consent or whether you would look to his mother as the most appropriate surrogate decision maker. The group home employee has no automatic legal authority to consent to treatment for any resident.

5. **(4)** Assisted suicide is still a criminal activity in most states (and in legal limbo in the others). Circumventing the client may seem to be an appealing option, but it substitutes paternalism for the autonomy we all claim as our due. A diagnosis of depression can hardly be made with inadequate data; the necessary information can only be determined by conferring with the client herself.

6. **(2)** Managed care organizations (MCOs) are one group of health care organizations affected by this law. All subscribers must be provided with the stated information at the time of enrollment. Advance directive documents, though extremely helpful in the health care setting, are never mandatory.

7. **(4)** These are the basic requirements for conducting research at health care facilities.

8. **(3)** The insurance carrier is thoroughly familiar with the processes of handling a claim. The insurance carrier will assist with every step of this fearsome activity; the first significant obligation the insurance carrier will meet is to put the nurse practitioner in touch with a lawyer. Conferring with the client or the

client's lawyer is never a wise move. Colleagues can only offer moral support at this stage; the lawyer is the professional of choice at this time. Never, never even think about altering a record; it can turn a defensible case into a indefensible one.

9. **(3)** Lobbying for underserved clients is an example of justice, which is the duty to treat all clients fairly, without regard to age, socioeconomic status, or other variables. Autonomy is the client's right to self-determination without outside control. Nonmaleficence is the duty to prevent or avoid doing harm, whether intentional or unintentional. Veracity is the duty to tell the truth.

10. **(4)** These are all valid reasons for protecting your assets in the event of litigation. There are opposing views regarding the need for professional liability insurance. Some professionals believe that if there are few assets to protect, insurance is an unnecessary expense. Nurses with professional liability coverage ("deep pockets") could be retained as defendants in a case for a longer period.

11. **(1)** Look to state law to define the circumstances under which confidential medical information may be disclosed. There may be additional requirements imposed by federal regulations (e.g., the handling of certain psychiatric records), but the bulk of the rule making on this issue is accomplished at the state level. There are exceptions to the requirement of client consent, such as communicable disease reporting to public health authorities and court-ordered record production. Third-party payers, although powerful with their fiscal controls, must produce some proof of client consent to acquire records. An diagnosis of acquired immunodeficiency syndrome (AIDS) does not shield a record from production, although many states have enacted extra levels of protection for this information. Again, knowledge of state laws is helpful.

12. **(3)** The Americans with Disabilities Act (ADA) does not protect this group of people. In fact, employers may test for illegal drug use; this is not considered a medical examination, which is ordinarily subject to specific requirements under the law.

13. **(4)** These are all ways to get satisfaction from a health plan. You could also offer to help explain clinical issues to plan personnel who may not be clinically oriented.

14. **(2)** The best immediate solution is to identify the item and remove it from service to avoid further client injury. Then the risk manager, in consultation with the facility's attorneys and/or insurers, will determine how to proceed with equipment analysis. Returning the item to the manufacturer removes it from your control and diminishes your opportunity to defend against a charge of user error. Immediate repair may fail to uncover the real cause of the client injury and impair successful defense of a claim. If the litigation potential is high, the parties may wish to pool their efforts (and costs) to conduct a third-party review of the equipment. If litigation is likely, then it is also likely that the manufacturer and others in the distribution chain will be co-defendants with the facility and its staff.

15. **(2)** The preferred level of education is a master's degree, not the associate degree conferred on the technical nurse. The legal issues are the province of the attorneys and the judge; the nurse is expected to be the expert in the clinical issues. Published authorship, on nursing issues, does add an aura of credibility, but specific work experience coupled with the educational credentials are more appealing.

16. **(3)** The Administrative Procedures Act (APA) describes the workings of federal agencies. The Patient Self-Determination Act (PSDA) deals with advance directives, and the Omnibus Budget Reconciliation Act (OBRA) of 1987 changed the rule dealing with long-term care.

17. **(4)** These and other elements combine to produce a program of systematic risk identification, analysis, treatment, and evaluation, with the overall goal of loss prevention.

18. **(4)** Liability insurance is acquired to protect the organization from suits arising from negligent acts of employees. Business interruption coverage is usually purchased in tandem with fire insurance. It reimburses an organization for losses sustained while the business is partially or completely shut down after a catastrophic event. The organization's management team (CEO and senior staff) is

insured against losses based on business judgment errors through directors and officers (D&O) coverage. Workers' compensation is the line of coverage that protects employees after on-the-job injuries. It is a no-fault system (negligence is not a factor) that covers employee medical bills and pays a percentage of wages while an employee is unable to work.

19. **(1)** The nurse practitioner was driving a personal vehicle, so her auto insurer is "primary"; that is, it responds first to a loss. Since the nurse practitioner was on company business, her injuries were sustained "within the course and scope of employment," so there is coverage under the employer's workers' compensation policy for your medical bills and wage replacement. Depending on the circumstances and policy definitions, there could be some "excess" or additional coverage available under the employer's auto policy, but in no event would that carrier be primarily responsible for her losses. This is not the type of incident that homeowner's insurance is intended to cover. The semitrailer, presumably in use as a business vehicle, would not be insured under a driver's personal auto policy.

20. **(4)** The intent of the NPDB is to improve the quality of health care by encouraging state licensing boards, hospitals and other health care entities, and professional societies to identify and discipline those who engage in unprofessional behavior and to restrict the ability of incompetent physicians, dentists, and other health care practitioners to move from state to state without disclosure or discovery of previous medical malpractice payment and adverse action history. Adverse actions can involve licensure, clinical privileges, professional society membership, and exclusions from Medicare and Medicaid.

21. **(3)** The forwarding facility needs to know whether the receiving facility has space for the new arrival and, more importantly, the ability to treat the particular illness for which the client needs therapy. A familiar example of a client transfer is that of the burn victim, for whom specialty care is mandatory and the locations of that specialty care are usually limited.

22. **(1)** Health care policy within the states is codified or enacted into law by the respective states' legislatures. The boards have significant input (hopefully) in the process, providing the research data and expert "testimony" that the legislatures need to make informed decisions. Nursing organizations should also be willing to provide background information and nurse experts to educate the lawmakers.

23. **(3)** The MCOs' cost-containment strategy is enhanced if providers practice within the treatment guidelines suggested by the plans. Providers who inform clients that a certain treatment regimen is the preferred alternative create difficulties if that alternative is excluded from coverage. MCOs usually clearly set out the exclusions in the plan documents, and member services personnel are expected to be able to explain the coverage to subscribers. Experimental treatment, if excluded, would be listed as such in the plan documents.

24. **(2)** These three are required to report deaths related to use of a medical device. Events occurring in the other settings are exempt from reporting requirements under this federal law.

25. **(2)** This is the most factual note; the writer does not apportion blame or assume liability. The other notes would be "red flags" for a chart reviewer. The mention of an incident report makes it virtually impossible to protect these documents from disclosure, especially in those jurisdictions that still afford some protection to these internal "early warning" documents that seek to alert risk management personnel to a potential claim.

26. **(3)** Clients are often unable to evaluate the quality of the care they receive, but they do react to the way in which the care is delivered. Perceptions by clients of rudeness or "uncaring" on the part of the provider often spur clients to pursue legal action. Clients tend to be more forgiving of less-than-optimal outcomes if they have been involved in the process and are treated with respect.

27. **(4)** Making one's own decisions is the basis for informed consent and the ethical underpinning of the PSDA. "Doing good" (Option #1) and its corollary "avoiding harm" (Option #3) are ethics principles usually cited as the basis for other health care activities, such as maintaining professional competency. Respect for persons is a more global ethical principle supporting much of a nurse's personal philosophy of caring.

28. **(3)** Usually phrased as *duty, breach, proximate cause, and damages*, these are the four

elements of proof required to prevail in a medical negligence action. Intentional acts are not synonymous with negligent acts. Duty presumes a professional relationship and obligation to provide services. The breach is the error or mistake ascribed to the provider that results in the harm to the client.

29. **(2)** A competent adult client is the person to whom you look for consent to treat. It is only when the client is unable to consent that surrogate decision makers are sought. Individual states' laws need to be checked for the selection and priority of surrogate decision makers.

30. **(1)** Lay jurors are not expected to know the clinical facts and circumstances involved in a professional negligence claim. The expert witness is needed to educate the jurors about those medical facts and to testify to the standard of care to be applied. Witnesses with direct involvement in the case are no less credible because of their involvement; their testimony, and personal bias if any, will be evaluated by the jurors in the context of their roles.

31. **(4)** With respect to nursing specialties, the standard of care is usually a national one. Facility policies, books, and journals are important to review; and physician input may be sought. In some cases, physicians may even be allowed to testify about the standard of care.

32. **(3)** One particular advantage of alternative dispute resolution is the flexibility of the system. In mediation, for example, the mediator can assist with crafting a solution package that meets all the needs of a party, including such things as an apology from the health care provider. Money isn't always the only answer. Insurers' goals, however, usually do focus on cash, with the goal of avoiding huge damage awards to plaintiffs. If a mediator is successful in facilitating case settlements, the costs are usually significantly lower than the costs of a court trial. Insurers with an eye on the bottom line are not averse to these advantages.

33. **(1)** Statutes of limitations set out each state's rules for the timing of the filing of lawsuits, including malpractice actions. These statutes are procedural laws in that they describe the "how to" parameters within which legal rights

may be exercised. Minority is considered a legal disability; other state laws usually define it and describe its effects. Rights to sue are not governed by statutes of limitations.

34. **(3)** Statutes may indeed differ from state to state with respect to the breadth of the protection, but most will protect a nurse who renders aid, without expectation of compensation, in a competent manner. Gross negligence will usually void the statutory protections.

35. **(1)** A professional appearance boosts your credibility as a witness. Inappropriate attire and gum chewing detract from the professional demeanor that you will want to project. Preparation is critical before your words are recorded and transcribed as part of the official litigation transcript. Review documents as noted, but refrain from bringing any materials with you to the deposition without your attorney's approval. Always ask for clarification of ambiguous questions. Speculation is not appropriate. Your professional work history is always requested, so a copy of your curriculum vitae (CV) is a useful tool to bring along to a deposition.

36. **(1)** Jousting in the client's medical record is never a good idea. It provides fodder for plaintiffs' lawyers but does not contribute to quality nursing care. If you have a conflict with another provider, deal with the provider directly, preferably in person. Another arena for resolving such disputes is the quality review process.

37. **(4)** All of these factors enter into an analysis of whether it is appropriate to accept a minor's consent to treatment. Another factor to consider is the type of treatment sought. Some states have statutes allowing minors to consent to specific therapies, such as treatment for venereal disease.

38. **(4)** Long-term care is a specialized area with layers of regulatory requirements, most stemming from the federal government. Nurses who work in this environment need to be vigilant about learning the rules and maintaining compliance. Ongoing, effective communication with regulators is essential.

39. **(4)** We have a tendency to get very careless with our information management and the way we interact with clients and their very

personal data. The often wide-open and very frantic front-desk atmosphere of an office does little to calm client fears that their information will be easily accessible to those without a need to know.

40. **(2)** Sexual preference is not a protected classification. The other options refer to groups for whom different federal laws provide varying degrees of protection. It is prudent to check with your business attorney to determine whether the policies you have drafted for your office are in compliance with federal guidelines. The Equal Employment Opportunity Commission (EEOC), which enforces the laws, publishes guidelines about the various statutes. These publications are available, either free or at minimal cost, from the agency. Some may be available on the Internet.

41. **(3)** This description seems to fit the criteria for a hostile environment, a form of sexual harassment. The harassment seems to be pervasive and longstanding; the women have complained, and apparently, no action has been taken. The isolated incident and single date request do not rise to the level of harassment. The participants did not find the actions objectionable, and job performance was not affected. In Option #2, although the potential was there for the nurse to use the prior relationship to either downgrade the employee or deny a benefit, this result did not occur.

42. **(4)** Advance directives are documents crafted by individuals who personally decide how they wish their future health care to be handled. The documents must be prepared while the signer is fully capable of understanding their content and importance. Since the wife in this scenario is already comatose, she has missed her opportunity to prepare an advance directive. This does not mean that the spouse is unable to decide on her medical treatment; it just means that a different consent process needs to be used.

43. **(3)** This option would create liability potential for the nurse practitioner under at least two legal theories (e.g., battery and false imprisonment). Obviously, Option #2 would be the first prong of a planned approach to convince this client that she needs the prescribed medical therapy. Option #4 would be the next choice. Court-ordered treatment is a consideration with a viable fetus.

44. **(1)** This is the overall goal of the ADA. It is not another entitlement program, and it cannot impose wheelchair ramp requirements on every building owner in America. Access ramps and interpreters may be required as a "reasonable accommodation" to qualified people in certain defined circumstances. There is no across-the-board mandate for these types of aid to the handicapped.

45. **(1)** The Supreme Court essentially deferred to the states to legislate on this topic. In most states, the activity is not permitted. In one of the states involved in the high court's case, a statute permitting assisted suicide is being challenged. Nurse practitioners need to look at their states' laws on this topic for guidance. The providers referenced in Options #2, #3, and #4 would act at their peril if their states' laws followed the current majority view.

46. **(1)** The purpose of a medical malpractice action is to make the claimant whole by the awarding of monetary compensation. The award compensates the claimant or plaintiff for the wrong (or tort) he/she has suffered at the hands of the defendant. On the criminal side, the state sues on behalf of society for violations of society's criminal laws. The punishment is fines, imprisonment, or both. Professional liability insurance usually excludes criminal and intentional acts, so coverage for these types of activities is unlikely.

47. **(4)** The full-blown jury trial is what alternative dispute resolution (ADR) seeks to avoid. Mediation and arbitration are the most well-known forms of ADR. Some jurisdictions use the settlement conference as a technique to attempt settlement after a lawsuit has been filed but before a trial begins. Another type of ADR is called *a summary jury trial*, which is a private, shortened version wherein the parties share some evidence and get a sense of the strengths and weaknesses of each side's position. There are also hybrids such as "med-arb" wherein a proceeding starts out as a mediation but, if the case is not settled, it is referred to an arbitrator for resolution.

48. **(3)** This is the so-called long tail of professional liability; there is always a time lag from the date of injury to the date a claimant files a malpractice action. In the case of an infant, that time lag can be many years because of the effect of the statute of limitations. This extends the period of potential risk to the nurse who

cares for children. Although there may be a sympathy factor involved when jurors decide damage awards, the judgment is usually proportional to the injury and not the age of the claimant. Insurance coverage for pediatric providers is no less available than that for other specialties; insurers adjust premiums to account for the level of risk.

49. **(4)** All clients are entitled to medical information in order to make an informed decision about treatment. Age, in and of itself, is not an exclusionary criterion. Providers may provide treatment in the other circumstances.

50. **(4)** If the human resources department has established guidelines for the handling of references, it would be wise to follow them. It is also an effective mechanism to deflect potentially problematic queries by passing requests to the department most equipped to handle them. Most employers will be very circumspect about the information released, often limiting the data to dates of employment only. In the absence of some protective state legislation, employers should be prudent about sharing comments on former employees' work histories.

51. **(3)** The purpose is to determine the appropriateness of the applicant for the job. Identifying health problems to prevent hiring an individual is discriminatory. Determination of mental status and disabilities may also be a part of the pre-employment physical exam but are not the primary purpose.

52. **(3)** The Occupational Safety and Health Administration (OSHA) requires that these records be held for 30 years after termination of employment.

53. **(3)** It is required by law that a report of any work-related injury be filed with the industrial commission of the state in which the injury occurred.

54. **(2)** The Occupational Safety and Health Act requires a report of any injury or illness that requires more than first aid treatment and/or involves loss of work time, limited work status, loss of consciousness, or death.

55. **(1)** The purpose is to record occupational injuries and illnesses, which would also include death reports and lost work days, which would also reveal dangerous working conditions.

56. **(4)** All of the conditions listed would qualify under the ADA and may require accommodation in the workplace.

57. **(4)** The crux of a bioethical dilemma is that the proposed solution(s) are not perfect and therefore create some aspect of moral conflict.